DISABILITY IN AMERICA

TOWARD A NATIONAL AGENDA FOR PREVENTION

Andrew M. Pope
and
Alvin R. Tarlov
Editors

Committee on a National Agenda for
the Prevention of Disabilities

Division of Health Promotion and
Disease Prevention

INSTITUTE OF MEDICINE

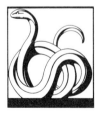

NATIONAL ACADEMY PRESS
Washington, D.C. 1991

NATIONAL ACADEMY PRESS • 2101 Constitution Avenue, N.W. • Washington, D.C. 20418

NOTICE: The project that is the subject of this report was approved by the Governing Board of the National Research Council, whose members are drawn from the councils of the National Academy of Sciences, the National Academy of Engineering, and the Institute of Medicine. The members of the committee responsible for the report were chosen for their special competencies and with regard for appropriate balance.

This report has been reviewed by a group other than the authors according to procedures approved by a Report Review Committee appointed by the members of the National Academy of Sciences, the National Academy of Engineering, and the Institute of Medicine.

The Institute of Medicine was chartered in 1970 by the National Academy of Sciences to enlist distinguished members of the appropriate professions in the examination of policy matters pertaining to the health of the public. In this, the Institute acts under both the Academy's 1863 congressional charter responsibility to be an adviser to the federal government and its own initiative in identifying issues of medical care, research, and education.

Support for this study was provided by the Centers for Disease Control (Contract no. 200-88-0690).

Library of Congress Cataloging-in-Publication Data

Institute of Medicine (U.S.). Committee on a National Agenda for
Prevention of Disabilities.
    Disability in America : toward a national agenda for prevention /
Andrew M. Pope and Alvin R. Tarlov, editors : Committee on a
National Agenda for the Prevention of Disabilities, Division of
Health Promotion and Disease Prevention, Institute of Medicine.
    p. cm.
    Report of a study undertaken by the Committee on a National Agenda
for the Prevention of Disabilities
    Includes bibliographical references and index.
    ISBN 0-309-04378-6
    1. Chronic diseases—United States—Prevention. 2. Handicapped—
United States. I. Pope, Andrew MacPherson, 1950- . II. Tarlov,
Alvin R. (Alvin Richard), 1929- . III. Title.
    [DNLM: 1. Handicapped. 2. Preventive Health Services—United
States. 3. Primary Prevention—methods—United States. 4. Public
Policy—United States. HV 1553 I59d]
    RA644.6.I58 1991
    614.5'99—dc20
    DNLM/DLC
    for Library of Congress   91-15496
                                                                         CIP

COMMITTEE ON A NATIONAL AGENDA FOR THE PREVENTION OF DISABILITIES

ARTHUR T. MEYERSON, Professor and Chairman, Department of Psychiatry and Mental Health Sciences, Hahnemann University School of Medicine, Philadelphia, Pennsylvania

DOROTHY P. RICE, Professor in Residence, Department of Social and Behavioral Sciences, School of Nursing, University of California, San Francisco

JULIUS B. RICHMOND, John D. MacArthur Professor of Health Policy, Emeritus, Harvard Medical School, Boston, Massachusetts

MAX J. STARKLOFF, President, Paraquad, Inc., St. Louis, Missouri

DEBORAH ANN STONE, David R. Pokross Professor of Law and Social Policy, Heller School, Brandeis University, Waltham, Massachusetts

S. LEONARD SYME, Professor of Epidemiology, Department of Biomedical and Environmental Health Sciences, School of Public Health, University of California, Berkeley

JOHN E. WARE, JR., Senior Scientist, The Institute for the Improvement of Medical Care and Health, New England Medical Center, Boston, Massachusetts

Institute of Medicine Staff

Andrew M. Pope, Study Director

Gary B. Ellis, Director, Division of Health Promotion and Disease Prevention

Alexandra N. Bernstein, Research Associate

Judith L. Estep, Administrative Secretary

Linda A. DePugh, Administrative Assistant

Cynthia Abel, Financial Associate

Preface

In 1985 the National Research Council and the Institute of Medicine released the landmark report *Injury in America*, which identified injury as the leading cause of death and disability among children and young adults and, indeed, the principal public health problem facing America. The primary measure used in the study to describe the public health significance of injury was "years of potential life lost" (before age 65). Because injury affects primarily young people, and because death and disability (defined in that report as the inability to work) are the significant outcomes associated with injury, the years of potential life lost to injury were revealed as a much larger public health issue than cardiovascular disease and cancer combined.

Disability in America builds on the *Injury* report to discuss not only disability caused by injury but also developmental disability, chronic disease and aging, and secondary conditions arising from primary disabling conditions. More important, this report focuses on preventing a potentially disabling condition from developing into disability and on minimizing the effects of such conditions on a person's productivity and quality of life. In one sense, disability frequently results from the failure of our successes—for example, success in saving the lives of low-birthweight babies and persons with traumatic injuries or chronic disease.

This report goes beyond the traditional medical model to consider and address the needs of people with disabling conditions after those conditions exist and after they have been "treated" and "rehabilitated." Prevention of the initial condition (primary prevention) is certainly important, but the emphasis in this report is on developing interventions that can prevent pathology from becoming impairment, impairment from becoming functional limitation, functional limitation from becoming disability, and any of these conditions from causing secondary conditions. Theoretically, each stage presents an opportunity to intervene and prevent the progression toward disability. Thus, the report sets forth a model developed by its authoring body, the Committee on a National Agenda for the Prevention of Disabilities, that describes disability not as a static endpoint but as a component of a process.

The report is organized loosely according to a life course perspective: it first discusses developmental disability, which is a group of conditions that begins during childhood; then injury-related disability, which affects primarily adolescents and young adults; and finally disability, which is often associated with chronic disease and aging. It also describes disability as a social issue and not just a physical condition. In other words, a person is not always disabled by paralysis but more commonly by the way he or she is treated by others and restricted from performing normal social roles. Moreover, although the spectrum of disabling conditions is broad, affecting every segment of society, individuals of low socioeconomic status feel its impact most heavily. Some disabling conditions barely make a difference in an individual's life; others, especially those that are most debilitating, can require continuous post-hospitalization care, assistive devices, attendant services, and work-site and home modifications—items and services that often are not covered by insurance programs. In these cases, those who can easily afford to pay for the most appropriate care do so; those who are impoverished use what is available through public programs; and those who are moderately well off must totally exhaust their own resources to become eligible for any assistance through public programs.

Disabilities affect not only the lives of the individuals who acquire them but everyone else as well. Their cost to the nation is great in terms of income supplements (to support those with chronically disabling conditions), medical and other health care expenditures, and lost productivity, which may result from disability, lack of retraining, or needed work-site modification. The emotional cost to family and friends of people with disabilities is incalculable.

To explore these issues and the range of available interventions, the Centers for Disease Control (CDC) in conjunction with the National Council on Disability (NCD) requested the Institute of Medicine to constitute an expert committee to develop a national agenda for the prevention of disabilities. The CDC is "the nation's prevention agency." The NCD, an independent federal agency, makes recommendations to the President, Congress, and other federal bodies on federal policy and programs that affect people with disabilities. It has become the principal national advocate for disability rights and improved services and has been largely responsible for the heightened national interest in preventing disabilities.

The NCD's efforts recently culminated in passage of the Americans with Disabilities Act, which bans discrimination against persons with disabilities in employment, transportation, public accommodations, telecommunications, and local and state government activities. This act also provides guidance for governmental policies and services, as well as for businesses and other organizations.

Other NCD initiatives have led to major steps forward in addressing disability prevention on the national level. For example, the 1986 NCD report *Toward Independence* was the impetus for establishing the Disabilities Prevention Program at CDC, which uses CDC's strengths in public health surveillance, epidemiology, technology transfer, and communication with state and local health departments to initiate and support state and local disability prevention programs and to increase the knowledge base necessary for developing and evaluating effective preventive interventions. The program currently focuses on developmental disability, head and spinal cord injury, and secondary conditions in people with physical limitations.

As seen in the CDC disabilities prevention program, there is increased awareness on the part of researchers, health care providers, and others of the need for an effective national disability prevention program to improve the quality of life of millions of Americans and reduce the cost of disability to the American public. A good deal of what is preventable could be prevented *now*—using what we already know about injury prevention, prenatal care, health promotion, and the care of disabling conditions to prevent secondary conditions. What is needed is better organization and coordination at the national level, coupled with improved collection of information on the incidence and prevalence of disability, the extension of disability prevention programs to all 50 states and the District of Columbia, and research into the most effective points of intervention.

Although this report addresses many issues related to disability prevention and the need for a National Disability Prevention Program, there is no detailed assessment of the costs of such a program. It is the committee's hope that an in-depth study of the costs of disability (and disability prevention) will follow this report, much as *The Cost of Injury* was prepared after *Injury in America*. Other topics that deserve additional attention vis-à-vis disability include mental health, chronic disease and aging, the ethics of disability prevention, access to assistive technology and personal assistance services, and gaps in health insurance, including medical underwriting practices. These topics are all related to health promotion and disability prevention and would be logical extensions of the current effort.

Many of the topics related to disability involve civil rights and social issues, and efforts to address them often engender controversy among knowledgeable persons with conflicting views. This was certainly the case with the work of this committee. Over a period of almost 2 years, we examined information, listened to testimony from experts, deliberated, debated, and formed working groups to write the individual chapters of the report. There was no suppression of any argument. Discussions were free-ranging and open, and voluminous amounts of information from various sources with differing perspectives were considered, analyzed, discussed, and debated. The contents of the report represent the committee's consensus on the issues it was charged to address, a consensus reached after a long, arduous process. Regrettably, one committee member (Deborah Stone) who attended few meetings and therefore did not have the benefit of the committee's deliberative process was unable to concur in the committee's views. Her dissenting statement and a response by the committee appear as Appendix B of this report.

The committee believes that disability prevention should be a high priority not only within the public health and allied health professions but also in the wider setting of American society. In addition, although it is important to learn how to prevent and ameliorate physical and mental conditions that can cause disability, it is equally important to recognize that a disabling condition is only a single characteristic of the person who has it. The time has come for the nation to address disability as an issue that affects all Americans, one for which an investment in education, access to preventive services and technology, and the development of effective interventions could yield unprecedented returns in public health, personal achievement, and national productivity.

> ALVIN R. TARLOV, Chair
> Committee on a National Agenda for
> the Prevention of Disabilities

Acknowledgments

The following colleagues in both the public and private sectors generously shared information, resource material, and expertise: M. J. Adams, Jr., Monroe Berkowitz, Betty Jo Berland, Scott C. Brown, Larry Burt, Jose Cordero, Philip Graitcer, Robert Griss, Lawrence Haber, James Harrell, Judith Heumann, Vernon Houk, Christopher Howson, Jack Jackson, Fred Krause, Daniel Levine, Saad Nagi, Godfrey Oakley, Sandra Parrino, Solomon Snyder, William Spencer, Thomas Stripling, William Taylor, Stephen Thacker, R. Alexander Vachon, Lois Verbrugge, Kent Waldrep, Deborah Wilkerson, Meyer Zitter, and Irving Zola. In addition to the efforts of the editors, Andrew Pope and Alvin Tarlov, Mark Bello deserves acknowledgment for his assistance and contributions in writing and editing. The committee also thanks Michael Stoto and Jane Durch for their analysis of disability data and contributions to Chapter 2 of the report, and Connie Rosemont for her assistance with references and last minute details. The committee also acknowledges the historical perspective of Michael Marge and his tireless efforts in promoting disability prevention and supporting this committee's work. The committee is grateful to Judy Estep for her cheerfulness and skill in "keeping the trains running" throughout most of the committee's tenure, and for the initial preparation of the manuscript. Randy Conner, Dorothy Majewski, and Rosena Ricks efficiently handled the final preparation of the manuscript for publication.

Contents

EXECUTIVE SUMMARY 1

1 INTRODUCTION 32
Disability: Definition and Concept, 34
Public Health and Disability Prevention, 37
Scope and Organization of the Report, 39

2 MAGNITUDE AND DIMENSIONS OF DISABILITY IN
THE UNITED STATES 41
Data Sources, 41
Prevalence of Disability, 45
Trends in the Prevalence of Disability, 53
Conditions Leading to Disability, 56
Life Table Perspective, 61
Economic Cost of Disability, 67
Conclusion, 73

3 A MODEL FOR DISABILITY AND DISABILITY
PREVENTION 76
Conceptual Framework, 76
Model of Disability, 83
The Need for Epidemiology, 95
Applying Traditional Prevention Strategies to Disability, 104

4 PREVENTION OF DEVELOPMENTAL DISABILITIES 109
Public Health Significance, 109
Approaches to Prevention, 122
Opportunities and Needs, 132

xi

5 PREVENTION OF INJURY-RELATED DISABILITY 147
   Injury in America: Magnitude of
      the Problem, 147
   Central Nervous System Injuries, 150
   Surveillance: Counting the Survivors and Assessing Their Needs, 156
   Primary Prevention: The Strategy of Choice, 159
   A Systems Approach to Acute Care and Rehabilitation, 164

6 PREVENTION OF DISABILITY ASSOCIATED WITH
   CHRONIC DISEASES AND AGING 184
   Magnitude of the Problem, 186
   Life Course Perspective on Disability and Its Prevention, 193
   Devising Approaches to Prevention, 195

7 PREVENTION OF SECONDARY CONDITIONS 214
   Model of Secondary Conditions, 215
   Components of a Comprehensive Prevention Program, 223
   Protocols for the Prevention of Secondary Conditions, 234

8 A COMPREHENSIVE APPROACH TO DISABILITY
   PREVENTION: OBSTACLES AND OPPORTUNITIES 242
   Demedicalization, 244
   National Health Promotion and Disease Prevention Objectives, 245
   Clinical Preventive Services, 247
   Federal Programs and Policies, 248
   The Need for Coordination, 258

9 RECOMMENDATIONS 267
   Organization and Coordination, 267
   Surveillance, 273
   Research, 277
   Access to Care and Preventive Services, 280
   Professional and Public Education, 284

REFERENCES 288

APPENDIXES 307
A. Disability Concepts Revisited: Implications for Prevention
   Saad Nagi, 309
B. Dissent and Response, 328
C. Committee Biographies, 340

INDEX 351

DISABILITY IN AMERICA

Executive Summary

Disability is an issue that affects every individual, community, neighborhood, and family in the United States. It is more than a medical issue; it is a costly social, public health, and moral issue.

- About 35 million Americans (one in every seven) have disabling conditions that interfere with their life activities.
- More than 9 million people have physical or mental conditions that keep them from being able to work, attend school, or maintain a household.
- More than half of the 4-year increase in life expectancy between 1970 and 1987 is accounted for by time spent with activity limitations.
- Disabilities are disproportionately represented among minorities, the elderly, and lower socioeconomic populations.
- Of the current 75-year life expectancy, a newborn can be expected to experience an average of 13 years with an activity limitation.
- Annual disability-related costs to the nation total more than $170 billion.

Disability is the expression of a physical or mental limitation in a social context—the gap between a person's capabilities and the demands of the environment. People with such functional limitations are not inherently disabled, that is, incapable of carrying out their personal, familial, and social responsibilities. It is the interaction of their physical or mental limitations with social and environmental factors that determines whether they have a disability. Most disability is thus preventable, which will not only significantly improve the quality of life for millions of Americans but also could save many billions of dollars in costs resulting from dependence, lost productivity, and medical care.

The pattern of conditions that cause disability is complex and difficult to summarize. For young adults, mobility limitations such as those caused by spinal cord injuries, orthopedic impairments, and paralysis are the most common causes. For middle-aged and older adults, chronic diseases, especially heart and circulatory problems, predominate as causes of limitation. Figure 1 shows the age-specific prevalence rates for activity limitation according to five groups of causes; Figure 2 shows the proportion in each age group ascribed to each of the groups of conditions.

Modern medicine's success in averting the death of many people who sustain life-threatening diseases and injuries often entails, as a consequence, the loss of at least some functional capacity. Indeed, the successful life-saving techniques of modern medicine are adding to the population of people with disabilities. For example, in the 1950s, only people with low-level paraplegia were generally expected to survive; today, even people with high-level quadriplegia are surviving and living lives of high quality. Indeed, one commentator has characterized the growing numbers of people with chronic conditions as the "failures of successes" achieved with medical technology. To help these individuals restore functional capacity, avert further deterioration in functioning, and maintain or improve their quality

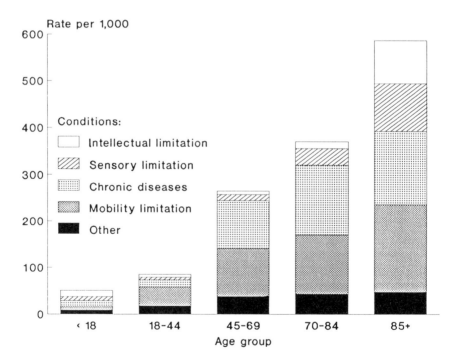

FIGURE 1   Prevalence of main causes of activity limitation, by age, 1983-1985.
Source: Calculated from LaPlante, 1988.

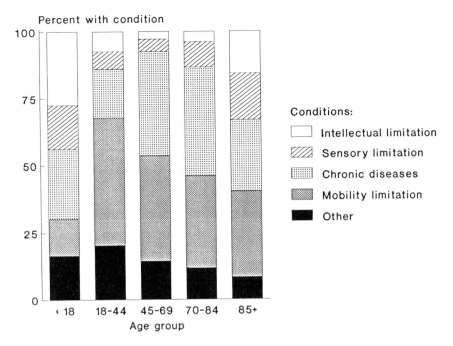

FIGURE 2   Percentage distribution of main causes of activity limitation, by age, 1983-1985. Source: Calculated from LaPlante, 1988.

of life, it is important to foster programs that emphasize rehabilitation and the prevention of secondary conditions. Partly for this reason the committee focused its report on prevention strategies for people who already have potentially disabling conditions, that is, on secondary and tertiary levels of prevention. In other words:

• What can be done to prevent an impairment or functional limitation that results from injury, a birth defect, or chronic disease from becoming a disability?
• What are the risks for developing a disability (or secondary condition), and how can they be controlled?
• How is quality of life affected by disabling conditions, and what can be done to improve it?

Good disability prevention strategies must be built on strong basic knowledge of the relationships between risk factors, disabling conditions, quality of life, and secondary conditions. Until now, approaches to the prevention of disability have been significantly limited by the narrowness of conceptual views and inadequate data. This report gives special attention to issues related to conceptual clarity and data needs and presents a model for studying the progression of conditions toward disability. The disability model described in this report should facilitate the development of improved surveillance systems, an epidemiology of disability, and more effective means of prevention.

Interfering with the development of effective prevention programs, however, is the lack of an effective public health surveillance network for monitoring the incidence and prevalence of disability, including predisposing risk factors. Without such a surveillance network, programs and policies intended to prevent disability will continue to be based on educated guesses rather than a solid data base that describes the sizable population of people that have either disabilities or a high risk of developing them. Furthermore, the fragmentation, gaps, and redundancies in the nation's disability-related programs—the focus of criticism in other quarters besides this report—will persist.

Although the current system for providing medical and social support to people with disabling conditions suffers from many inadequacies, most of the elements required for longitudinal care, as recommended by this committee, are likely to be in place. Additional financial resources may not be needed for many of the prevention measures noted here so much as a commitment to coordination, program planning, and service delivery to form a network that is readily accessible by consumer populations.

TOWARD A COMPREHENSIVE APPROACH TO DISABILITY PREVENTION

Despite an officially stated national goal of independence and equality of opportunity for people with disabilities, current approaches to preventing disability and improving the lives of people with disabling conditions lack conceptual clarity and unity of purpose. Reducing the prevalence and incidence of disability poses challenges on many fronts and requires coherent, comprehensive responses rather than the piecemeal actions that now characterize medical, rehabilitative, and social programs related to disability. In short, disability prevention requires new thinking, new collaborations among researchers, new relationships between agencies and organizations, both public and private, new approaches to delivering services, and new societal attitudes.

In developing its framework for a national disability prevention program, the committee sought to identify issues and needs that cut across the major categories of health conditions that can result in disability. It developed a model for disability and disability prevention (see Chapter 3) based on the work of Saad Nagi and the World Health Organization, and expanded it to include risk factors and quality of life. The committee then reviewed current knowledge in four major areas; developmental disabilities (Chapter 4);

injury-related disabilities, specifically those related to spinal cord injury and traumatic brain injury (Chapter 5); disabilities associated with chronic diseases and aging (Chapter 6); and secondary conditions associated with primary disabling conditions (Chapter 7). Needs and challenges specific to each category of disability are identified in the individual chapters.

Time and resources did not permit a review of all areas of disability. Mental health conditions, for example, are discussed only briefly as secondary conditions and, to a lesser extent, as primary conditions. Chapter 8 discusses the obstacles to and opportunities for a comprehensive approach to disability prevention, and Chapter 9 presents the committee's recommendations for a national agenda for the prevention of disability. A summary of Chapters 3-7 appears below, beginning with a discussion of the committee's model and followed by the committee's recommendations for a national agenda for the prevention of disability (Chapter 9 in its entirety).

A Model of Disability

There are two major conceptual frameworks in the field of disability: the International Classification of Impairments, Disabilities, and Handicaps (ICIDH), and the "functional limitation," or Nagi, framework, which is not accompanied by a classification system. The ICIDH is a trial supplement to the World Health Organization's International Classification of Diseases; it has stimulated extensive discussions of disability concepts, received both positive and negative reviews in the literature, and is used widely around the world. Several European countries including France and the Netherlands have adopted the ICIDH and use it extensively in administrative systems and clinical settings. As a classification system that has received broad international sponsorship the ICIDH deserves considerable attention, and the WHO is to be commended for its efforts in developing a system that has met with such success. As has been pointed out in the literature, however, the ICIDH is neither a classification of persons nor a research tool.

The original intent of the ICIDH classification system was to provide a framework to organize information about the consequences of disease. As such, it has been considered by some as an intrusion of the medical profession into the social aspects of life—a "medicalization of disablement." The WHO is planning to revise the ICIDH in the near future, which will provide opportunities for significant improvements.

Both frameworks (i.e., the ICIDH and the Nagi or functional limitation framework) have four basic concepts. In the ICIDH the four concepts are disease, impairment, disability, and handicap. In the Nagi framework, the four concepts are pathology, impairment, functional limitation, and disability. Both frameworks recognize that whether a person performs a socially expected activity depends not simply on the characteristics of the person but also on the larger context of social and physical environments. Conceptual clarity, however, seems to be a problem with some of the classifications in the ICIDH. As discussed in the literature, some of the ICIDH classifications are confusing; for example, certain social role limitations (e.g., family role, occupational role) are classified as "behavior disabilities," instead of "occupation handicaps" or "social integration handicaps." Another example cited is the distinction between "orientation handicaps" and disabilities associated with self-awareness, postural, or environmental problems.

In considering the options for a conceptual framework, the committee was faced with the fact that the ICIDH includes the term "handicap" in its classification. Traditionally, *handicap* has meant limitations in performance, placing an individual at a disadvantage. Handicap sometimes has been used to imply an absolute limitation that does not require for its actualization any interaction with external social circumstances. In recent years, the term has fallen into disuse in the United States, primarily because people with disabling conditions consider handicap to be a negative term. Yet the shadow of "handicap" as a commonly used term hovers behind the concept of quality of life, and has the effect of reducing quality of life even though impairment, functional limitation, and disability do not necessarily do so. Much as the term "cripple" has gone out of style, handicap seems to be approaching obsolescence, at least within the community of people with disabilities in the United States.

The committee concurs with those who have noted internal inconsistencies and a lack of clarity in the ICIDH concepts of disability and handicap, and it notes the need for its pending revision. It prefers not to use handicap in this report and offers an alternative framework that does not focus on the consequences of disease. The committee's alternative framework draws on the widespread acceptance and success of the ICIDH and the conceptual clarity and terminology of the Nagi framework, and then adds risk factors and quality of life into a model of the disabling process. Committee members found that this framework and model improved their understanding of the relationships among and between components of the disabling process and helped them identify strategic points for preventive intervention. It is hoped that this framework will be considered as a viable alternative in the revisions of the WHO ICIDH.

The conceptual framework used in this report is composed of four related but distinct stages: pathology, impairment, functional limitation, and disability. In the course of a chronic disorder, one stage can progress to the next. But depending on the circumstances, progressively greater loss of function need not occur, and the progression can be halted or reversed. Thus disability prevention efforts can be directed at any of the three stages that precede disability, as well as at the disability stage itself, where efforts can focus on reversal of disability, restoration of function, or prevention of

PATHOLOGY →	IMPAIRMENT →	FUNCTIONAL LIMITATION →	DISABILITY
Interruption or interference of normal bodily processes or structures	Loss and/or abnormality of mental, emotional, physiological, or anatomical structure or function; includes all losses or abnormalities, not just those attributable to active pathology; also includes pain	Restriction or lack of ability to perform an action or activity in the manner or within the range considered normal that results from impairment	Inability or limitation in performing socially defined activities and roles expected of individuals within a social and physical environment

Level of reference

Cells and tissues	Organs and organ systems	Organism— action or activity performance (consistent with the purpose or function of the organ or organ system)	Society— task performance within the social and cultural context

Example

Denervated muscle in arm due to trauma	Atrophy of muscle	Cannot pull with arm	Change of job; can no longer swim recreationally

FIGURE 3   An overview of the concepts of pathology, impairment, functional limitation, and disability.

complications (secondary conditions) that can greatly exacerbate existing limitations or lead to new ones. Figure 3 summarizes the four stages of the framework.

As mentioned above, the committee's model for disability builds on the conceptual frameworks of Nagi and the WHO, placing disability within the appropriate context of health and social issues (Figure 4). It depicts the interactive effects of biological, environmental (physical and social), and lifestyle and behavioral risk factors that influence each stage of the disabling process; the relationship of the disabling process to quality of life; and the stages of the disabling process that often precede disability. A brief description of the components of the model follows.

Risk Factors

Risk factors are biological, environmental (social and physical), and lifestyle or behavioral characteristics that are causally associated with health-related conditions. Identifying such factors can be a first step toward determining a mechanism of action in the disabling process and then developing preventive interventions. The disability research and service communities have not yet adopted a systematic, comprehensive conceptual model for understanding disability risk factors. A model that incorporates biological, environmental (physical and social), and lifestyle and behavioral risk factor categories will help move the disability research and service communities nearer to a more unified understanding of disability and disability prevention.

Quality of Life

The quality of life concept subsumes many aspects of personal well-being that are not directly related to health. It is becoming increasingly clear, however, that health is the product of a complex array of factors, many of which fall outside the traditional province of health care. Similarly, the health of the nation's citizens has commercial, economic, and social importance. Thus quality of life is assuming greater importance and acceptance, and its enhancement, in addition to curing disease or improving survival, is becoming an accepted goal of the health-related professions.

As depicted in Figure 4, quality of life affects and is affected by the outcomes of each stage of the disabling process. Within the disabling process, each stage interacts with an individual's quality of life. There is no universal threshold—no particular level of impairment or functional limitation—at which people perceive themselves as having lost their personal autonomy and diminished the quality of their lives. Yet perceptions of personal independence and quality of life are clearly important in determining how individuals respond to challenges at each of the four stages of the disabling process. Similar theoretical models for health status and quality of life have been described by others.

The Disabling Process

At the center of the model is the disabling process. Although it seems to indicate a unidirectional progression from pathology to impairment to functional limitation to disability, and although a stepwise progression often occurs, progression from one stage to another is not always the case. An individual with a disabling condition might skip over components of the model, for example, when the public's attitude toward a disfiguring impairment causes no functional limitation but imposes a disability by affecting

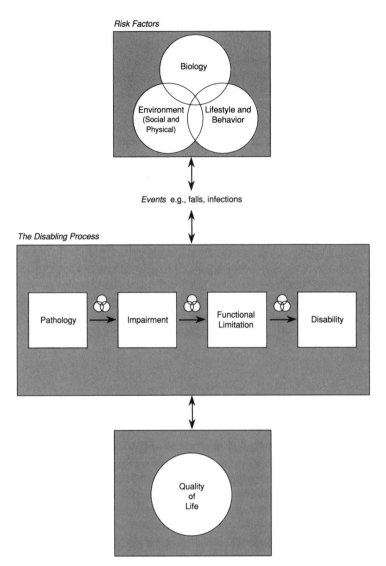

FIGURE 4 Model of disability showing the interaction of the disabling process, quality of life, and risk factors. Three types of risk factors are included: biological (e.g., Rh type); environmental (e.g., lead paint [physical environment], access to care [social environment]); and lifestyle and behavior (e.g., tobacco consumption). Bidirectional arrows indicate the potential for "feedback." The potential for additional risk factors to affect the progression toward disability is shown between the stages of the model. These additional risk factors might include, depending on the stage of the model, diagnosis, treatment, therapy, adequacy of rehabilitation, age of onset, financial resources, expectations, and environmental barriers.

social interaction. Also, the effects of specific stages in the model can be moderated by such interventions as assistive devices. Similarly, environmental modification (e.g., elimination of physical obstacles and barriers) is an important form of disability prevention, as is such landmark antidiscrimination legislation as the recently enacted Americans with Disabilities Act.

A variety of personal, societal, and environmental factors can influence the progression of a disabling condition from pathology to disability. They can also affect the degree of limitation or disability a person experiences and the occurrence of secondary conditions. A few of these factors are health status, psychological state, socioeconomic status, educational attainment and vocational training, climate, and the presence of multiple conditions and disabilities.

As indicated in the model, quality of life is an integral part of the disabling process. Research indicates that a person's perception of quality of life influences his or her responses to potentially disabling conditions and therefore outcomes. In turn, each successive stage in the disabling process poses an increasing threat of diminished quality of life. Measures that reduce this threat—for example, providing assistive technology that enables an individual to remain autonomous in at least some roles or modifying the work site to accommodate a person's limitations—can be effective interventions for preventing disability.

Thus disability is the product of a complex interactive process involving biological, behavioral, and environmental (social and physical) risk factors, and quality of life. Although disability always begins with a pathological condition, it is not inevitable even for people with incurable diseases or injury-caused conditions that carry the highest risks. There are usually, if not always, many points in the progression to disability at which to intervene and improve the quality of life for people with potentially disabling conditions.

The next four sections briefly discuss some of the information from each of the focus chapters. In the full report, these chapters each cover the magnitude of disability related to that category of disability, data needs, and prevention strategies. Although some primary prevention measures are described and discussed, the emphasis in the chapters and in these sections is on prevention for people who already have potentially disabling conditions (i.e., secondary and tertiary prevention).

Developmental Disabilities

Developmental disabilities affect about 4 percent of the population under age 21 and are caused by a variety of conditions, including cerebral palsy, seizure disorders, mental retardation, hearing and vision impairments, autism, structural birth defects (e.g., spina bifida) that cannot be corrected by surgery, and social and intellectual deprivation. These conditions, which usually persist throughout an individual's lifetime, are diagnosed in an estimated 80,000 children each year. Because of their early onset, developmental disabilities account for a large percentage of the cumulative total of disability years[1] for all age groups. In 1984, federal, state, and local governments spent an estimated $16.5 billion on programs and services for children with developmental disabilities. Not included in this cost estimate are programs and services for the additional 5-10 percent of all children who have learning disorders and require special education services.

Research has led to a number of important measures for preventing potentially disabling conditions that are acquired during childhood or that are the product of events during prenatal development. For example, lead screening followed by environmental lead abatement programs can reduce the incidence of lead toxicity. The removal of lead from gasoline has significantly reduced environmental exposure to lead. In the late 1970s an estimated 1.5 million children ages 6 months to 5 years had blood lead levels greater than or equal to 25 µg/dl. It has also been estimated that, in 1984, 200,000 children (ages 6 months to 5 years) in standard metropolitan statistical areas (SMSA) had blood lead levels greater than or equal to 25 µg/dl. Recent studies indicate, however, that adverse effects on the fetus and child probably begin at blood lead levels of 15 µg/dl and below. A lower recommended threshold (currently 25 µg/dl) will probably be set, and more aggressive measures are being advocated for removing lead from the environment.

Interventions to prevent many birth defects and developmental disabilities have not yet been developed. Even when the means are known, they are often not adopted. For example, abstinence from alcohol during pregnancy prevents fetal alcohol syndrome, which can result in mental retardation, growth deficiency, facial abnormalities, and other conditions. The prevalence of fetal alcohol syndrome in the general population is estimated to be 1.7 cases per 1,000 births, but much higher rates have been reported for certain groups.

Injury-Related Disabilities

About 57 million Americans sustain injuries each year at a total lifetime cost of $158 billion. For every death caused by injuries—about 142,000 annually—16 people are hospitalized and 381 additional people incur injuries that do not require inpatient treatment. About $108 billion in economic costs, more than two-thirds of the total estimated lifetime cost of injuries, stem from nonfatal injuries.

---

[1]A "disability year" is a year of life lived with a defined disability. Similar to "years of potential life lost," disability years provide an indicator of public health significance.

In this report, the committee focused on head injuries and spinal cord injuries, which can cause significant physical, neurological, and psychosocial deficits and result in economic costs per person that are among the highest for injury-caused pathologies and impairments. Each year, about 1.3 million people suffer head injuries, and 70,000 to 90,000 of these individuals sustain moderate to severe traumatic brain injuries. Total annual medical costs for people who sustain head injuries were estimated to be $12.5 billion in 1982. At highest risk of sustaining traumatic brain injuries are people between the ages of 15 and 24, especially males. Demographic studies indicate that the incidence of traumatic brain injury is greatest for nonwhite urban populations and lowest for white populations living in suburban and rural areas. Motor vehicle collisions and falls are the leading causes of such injury. To the extent that they are discernible, trends over the past 10 years indicate that improvements in emergency medical services and acute management of head injuries have substantially increased the proportion of people who survive these injuries.

Each year, between 10,000 and 20,000 people sustain spinal cord injuries. Estimated lifetime costs for consequent medical treatment for such injuries range from $210,400 to $751,900, depending on the extent of injury. The most common major impairments are muscle paralysis and loss of sensation. Older adolescent males and young men are at greatest risk of spinal cord injury. Motor vehicle collisions and falls are the leading causes, followed by acts of violence, especially those involving firearms. In the 1950s, only people with low-level paraplegia were generally expected to survive; today, even people with high-level quadriplegia survive and live lives of high quality. A national study found that quadriplegia continues to be the outcome for half of all people who sustain spinal cord injuries; however, the proportion of people with quadriplegia who have neurologically incomplete lesions and therefore retain some motor control and sensation increased from 38 percent in 1973 to 54 percent in 1983.

Disabilities Associated with Chronic Disease and Aging

The prevalence of chronic disease—incurable, long-lasting pathologies such as osteoarthritis, cancer, heart disease, and diabetes—has increased to near-epidemic proportions in the United States. Almost half of all working-age people have one or more chronic conditions. An estimated 80 percent of the elderly have a chronic condition, and about 40 percent have some form of activity limitation due to chronic conditions.

Chronic conditions increase a person's risk of disability, although the degree of risk varies among conditions. Indeed, the most prevalent conditions, such as sinusitis, hypertension, and hearing impairment, generally pose low risks of activity limitation, whereas the least prevalent conditions, such as multiple sclerosis and lung or bronchial cancer, pose very high risks of disability. Thus conditions that frequently result in disability may be more appropriate targets for primary prevention strategies, and those that pose lower risks of developing into disability may be more appropriately addressed by secondary or tertiary prevention strategies.

Many chronic conditions are associated with the aging process, which contributes to the widely held stereotype that aging is synonymous with a decline in functional capacity. An increasing body of research contradicts this stereotype, demonstrating that the physical and mental health status of elderly people can improve as well as deteriorate. Studies show, for example, that the adoption of health-promoting practices even late in life is beneficial. Potentially debilitating problems such as those associated with incontinence and osteoporosis are amenable to skillful rehabilitation. Prospects are good for increasing the number of disability-free years in the average life span, but much more research on the aging process, on potentially effective interventions, and on the delivery and coordination of services is needed.

Secondary Conditions Associated with Disability

People with disabling conditions are often at risk of developing secondary conditions that can result in further deterioration in health status, functional capacity, and quality of life. Secondary conditions by definition are causally related to a primary disabling condition and include decubitus ulcers, contractures, physical deconditioning, cardiopulmonary conditions, and mental depression. Considerable research has been done on the etiology and prevention of certain secondary conditions (e.g., pressure sores); in general, however, secondary conditions have received very little attention from researchers and health care and social service providers, despite the causal relationship that makes many of them easily predictable.

Much of what is known about the prevention of many secondary conditions is incidental and often results from deduction based on individual or clinical experience. There is a clear need for systematic evaluations of currently used interventions, as well as for research devoted to developing treatment protocols for people with specific types of disabilities. Such protocols would list assessment and treatment strategies for patients whose conditions matched prespecified characteristics, addressing not only medical needs but also environmental (social and physical) and behavioral risk factors associated with secondary conditions. Implementation of the protocols, of course, will require the participation of a wide spectrum of professionals in medical and nonmedical fields, as well as the people with disabling conditions themselves, their families, personal attendants, and advocates.

Also requiring greater attention, in both research and service delivery, is the role of assistive technology. Such technology promotes personal independence, facilitates the performance of tasks related to personal, familial, and social roles, and helps prevent debilitating, costly secondary conditions. However, outmoded concepts held by public and private insurance programs of what is "medically necessary" often result in restriction or denial of coverage for assistive technologies. This problem indicates the need for improved programs of research and services that focus on secondary and tertiary prevention of disability—in the committee's model, halting progress toward disability and preventing secondary conditions.

RECOMMENDATIONS

As described and discussed throughout the report, the social and environmental aspects of disability and disability prevention are of critical importance and help to define limitations in the role of medicine in disability prevention. Indeed, the major disability-related roles for the fields of public health and medicine involve the prevention, early detection, diagnosis, treatment, and rehabilitation of potentially disabling conditions. Once such a condition is identified, however, the means of disability prevention go beyond rehabilitative restoration of function to include important social and economic factors.

Increasing attention to and understanding of the broad range of issues related to disability in this country recently resulted in the Americans with Disabilities Act signed into law by President Bush on July 26, 1990. That same impetus, amplified by the desire for accessible, affordable quality health care for all, led to the committee's finding that there is an urgent need for a well-organized, coordinated national disability prevention program. An agenda for such a program is presented on the next page. The agenda includes the program's stated goal and five strategies for its achievement: organization and coordination of the national program, surveillance, research, access to care and preventive services, and professional and public education. The full set of recommended measures to support each strategy is presented in Chapter 9; some of them are listed below (their numbers correspond to the numbers in Chapter 9).

Organization and Coordination

There are a number of disability-related programs in the federal government, but currently no one agency has been charged with leadership responsibilities that focus on prevention. The committee's recommendations below suggest mechanisms to organize and coordinate a national disability prevention program and to provide input from the diverse groups affected by disability.

A NATIONAL AGENDA FOR THE PREVENTION OF DISABILITY

GOAL

To reduce the incidence and prevalence of disability in the United States, as well as the personal, social, and economic consequences of disability in order to improve the quality of life for individuals, families, and the population at large.

STRATEGIES

Organization and Coordination—Establish leadership and administrative responsibility for implementing and coordinating the National Agenda for the Prevention of Disability within a single unit of the federal government. Implementation of the agenda should be guided by a national advisory committee, and progress should be critically evaluated periodically. In addition to federal leadership, achieving the goals of the agenda will require the strong, sustained participation of the state, local, and private sectors.

Surveillance—Develop a conceptual framework and standard definitions of disability and related concepts as the basis for a national disability surveillance system. Such a system should be designed to (1) characterize the nature, extent, and consequences of disability and antecedent conditions in the U.S. population; (2) elucidate the causal pathways of specific types of disability; (3) identify promising means of prevention; and (4) monitor the progress of prevention efforts.

Research—Develop a comprehensive national research program on disability prevention. The research should emphasize longitudinal studies and should focus on preventive and therapeutic interventions. Special attention should be directed to the causal mechanisms whereby socioeconomic and psychosocial disadvantage lead to disability. Training young scientists for careers in research on disability prevention should become a high priority.

Access to Care and Preventive Services—Eliminate the barriers to access to care, especially for women and children, to permit more effective primary prevention and prevent progression of disability and the development of secondary conditions. Existing programs of proven effectiveness should be expanded, and new service programs should be introduced. Returning persons with disabling conditions to productive, remunerative work is a high priority.

Professional and Public Education—Educate health professionals in the prevention of disability. Foster a broad public understanding of the importance of eliminating social, attitudinal, and environmental barriers to the participation of people with functional limitations in society and to the fulfillment of their personal goals. Educate health professionals, people with disability, family members, and personal attendants in disability prevention and preventing the development of secondary conditions.

Leadership of the National Disability Prevention Program

The congressionally mandated role of the National Council on Disability (NCD) is to provide advice and make recommendations to the President and to Congress with respect to disability policy. In keeping with its charter, the council has been and should continue to be an effective leader in developing disability policy in such areas as education, health care services, and civil rights.

In 1986 the NCD identified the need for a national program for disability prevention and recommended to the President and Congress that such a program be established in the Centers for Disease Control (CDC). In 1988 CDC initiated the Disabilities Prevention Program to build capacity in disability prevention at the state and local levels, establish systems of surveillance for disabilities, use epidemiological approaches to identify risks and target interventions, and provide states with technical assistance. It is the only federal program that has been charged specifically with disability prevention. Its initial focus has been prevention of the more readily identifiable injuries and developmental disabilities, and the secondary conditions that are often associated with them.

The committee endorses the emerging federal leadership in disability prevention at CDC. The agency's traditional strengths—epidemiology, surveillance, technology transfer, disease prevention, and communication and coordination with state, local, and community-based public health activities—are consonant with the needs of a national program. Moreover, CDC has demonstrated its leadership in the development and effective implementation of interventions in numerous specific public health situations, in quality control for screening programs and their implementation, in the development of school and other public health curricula, and in the evaluation of public health service delivery programs.

Given the magnitude of the public health problem disability presents and the large number of various types of disability-related public and private programs, there is a need for expansion and coordination of disability prevention activities. The committee's recommendations, which appear below, have been formulated to address that need and provide a framework for future program development.

The CDC Disabilities Prevention Program is a good first step in the development of such a framework. In addition, the informal relationship that currently exists between it and the National Council on Disability appears to be a mutually beneficial one that has strengthened federal disability prevention activity during its infancy. To the extent that such a relationship remains beneficial to developing a national program for disability prevention, it should continue.

RECOMMENDATION 1:   Develop leadership of a National Disability Prevention Program at CDC

To advance the goal and carry out the strategies of the national agenda, the committee recommends that the CDC Disabilities Prevention Program be expanded to serve as the focus of a National Disability Prevention Program (NDPP). In assuming the lead responsibility for implementing the national agenda for the prevention of disability over the life course, the NDPP should coordinate activities with other relevant agencies, emphasizing comprehensive surveillance, applied research, professional and public education, and preventive intervention with balanced attention to developmental disabilities, injuries, chronic diseases, and secondary conditions.

As the national program develops, with its emphasis on prevention of disability throughout the life course, it should focus on identifying and modifying the biological, behavioral, and environmental (physical and social) risk factors associated with potentially disabling conditions, as well as monitoring the incidence and prevalence of the conditions themselves. The program should be conducted in cooperation and in partnership with state health agencies and other public agencies. A major component of the program should be the development at the state level of a sharply increased capacity to prevent disability.

A disability prevention program of the scope and ambition envisioned by the committee will require much more than can be accomplished by governments acting alone. The active participation of all segments of society is required.

RECOMMENDATION 2:   Develop an enhanced role for the private sector

The NDPP should recognize the key role of the private sector in disability prevention, including advocacy groups, persons with disabilities, business and other employers, the insurance industry, academia, the media, voluntary agencies, and philanthropies. Indeed, the potential contributions of the private sector in achieving the program's goals cannot be emphasized too strongly. Its role encompasses the provision of employment opportunities, modification of the workplace, research in and development of assistive technology, provision of appropriate insurance, and development of a national awareness program.

One way to involve the private sector might be to establish an independent forum on disability policy for the promotion, coordination, and resolution of disability-related issues that would facilitate prevention. Addressing many of these issues requires the collaborative support and involvement of a broad array of scientists and informed leaders from both the private and public sectors. The purpose of the forum would be to improve policymaking through a continuing dialogue among individuals and groups that play a significant role in shaping policy and public opinion. Areas for consideration might include access to assistive technology and personal assistance services, gaps in health insurance coverage, family leave policies, and implementation issues related to the Americans with Disabilities Act.

Advisory Committee

As stated throughout the full report, disability is a public health and social issue. Thus a national disability prevention program will be centrally dependent on public attitudes toward people with disabilities and on the way community activities are organized, which includes access to housing, public transportation, and the workplace. Equally important is the reduction of prejudice and discrimination toward people with disabilities. An agenda for disability prevention will require cooperation among all levels of government; the health, social services, and research professions; business; educational institutions; churches; and citizens' organizations throughout the country.

RECOMMENDATION 3:   Establish a national advisory committee
An advisory committee for the NDPP should be established to help ensure that its efforts are broadly representative of the diverse interests in the field. The advisory group should include persons with disabilities and their advocates; public health, medical, social service, and research professionals; and representatives of business, insurance, educational, and philanthropic organizations, including churches. The role of the advisory committee would be to advise CDC on priorities in disability prevention research and the nationwide implementation of prevention strategies, as well as to assess progress toward the goal of the national agenda for the prevention of disability. The advisory committee should be appointed by the Department of Health and Human Services and meet at least three times a year. In keeping with its role in regard to disability policy, the National Council on Disability should be a permanent member of this committee.

Interagency Coordination and Periodic Review

The fragmentation of disability-related activities and the lack of continuity of care are highly disruptive to preventive efforts. Part of the problem derives from the fact that essential services are funded and provided by various agencies and by different levels of government without a clear focus of authority and responsibility, leading to gaps in services. The lack of coordination of health and medically related rehabilitation activities and social services is a long-standing problem that is not easily rectified. Improvements will require energy and direction, a focus on prevention, and a clear strategy for coordination, cooperation, and integration among several federal programs as they are administered at the local level. These federal programs include those concerned with health care (Health Care Financing Administration), disability benefits (Social Security Administration and the Department of Veterans Affairs), vocational rehabilitation (Department of Education), community support (National Institute of Mental Health), and housing (Department of Housing and Urban Development). Thus responsibility for planning, coordination, and evaluation of these activities should be highly placed in the federal government (e.g., in the Office of the Secretary of the Department of Health and Human Services) to facilitate the type of coordinated leadership at the federal level necessary to ensure cooperation at the local level.

RECOMMENDATION 4:   Establish a federal interagency council
A standing Interagency Council on Disability Prevention should be established by the Secretary of Health and Human Services. The interagency council should be charged with examining and developing conjoint activities in disability prevention and with identifying existing policies that inhibit disability prevention and rehabilitation. More specifically, the interagency council should be convened semiannually to identify, examine, and foster enhanced disability prevention strategies by (1) recommending the elimination of conflicting public policies and coordinating and integrating programs, (2) developing new policy initiatives, (3) improving service delivery, and (4) setting research priorities. The interagency council should have a permanent staff and issue public reports to the Secretary of Health and Human Services, Congress, and the National Council on Disability.

The members of the interagency council should be high-level administrators drawn from the major agencies involved in the various aspects of disability, which include the following: Centers for Disease Control; Health Care Financing Administration; Alcohol, Drug Abuse, and Mental Health Administration; National Institute on Disability and Rehabilitation Research; Health Resources and Services Administration (HRSA), including the Maternal and Child Health Bureau; Agency for Health Care Policy and Research; Social Security Administration; National Institutes of Health; Consumer Product Safety Commission; Bureau of the Census; and other agencies within the Departments of Health and Human Services, Housing and Urban Development, Education, Transportation, Labor, Defense, Veterans Affairs, and others as appropriate.

Surveillance

Although information on the incidence and prevalence of disability is available, it is organized in so many different ways that accurate, useful analysis is impeded. Estimates of the prevalence of disability vary by more than 100 percent. One difficulty is the conceptual confusion surrounding disability and its antecedent conditions. Until there is a consistently applied, widely accepted definition of disability and related concepts, the focus for preventive action and rehabilitation will remain uncertain.

Conceptual Framework

Conceptual confusion regarding disability is not limited to the United States, as indicated by the World Health Organization's development of the International Classification of Impairments, Disabilities, and Handicaps. The WHO classification scheme, which seeks to establish uniformity in the use of important concepts, is an important step toward international comparative studies of disability. The committee, however, saw a need to develop its own system and in this report presents a conceptual framework and model derived from the works of Nagi and the WHO that differs from both primarily in that it incorporates risk factors and quality of life. What is needed now is international agreement on a logical, conceptual system that would result in comparable disability statistics across nations. Existing frameworks represent only the initial steps in a process of conceptual refinement and evaluation.

RECOMMENDATION 6:   Develop a conceptual framework and standard measures of disability
The CDC, which is responsible for surveillance of the nation's health, should design and implement a process for the development and review of conceptual frameworks, classifications, and measures of disability with respect to their utility for surveillance. This effort should involve components of the private sector that collect disability data, as well as federal agencies including the National Institutes of Health; Alcohol, Drug Abuse, and Mental Health Administration; National Council on Disability; Office of Human Development Services (a component of the Department of Health and Human Services); Agency for Health Care Policy and Research; Health Care Financing Administration; Bureau of the Census; Department of Veterans Affairs; Social Security Administration; and HRSA's Maternal and Child Health Bureau. The objective should be consensus on definitions, measures, and a classification and coding system of disability and related concepts. These elements should then be adopted by all local, state, federal, and private agencies that gather data and assemble statistics on disability. Collaboration

with the WHO and other international agencies should be encouraged in developing a classification system to obtain comparable disability data across nations.

A National Disability Surveillance System

Despite its significance as a public health and social issue, disability has received little attention from epidemiologists and statisticians; consequently, surveillance of disabling conditions is inadequate in many ways. When disability is a focus of attention, surveillance is more often concerned with counting the number of people affected than with investigating its causes and secondary conditions. Without knowledge of the conditions and circumstances that can lead to disability, the problem in its many manifestations cannot be fully understood, nor can effective prevention strategies be systematically developed.

Disability prevention will require expanded epidemiological studies and surveillance to identify risk factors, the magnitude of risk, and the degree to which risk can be controlled. Because disability is the product of a complex interaction among behavioral, biological, and environmental (social and physical) factors, epidemiological investigations must encompass a broad range of variables that influence the outcomes of mental and physical impairment. Current surveillance systems are condition specific, permitting identification, for example, of the risk factors associated with injuries. None of them, however, track the risk factors associated with the progression from pathology to impairment to functional limitation to disability. Nor is there sufficient research on the range of consequences associated with specific behaviors and circumstances.

Congenital and developmental conditions, injuries, and chronic diseases that limit human activity do not occur randomly within the general population. Epidemiological principles can be used to identify high-risk groups, to study the etiology, or causal pathways, of functional limitations and disabilities, and to evaluate preventive interventions. More specifically, epidemiology and surveillance could play an increased role in the prevention of disability by (1) accurately determining the dimensions of the populations of people with disabilities, (2) identifying the causes of disabilities, (3) guiding the development and selection of preventive interventions, and (4) evaluating the implementation of interventions.

RECOMMENDATION 7: **Develop a national disability surveillance system**
A national disability surveillance system should be developed to monitor over the life course the incidence and prevalence of (1) functional limitations and disabilities; (2) specific developmental disabilities, injuries,

and diseases that cause functional limitations and disability; and (3) secondary conditions resulting from the primary disability. The system should also monitor causal phenomena, risk factors, functional status, and quality of life, and provide state-specific data for program planning and evaluation of interventions. This system should be developed in cooperation with a broad range of federal agencies and private organizations and be implemented as part of the National Disability Prevention Program.

Research

A wide variety of disability risk factors are associated with the spectrum of diseases and injuries that can lead to disability. These risk factors affect not only the occurrence of the initial event but also the progression of pathologies to impairments, functional limitations, and disabilities. To the extent that risk factors can be eliminated or moderated, the incidence of initial disabling conditions and the progression toward disability can be limited. Much more needs to be known, however, and such knowledge can be acquired only through a broad range of research activities.

Coordinated Research Program

RECOMMENDATION 11:   Develop a comprehensive research program
A coordinated, balanced program of research on the prevention of disability associated with developmental disabilities, injury, chronic disease, and secondary conditions should be an essential component of the National Disability Prevention Program. Emphasis should be placed on identifying biological, behavioral, and environmental (physical and social) risk factors over the life course that are associated with disability and secondary conditions and on developing effective intervention strategies. A continuing effort should be made to incorporate functional assessment and quality of life indicators into the research agenda and surveillance measures.

Longitudinal Studies

The process of developing a disabling condition, as well as the associated potential for secondary conditions, is complex and longitudinal. Yet most available data on disability are cross-sectional, making it impossible to accurately gauge the course of disability in relation to varying risk factors or the impact of timely interventions on the development of disability. There is thus a great need for longitudinal studies that effectively describe the course of disability and identify the most strategic points for effective intervention.

RECOMMENDATION 12:   Emphasize longitudinal research
A research program of longitudinal studies should be developed to determine the course of conditions and impairments that lead to disability and to identify the strategic points of preventive intervention. The research should emphasize the prevention of secondary conditions, improved functional status, and improved quality of life. In addition, because rapid changes are occurring for people with disabling conditions in terms of health services, public attitudes, and opportunities for social participation, cohort studies are needed to assess the effects of these changes over the life course.

Relationship of Socioeconomic Status

Deeper understanding of the biological underpinnings of pathologies, impairments, and functional limitations is an obvious need, and this knowledge is being pursued in a variety of biomedical research programs, such as those sponsored by the National Institutes of Health and the Alcohol, Drug Abuse, and Mental Health Administration. Far less effort has been devoted to the influence of behavioral, physical and social environmental, and social factors on the development of disability. One transcendent problem, for example, is the high rate of disability among people of low socioeconomic status. Most studies of disability attempt to control statistically for socioeconomic status because it is a powerful risk factor. Moreover, because socioeconomic status has sometimes been considered to be   incidental to research investigations, the relationship between disability and socioeconomic status has rarely been addressed directly.

RECOMMENDATION 13:   Conduct research on socioeconomic and psychosocial disadvantage
Research should be conducted to elucidate the relationship between socioeconomic and psychosocial disadvantage and the disabling process. Research that links the social and biological determinants of disability should result in improved understanding of the complex interactions leading to disability, an understanding that would help in developing new prevention strategies.

Interventions

There is a clear need to incorporate existing knowledge more efficiently into disability prevention. A concomitant need is to ascertain the effectiveness of current approaches in the wide variety of situations in which disability occurs. All areas of prevention require critical evaluations of the effectiveness of the tools and methods used in the prevention of disability and secondary conditions.

The federal government spends about $60 billion annually for medical coverage and to supplement the incomes of people with disabilities; it spends a relatively small amount on research to identify practices and technologies that can prevent the initial occurrence of disability or limit complications among people with disabilities to help them lead more productive lives. Moreover, the federal funding agencies that support biomedical research have not made prevention a high priority, and there has been little effort devoted to developing research programs on the prevention of disability and secondary conditions.

RECOMMENDATION 14: Expand research on preventive and therapeutic interventions
Research on the costs, effectiveness, and outcomes of preventive and therapeutic interventions should be expanded. The expanded research program should also include acute care services, rehabilitative and habilitative services and technologies, and longitudinal programs of care and interventions to prevent secondary conditions. The National Institute on Disability and Rehabilitation Research, the Department of Veterans Affairs, the National Institutes of Health, the Alcohol, Drug Abuse, and Mental Health Administration, and the Agency for Health Care Policy and Research should join with CDC to develop cooperative and collaborative research programs in the biological, behavioral, and social sciences as they relate to disability prevention. These programs should also emphasize the translation of new findings into national prevention efforts that inform and educate people with disabilities, their families, personal attendants, and advocates, as well as clinical practitioners. Consideration should be given to approaches used in other countries (e.g., the Netherlands, Sweden, England, and France), where disability prevention is viewed from a broad perspective that includes social and ethical implications and socioeconomic costs.

Access to Care and Preventive Services

Many persons with disabilities are not covered by Medicare or Medicaid and have little access to private coverage because they either are unemployed or have been rejected for insurance because of their disabilities. Thus the problem of access to care is even greater for people with disabilities than for the general American population. Moreover, persons with disabilities and those at risk of disability are disproportionately poor, making it difficult for them to purchase insurance, make required copayments, or purchase essential services and equipment for their rehabilitation. In addition, poverty compounds the difficulties faced by those with disabilities in gaining recognition of their needs (which are often complicated by the social circumstances associated with poverty) and in developing satisfactory relationships with health providers.

Accessible, Affordable Quality Care

The committee recognizes that the problems of access to health care are deeply embedded in the organization of the U.S. health insurance system and its relationship to employment and other issues. The committee is also aware that resolution of many of the problems identified in this report will require a fundamental restructuring of the financing and organization of the nation's health services. This committee was not charged with addressing these larger issues; nevertheless, its members feel strongly that the gaps in the nation's present system contribute to an unnecessary burden of disability, loss of productivity, and lowered quality of life, and that the United States must make basic health services accessible to all.

Thirty to forty million Americans, including millions of mothers and children, do not have health care insurance or access to adequate health services. Even those Americans who have health care insurance are rarely covered for (and have access to) adequate preventive and long-term medical care, rehabilitation, and assistive technologies. These factors demonstrably contribute to the incidence, prevalence, and severity of primary and secondary disabling conditions and, tragically, avoidable disability.

Recently, the U.S. Bipartisan Commission on Comprehensive Health Care (the Pepper Commission) recommended a universal insurance plan that emphasizes preventive care and identifies children and pregnant women as the groups whose needs should be addressed first. In addition, the American Academy of Pediatrics (AAP) has developed a specific proposal to provide health insurance for all children and pregnant women. The AAP proposal presents several principles relative to ensuring access to health care, as well as estimates of program costs and a package of basic benefits. Many aspects of the proposal could have favorable effects on the cost of health care (e.g., prenatal care should lower expenditures for intensive care of newborns and subsequent disabling conditions).

The committee believes that a system that provided accessible, affordable quality health care for all would have an enormous beneficial effect on the prevention of disability. Yet the economic and political hurdles to that end are formidable, and a near-term solution is not in sight. A first step that has been proposed is to provide quality health care services for all mothers and children (up to age 18). These services have a high probability of preventing disability; however, assessing or evaluating their cost implications was not part of the charge to this committee.

RECOMMENDATION 16: **Provide comprehensive health services to all mothers and children**
Preventing disability will require access by all Americans to quality health care. An immediate step that could be taken would be to ensure the availability of comprehensive medical services to all children up to the age of 18 and to their mothers who are within 200 percent of the poverty level; in addition, every pregnant woman should be assured access to prenatal care. When provided, these services should include continuous, comprehensive preventive and acute health services for every child who has, or is at risk of developing, a developmental disability. In certain circumstances—for example, providing prenatal care for the prevention of low birthweight—the economic consequences have been shown to be favorable, but they need to be explored further in other areas of health care delivery.

Research on prenatal care has demonstrated that comprehensive obstetric care for pregnant women, beginning in the first trimester, reduces the risk of infant mortality and morbidity, including congenital and developmental disability. Researchers also have documented that women who have the greatest risk of complications during pregnancy—teenagers and women who are poor—are also the least likely to obtain comprehensive prenatal care. Furthermore, in its 1985 report, *Preventing Low Birthweight*, the IOM showed conclusively that, for each dollar spent on providing prenatal care to low-income, poorly educated women, total expenditures for direct medical care of their low-birthweight infants were reduced by more than $3 during the first year of life.

RECOMMENDATION 17: **Provide effective family planning and prenatal services**
Educational efforts should be undertaken to provide women in high-risk groups with the opportunity to learn the importance of family planning services and prenatal care. Access to prenatal diagnosis and associated services, including pregnancy termination, currently varies according to socioeconomic status. The committee respects the diversity of viewpoints relative to those services but believes they should be available to all pregnant women for their individual consideration as part of accessible, affordable quality care.

Even among privately or publicly insured people with disabilities, access to needed services is often a problem. Coverage may be limited by an arbitrarily defined "medical necessity" requirement that does not permit reimbursement for many types of preventive and rehabilitative services and assistive technologies. Insurance policies tend to mirror the acute care orientation of the U.S. medical system and generally fail to recognize the importance and value of longitudinal care and of secondary and tertiary prevention in slowing, halting, or reversing deterioration in function. The presumption, which has never been thoroughly evaluated, is that rehabilitative and attendant services, assistive technology, and other components of longitudinal care are too costly or not cost-effective.

Access to health care, particularly primary care, is a major problem for persons with disabilities. Many report that they have great difficulty finding a physician who is knowledgeable about their ongoing health care needs. They also have problems obtaining timely medical care and assistive technology that can help prevent minor health problems from becoming significant complications. National data indicate that, relative to the general population, persons with disabilities, regardless of age, have high rates of use of health care services such as hospital care.

The problem of access to care for persons with disabilities transcends the availability of insurance or a regular relationship with a health professional (although for many large gaps exist in both these areas). More important is that the person have access to appropriate care during the full course of a disabling condition. Such care should be provided in a way that prevents secondary conditions and maximizes the person's ability to function in everyday social roles. It must have continuity and not be restricted by arbitrary rules that limit services necessary for effective rehabilitation and participation in society. Persons with disabilities often face enormous impediments to obtaining the coordinated services they need to prevent secondary conditions and improve their opportunity for successful lives. Such impediments include (1) lack of support from insurance and other funding agencies, (2) lack of locally available services, and (3) absence of local coordinating mechanisms.

RECOMMENDATION 18: Develop new health service delivery strategies for people with disabilities
New health service delivery strategies should be developed that will facilitate access to services and meet the primary health care, health education, and health promotion needs of people with disabling conditions. These strategies should include assistive technologies and attendant services that facilitate independent living.

Access to Vocational Services

Vocational services are crucial to ensure that return-to-work goals are achieved. These services may include counseling and work readiness evaluations, job training, job placement, work-site modification, and postemployment services (e.g., Projects with Industry) to ensure satisfactory adjustment and assistance in sustaining employment.

RECOMMENDATION 22:   Provide comprehensive vocational services
Vocational services aimed at reintegrating persons with disabilities into the community and enabling them to return to work should be made financially and geographically accessible.

Professional and Public Education

The prevention of disability requires not only access to care and restructuring of services but also a radically different mind-set among many health and other professionals (e.g., psychologists, sociologists, educational specialists) and the general public. As the committee observes throughout its report, the attitudes and behavior of health professionals and the public could either facilitate effective coping and productive lives for persons with disabilities or erect obstacles in their path. For example, many secondary conditions are preventable, but health professionals often are not familiar with the intervention strategies that can be used, and may provide inappropriate care as a result.

Education of Professionals

The committee notes that the field of physical medicine and rehabilitation is one of only a few medical specialties with a shortage of physicians. This situation is not surprising because rehabilitation has had a low priority in medical schools and residency training programs, and many do not even offer courses on disability and rehabilitation. Similarly, personnel shortages exist in physical therapy, speech therapy, occupational therapy, and all allied health and nursing disciplines dealing with disability. Yet the problem goes well beyond these shortages. Even if the numbers of practitioners in these specialties were substantially increased, many problems would remain (e.g., there are few incentives for practicing the types of longitudinal care this committee advocates, and health professionals who follow these careers historically have had little recognition and prestige within their professional groups). In addition, longitudinal care, which has its own special appeal, is also "patient intensive" and requires complex teamwork, two factors that may outweigh its rewards in the minds of many health professionals.

Steps must be taken to ease the current shortage of knowledgeable physicians, allied health professionals, and others (e.g., psychologists, sociologists, educational specialists) working in disability prevention. In fact, all specialties should have a better understanding of the process of disability and appropriate modes of preventive intervention. The longitudinal care described in this report is sometimes provided by specialists in physical medicine and rehabilitation, but most typically it will be provided by general internists, family physicians, psychiatrists, psychologists, social workers, and others. Any long-term strategy must address the education of a broad range of these professionals as part of a national agenda for the prevention of disability.

RECOMMENDATION 23: **Upgrade medical education and training of physicians**
Medical school curricula and pediatric, general internal medicine, geriatric, and family medicine residency training for medical professionals should include curricular material in physical medicine, rehabilitation, and mental health. In addition, such curricula should address physiatric principles and practices appropriate to the identification of potentially disabling conditions of acute illness and injury. Appropriate interventions, including consultation and collaboration with mental health and allied health professionals, social workers, and educational specialists, and the application of effective clinical protocols should also be included.

RECOMMENDATION 24: **Upgrade the training of allied professionals**
Allied health, public health, and other professionals interested in disability issues (e.g., social workers, educational specialists) should be trained in the principles and practices of disability prevention, treatment planning, and rehabilitation, including psychosocial and vocational rehabilitation.

Education of Persons with Disabilities and Their Families, Personal Attendants, and Advocates

People with disabilities and their families, personal attendants, and advocates should be better informed about the principles of disability prevention. Such education would contribute significantly to the prevention of disability and secondary conditions—those brought about by poor self-care as well as those induced by a lack of needed social and other support services, architectural inaccessibility, unequal educational and employment opportunities, negative attitudes toward disability, changes in living environments, and greater exposure to disruptive, frustrating events.

Independent living centers, which are controlled and staffed by persons with disabilities, are designed to deal with the prevention of secondary conditions and to be a source of information on the practical aspects of daily living with a disability. Because these centers are usually staffed by persons with disabilities who are living independently, they offer advice based on first-hand experience of the motivation and ingenuity needed to pursue an independent lifestyle. Being able to share experiences with peers who are independent brings to light those coping mechanisms that aid in preventing secondary conditions. Independent living centers are also effective advocates for attitudinal and architectural changes in society that would improve accessibility, stimulate social interaction and productivity, and facilitate an active, quality lifestyle.

RECOMMENDATION 27: Provide more training opportunities for family members and personal attendants of people with disabling conditions
Persons with disabilities, their families, personal attendants, and advocates should have access to information and training relative to disability prevention with particular emphasis on the prevention of secondary conditions. Independent living centers and other community-based support groups provide a foundation for such training programs and offer a source of peer counseling.

A list of the committee's recommendations for a national agenda for the prevention of disabilities follows.

LIST OF RECOMMENDATIONS

A NATIONAL AGENDA FOR THE PREVENTION OF DISABILITY

ORGANIZATION AND COORDINATION
Develop leadership of National Disability Prevention Program at CDC
Develop an enhanced role for the private sector
Establish a national advisory committee
Establish a federal interagency council
Critically assess progress periodically

SURVEILLANCE
Develop a conceptual framework and standard measures of disability
Develop a national disability surveillance system
Revise the National Health Interview Survey
Conduct a comprehensive longitudinal survey of disability
Develop disability indexes

RESEARCH
Develop a comprehensive research program
Emphasize longitudinal research
Conduct research on socioeconomic and psychosocial disadvantage
Expand research on preventive and therapeutic interventions
Upgrade training for research on disability prevention

ACCESS TO CARE AND PREVENTIVE SERVICES
Provide comprehensive health services to all mothers and children
Provide effective family planning and prenatal services
Develop new health service delivery strategies for people with disabilities
Develop new health promotion models for people with disabilities
Foster local capacity building and demonstration projects
Continue effective prevention programs
Provide comprehensive vocational services

PROFESSIONAL AND PUBLIC EDUCATION
Upgrade medical education and training of physicians
Upgrade the training of allied professionals
Establish a program of grants for education and training
Provide more public education on the prevention of disability
Provide more training opportunities for family members and personal
  attendants of people with disabling conditions

1

Introduction

About 35 million Americans—one person in seven—have physical or mental impairments that interfere with their daily activities (National Center for Health Statistics, 1989a). The functional limitations of more than 9 million of these people are so severe that they cannot work, attend school, or maintain a household. By these two measures alone, disability ranks as the nation's largest public health problem, affecting not only individuals with disabling conditions and their immediate families, but also society at large. Many medically, socially, and economically important issues call attention to the need for developing an effective national disability prevention program. One is modern medicine's progress in prolonging life, or, more accurately, averting deaths. For example, the odds of survival for low-birthweight babies have increased steadily during the past several decades. The age-adjusted rate of deaths caused by injuries has fallen precipitously, from 57.5 deaths per 100,000 injuries in 1950 to 35.2 deaths per 100,000 injuries in 1986 (National Center for Health Statistics, 1989a). Medical victories, however, do not always translate into absolute victories. The outcome of surviving prematurity, injury, heart attack, or stroke may be disabling conditions that can result in a diminished quality of life and the need for continuing supportive services. Because assessments of the nation's health are based largely on mortality statistics, U.S. society rarely reckons with the full consequences of extending lives. As the number of people who survive life-threatening conditions increases, quality of life issues must be given fuller consideration in health and social policy decisions.

The need to intensify the search for effective strategies for disability prevention is heightened by the aging of the population. By the year 2020, people over age 65 will number 51.4 million and constitute 17.3 percent of the population, as compared with 31.7 million and 12.7 percent in 1990.

The risk of developing cardiovascular disease, rheumatoid arthritis, and many other chronic diseases increases with age, as does the likelihood of disability caused by these conditions. If these chronic conditions cannot be prevented, then the focus of medical care and support services should be on the prevention of associated conditions with the purpose of increasing the number of disability-free years in the lengthened life span.

Beyond the demonstrated need for a national disability prevention program, circumstances suggest that the beginning of the 1990s is an especially appropriate time to develop such a program. For example, two decades of efforts by disability-rights groups to increase public awareness paved the way for passage of the Americans with Disabilities Act, which bans discrimination in employment and the provision of services. This legislation affirms the goals of equal opportunity and independence for Americans with physical and mental disabilities and acknowledges the importance of their participation in the affairs of society. The act includes protection against discrimination on the basis of disability in public and private transportation, public accommodations, employment, telecommunications, and local and state government activities.

The Americans with Disabilities Act will have several beneficial effects. For example, the expected increase in the employment of people with disabling conditions should result in their enjoying higher standards of living and fuller integration into society; in addition, more individuals will have jobs commensurate with their skills and training and will receive employer-provided health benefits. Collectively, these effects should help reduce the incidence of many secondary conditions, including depression, that commonly result from discrimination and the social and economic barriers now encountered by people with disabling conditions.

Also cause for optimism in disability prevention efforts is research progress toward understanding the biological, behavioral, and environmental (physical and social) risk factors of disability. New understanding of risk factors can be translated into intervention strategies to prevent or mitigate developmental conditions, injuries, chronic diseases, and secondary conditions that increase the risk of disability. Moreover, accumulating experience shows that continuing deterioration of physical or mental health and increasing dependency need not be the outcomes of chronic diseases and functional limitations. Opportunities are increasing to reverse, interrupt, or at least slow the progression to disability, as well as to prevent the development of secondary conditions in people who already have a potentially disabling condition. A few advances in this area have been dramatic. For example, in 1990 researchers reported that administering the steroid methylprednisolone within eight hours of the occurrence of a spinal cord injury can significantly reduce the severity of resulting functional limitations (Bracken et al., 1990). Thus a person who once would have been fully paralyzed in the legs might now retain sufficient functioning to walk with the aid of crutches and braces.

Failure to seize emerging opportunities and develop a comprehensive strategy for disability prevention is tantamount to allowing the health and quality of life of a large portion of the U.S. population to deteriorate. A growing number of health and social service professionals, policymakers, and members of the public deem such an outcome unacceptable.

In 1986, building on the work of Marge (1981), the National Council on Disability (NCD) identified and underscored the need for a national effort to prevent disability and recommended to the President and Congress that such a program be established at the Centers for Disease Control (CDC). In 1988 CDC initiated the Disabilities Prevention Program, which is designed to build capacity in disability prevention at the state and local levels, establish systems of surveillance for disabilities, use epidemiological approaches to identify risks and target interventions, and provide states with technical assistance. It is the only federal program that has been charged specifically with disability prevention. Its initial focus has been prevention of the more readily identifiable injuries and developmental disabilities, and the secondary conditions that are often associated with them.

This report, prepared by the Institute of Medicine's Committee on a National Agenda for the Prevention of Disability at the request of the CDC and the NCD, responds to the challenge to create a blueprint for a comprehensive national undertaking to reduce substantially the incidence and prevalence of disability in the United States. The report addresses many of the public health and social issues that intersect under the heading of disability. It describes a conceptual model of the characteristics and determinants of disability and outlines measures for creating a national program for disability prevention.

The remainder of this chapter describes briefly the definition and concept of disability used in this report, the application of public health concepts to disability prevention, and the report's scope and organization.

DISABILITY: DEFINITION AND CONCEPT

Although understanding of the medical, behavioral, social, and economic aspects of disability is growing, terminology continues to breed confusion, even among professionals in disability-related fields. For example, the failure of data collection agencies to use consistent definitions of disability and related concepts results in varied estimates of the prevalence of disability. Such confusion and inconsistency are common in emerging fields. Given the nascent state of disability prevention in general and of the epidemiology of disability in particular, confusion and inconsistency are understandable. But they pose obstacles to surveillance efforts and to efforts to elucidate the many factors that underlie the disabling process and the occurrence of secondary conditions. They also impede the design and evaluation of preventive interventions. As one aspect of its work, the committee has attempted to improve conceptual clarity and sharpen the definitions of terms.

The term *disability* as used in this report refers to limitations in physical or mental function, caused by one or more health conditions, in carrying out socially defined tasks and roles that individuals generally are expected to be able to do (see Appendix A, this volume). The term *health condition* includes *pathology*, or active disease, as well as *impairment*, which refers to losses of mental, anatomical, or physiological structure or function owing to injury, active disease, or residual losses from formerly active disease. The term *disabling condition* refers to any physical or mental health condition that can cause disability.

Health conditions differ in the degree to which they precipitate disability, but all physical and mental health conditions that have a measurable association with or likelihood of causing disability are *potentially* disabling conditions. A *secondary condition* is any additional physical or mental health condition that occurs as a result of having a primary disabling condition. Secondary conditions quite often increase the severity of an individual's disability and are also highly preventable. An illustration of these terms applied to a hypothetical case is provided in the box below. The phrases *disability prevention* and *prevention of disability* are meant to include the prevention of potentially disabling health conditions and their progression toward disability, the prevention or reduction of disability itself, and the prevention of secondary conditions. Chapter 3 discusses these terms in greater detail in the context of a model of the disabling process developed by the committee.

AN ILLUSTRATION OF DISABILITY TERMS

Paraplegia is an example of a disabling condition. In a hypothetical scenario, a man is in an automobile crash and sustains fractured lumbar vertebrae and permanent crush-injury of the spinal cord (pathologies), which result in flaccid paralysis of the muscles of the lower limbs (paraplegia, an impairment). Consequently, he cannot walk or drive his car (functional limitations). Public transportation, sidewalks, washrooms, and work environments do not accommodate his wheelchair. As a result, he is now deprived of employment and social and cultural activities (disability). Because he is unemployed, he loses his health insurance and cannot afford to purchase an individual policy. He develops pressure sores from his wheelchair and becomes depressed (secondary conditions), which could have been prevented if he had insurance to cover appropriate educational and rehabilitative services.

In common parlance, *disability* is a value-laden, stereotyping term that categorizes people according to their impairments. People who have reduced ability to perform expected activities—that is, those who are said to have "disabilities"—are often viewed as permanently sick. Such a perception deprives many people with disabilities of the opportunities that should accompany their membership in society. The disability-rights and independent-living movements have struggled to overcome this stereotyping. We concur with their argument against the use of the phrase *disabled people*, preferring instead *people with disabilities*, and hasten to point out that a person's identity is the product of a host of characteristics and that disabling conditions are but a few of them. The message in this seemingly subtle preference for language is important: external factors, like stereotypes, impose obstacles to the performance of chosen roles. In fact, it is external factors like these that can transform a functional limitation into a disability.

Thus disability is not inherent in a person, nor is it determined solely by biological factors—losses or abnormalities of psychological, physiological, or anatomical structures or functions. To view disability strictly as a biological phenomenon is to categorize it as a medical entity and to ignore the complexity of factors that in combination determine whether a physical or mental impairment will progress to a functional limitation and then to disability (the inability to perform expected social and personal roles and tasks). An accurate understanding of disability requires explicit recognition of the roles of the environment and public attitudes in determining whether functional limitations become disabilities. For example, a concert pianist or a typist who loses a finger faces a more challenging rehabilitation than a computer programmer, schoolteacher, or truck driver, whose work depends far less on having a full set of agile fingers.

Disability is not an unavoidable consequence of a chronic disease, an impairment, or even a functional limitation. The sophistication with which the health care system responds to an initially occurring disease, injury, or condition—in terms of medical care, assistive technology, and an array of related social support services—will affect the extent of the individual's functional limitation and the potential for progression to disability and secondary conditions. Whether disability results, and the level of severity if it does, depends on the many factors detailed in this report. These factors transcend aspects of medical care and extend to social determinants of the quality of life, including access to facilities and opportunities in everyday settings and the receptiveness of the community to persons with disabilities. Describing disability prevention in medical terms poses the danger of perpetuating the misconception that disability is purely a medical problem, confined to the domains of primary health care. Such an orientation ignores the importance of social integration and quality of life in influencing the disabling process. Major responsibility for disability prevention must rest with society as a whole. The perceptions of the public and the willingness of society to accommodate the specific needs of people with disabilities often determine whether those individuals can carry out their chosen roles in life and be productive members of society, or whether their conditions become disabilities.

PUBLIC HEALTH AND DISABILITY PREVENTION

The public health concepts of primary, secondary, and tertiary prevention are applied to disability prevention as follows. Primary prevention seeks to avert the onset of pathologic processes by reducing susceptibility, controlling exposure to disease-causing agents, and eliminating, or at least minimizing, behaviors and environmental factors that increase the risk of disease or injury that can cause disabling conditions. Secondary prevention is the early detection of a potentially disabling condition, followed by the implementation of interventions that are designed to halt, reverse, or at least retard the progress of that condition. Secondary prevention becomes especially important as the population ages, given that the prevalence of chronic conditions increases with age as does the risk of disability associated with these conditions. Tertiary prevention concentrates on reducing the effects of an existing condition. In tertiary preventive strategies habilitative and rehabilitative measures, which include counseling, vocational training, environmental adaptations, and mobility training, are employed to restore as much functioning as possible. Tertiary measures are also intended to prevent the occurrence of secondary conditions, such as muscle atrophy, obesity, ulcers, and contracture—an area of major interest in this report.

Disability prevention measures described in this report are designed to reduce the incidence and prevalence of potentially disabling conditions in the U.S. population. The targets of these measures are high-risk groups that, because of behavioral, environmental, biologic, economic, dietary, or other factors, are more likely than the rest of the population to develop a disability. Risk factors are many and varied, and their identification is a major focus of epidemiological research, which helps to identify the often complex chain of events that can lead to disability and secondary conditions. For some disabling conditions, this chain of events begins before birth. Lack of good prenatal care beginning early in pregnancy, for example, increases the risk of prematurity and low birthweight, which in turn increases the risk of developmental disability, such as mental retardation. Because women who are socially disadvantaged and those who live in rural areas have the most difficulty obtaining obstetrical services, they are an obvious target group for preventive measures designed to increase access to and use of prenatal care.

Another example is disabilities resulting from injuries sustained in traffic collisions. These also lend themselves to focused prevention strategies, such as seat belt laws and passive restraints, stringent drunk-driving laws and enforcement, and educational programs to encourage bicyclists to wear helmets. The obvious target population is teenagers and young adults, for whom traffic injuries are the leading cause of mortality and morbidity.

As these two examples illustrate, disabling conditions are not the products of random events. Early identification of risk factors followed by measures to eliminate or reduce them are the cornerstones of all successful prevention strategies. In this regard, disability prevention meshes well with the public health model of disease prevention, as typified by vaccination programs that immunize at-risk populations against certain infectious agents. Obviously, greater emphasis on efforts to identify risk factors across a broad range of areas and subsequently to develop intervention measures to reduce the occurrence of diseases, injuries, and other potentially disabling conditions must be a fundamental part of a national agenda for disability prevention. Clearly, there are hundreds of important health conditions that pose the risk of disability and that are, in some measure, preventable. Many of these conditions, their risk factors, and means of primary prevention have been previously addressed.[1] Primary prevention strategies are also discussed in this report, but additional emphasis is placed on the needs of people who already have potentially disabling conditions, that is, secondary and tertiary prevention—a relatively unattended area of prevention.

A Life Course Perspective

One of the major goals of disability prevention is to maximize an individual's functioning, well-being, and quality of life throughout the life course. This goal incorporates the strategies of health promotion, disease prevention, and chronic illness management to prevent disability. Within a life course framework for disability prevention, the three strategies—health promotion, disease prevention, and chronic illness management—are complementary. Health

---

[1] Many study groups have reviewed current knowledge on risk factors and preventive activities as they relate to specific conditions, such as heart disease, cancer, stroke, and injuries. Examples are *Diet and Health: Implications for Reducing Chronic Disease Risk* (National Research Council [NRC], 1989), *Diet, Nutrition and Cancer* (NRC, 1982), *Injury in America* (NRC, 1985), *The Surgeon General's Report on Nutrition and Health* (U.S. Department of Health and Human Services [HHS], 1989c), *Surgeon General's Workshop: Health Promotion and Aging* (U.S. HHS, 1988b), *Healthy People: The Surgeon General's Report on Health Promotion and Disease Prevention* (U.S. Department of Health, Education, and Welfare, 1979), *Closing the Gap: The Burden of Unnecessary Illness* (Amler and Dull, 1984), *Guide to Clinical Preventive Services* (U.S. HHS, 1989a), *Unnatural Causes: The Three Leading Killer Diseases in America* (Maulitz, 1989), and *Healthy People 2000: National Health Promotion and Disease Prevention Objectives* (U.S. HHS, 1990).

promotion helps people develop lifestyles to maintain and enhance their well-being through both community and individual measures. Disease prevention protects people from the consequences of a threat to health, such as a disease or environmental hazard (U.S. Department of Health, Education, and Welfare, 1979). Chronic illness management includes not only medical care and rehabilitation but also psychological, social, occupational, and environmental interventions to minimize or control potential disability. After the onset of a potentially disabling condition, the focus of disability prevention becomes one of retarding the progression toward disability and preventing the development of secondary conditions.

Recognizing the interactive nature of the process that can lead to disability, a life course perspective on disability prevention should address not only the factors that are directly related to health but also the other influences that determine quality of life, because good health, as well as poor health, is the result of interactions among biological, behavioral, and environmental (social and physical) factors. It is clear, for example, that inadequate housing, lack of education, and other problems that are the traditional concerns of social service agencies are also powerful influences on success or failure in preventing disability. Thus a comprehensive approach to the design and delivery of health and social services throughout the life course is an integral element of disability prevention.

SCOPE AND ORGANIZATION OF THE REPORT

In the 1985 publication *Injury in America*, the National Research Council and the Institute of Medicine identified death and disability caused by injury as one of the most important public health issues in the United States (National Research Council, 1985). This report expands on that effort by addressing a broader range of preventable disabling conditions and by considering approaches to ensure that people with disabling conditions have the opportunity to participate fully in society.

Injury prevention is perhaps the most developed area within the entire province of disability prevention. Yet the scope of effort in this area—in terms of surveillance and data collection, research, and the development and evaluation of interventions—is limited when compared with the magnitude of the need. In other areas of disability prevention, the disparity is even greater. Consequently, the scientific foundation on which prevention efforts must build is small. This is not to say that disability prevention efforts undertaken in these areas are not worthwhile. To the contrary, there is a great need for research and evaluation in disability prevention, and this report proposes an agenda for these activities. However, time and resources did not permit the committee to review current understanding in all areas of disability. One notable omission is mental health. In a recent analysis of

67 chronic health conditions or groups of health conditions, mental health conditions ranked as the ninth leading cause of activity limitation (LaPlante, 1989a). Moreover, depression and other mental health conditions are critically important determinants of the progression to physical disability, a point noted throughout this report. Given their importance, mental health conditions that lead to disability or that are involved in physical disability merit more in-depth study than was possible here.

In this report, the committee addresses the topic of disability prevention from general and specific perspectives, focusing most of their attention on the prevention needs of people with disabling conditions, that is, secondary and tertiary prevention. Chapter 2 describes the magnitude and dimensions of disability in the United States. Chapter 3 describes the committee's conceptual approach to disability, assesses the adequacy of existing data collection and surveillance systems for addressing this important public health issue, and describes how the tools and principles of epidemiology can be used to study health-related limitations in human activity and to develop preventive interventions.

In the four succeeding chapters, the committee concentrates on four major areas of disability: developmental disabilities (Chapter 4); injury-related disabilities, specifically those related to spinal cord injury and traumatic brain injury (Chapter 5); disabilities associated with chronic diseases and aging (Chapter 6); and secondary conditions associated with primary disabling conditions (Chapter 7). In each of these chapters, the public health significance of each is assessed, current medical and social approaches to prevention are discussed, and research needs are identified.

Chapter 8 reviews government and private-sector programs concerned with disability prevention and describes and assesses the overall effectiveness of existing service programs and their guiding policies. Obstacles to and opportunities for achieving a more integrated and effective program are discussed. In the first eight chapters of the report, committee "findings"—statements thought to be of particular importance—are printed in bold type and indented.

The concluding chapter (Chapter 9) presents the committee's overarching conclusions and recommendations. Together, they constitute a framework for assembling a national agenda for the prevention of disability. The recommendations are organized into five groups: organization and coordination of a national program for the prevention of disability, surveillance, research, access to care and preventive services, and professional and public education.

Finally, there are 3 appendixes in the report. Appendix A is a paper that was written for this committee by Saad Nagi. It describes disability concepts and offers an assessment of existing frameworks. Appendix B contains a dissenting statement from one committee member, Deborah Stone, and a response to her dissent by the other 22 members of the committee. Appendix C contains brief biographical sketches of the committee members.

2

Magnitude and Dimensions of Disability in the United States

Disability is a serious public health and social issue in the United States. About 35 million Americans experience activity limitations owing to chronic health problems or impairments, and many of them are deprived economically and socially because of these limitations. They incur high health care costs and have special problems in accessing health care. Despite the apparent magnitude of the problem, however, few comprehensive assessments of the prevalence and nature of disability in the United States are available (Rice and LaPlante, 1988a).

Data on disability come from a wide variety of data systems, each of which collects data for its own purposes, requiring different standards and definitions. These different purposes provide for a rich diversity of information on disability in the United States, but the resulting differences in definitions and statistical practices make it difficult to assess the full public health and social impacts of disability in a comprehensive way (National Research Council, 1990).

This chapter reviews data from several of these systems. Comparing and synthesizing those data, it presents an analysis of the dimensions of disability in the United States, now and in the past, and describes the prevalence of disability and its associated chronic health conditions in the population. The focus is on the broad dimensions of disability rather than on special problems or populations. Similarly, this analysis focuses on the prevalence of disabling conditions, not on the causes of these limitations. This is followed by a brief discussion of the economic costs of disability.

DATA SOURCES

Students of disability-related issues continue to debate the best statistical system for assessing and analyzing the dimensions of disability (National

Research Council, 1990). As defined and described throughout this report, much of "disability" is a social issue, going beyond biological or functional limitations and relating to people's ability to perform their expected social roles. This chapter, however, attempts to avoid the debate about how disability should be defined and measured, and simply reports on the data that are available.

The National Health Interview Survey (NHIS) is a population survey that has been conducted continuously by the National Center for Health Statistics for almost 30 years (National Center for Health Statistics, 1989a). The NHIS data, particularly the data on "activity limitation," provide a reasonably consistent national picture over a long period of time, and hence are used as the framework of the synthesis in this chapter. These data are supplemented, where appropriate, by data from other surveys described below.

The National Health Interview Survey (NHIS)

The NHIS is designed to collect representative data on the civilian noninstitutionalized population living in the United States. Among those excluded from the scope of the NHIS are residents of nursing homes, members of the armed forces, prisoners, and U.S. citizens living abroad. In 1988, the survey reached a sample of 122,310 persons in 47,485 households. The use of households to locate survey respondents means that the NHIS tends to underrepresent that portion of the population, the homeless, for example, that do not live in households. To the extent possible, adults are interviewed directly. Proxy respondents provide information for all children in the household and for those adults who cannot be interviewed in person (National Center for Health Statistics, 1989a).

The NHIS data on activity limitation are obtained through questions that establish whether an "impairment or health problem" prevents or limits activities and whether that impairment or health problem is chronic. Respondents are further classified according to the degree of activity limitation: (1) limited, but not in "major activity" (the least severely limited category); (2) limited in amount or kind of "major activity"; or (3) unable to carry out "major activity" (the most severely limited category). "Major activity" is defined as the predominant social role expected of a person of a given age. According to the current definition, the major activities are "playing" for children under age 5, "attending school" for children ages 5-17, "working or keeping house" for adults ages 18-69, and "living independently" for adults age 70 and over. As discussed below in the section on trends, however, these definitions have changed over time (National Center for Health Statistics, 1989a).

A chronic condition is one that has existed for at least three months or one such as arthritis or heart disease that would normally continue for at least three months. Respondents who have more than one limiting condition are asked to identify one of them as the main cause of their limitation. Identification of these causes depends on the respondents' understanding of their conditions, their perceptions of how limiting they are, and their willingness to report them. In a separate set of questions, the NHIS also collects data on the overall prevalence of specific chronic conditions, without regard to whether the condition causes any activity limitation (National Center for Health Statistics, 1989a). This distinction between presence of a condition and limitation caused by a condition is consistent with the distinction that has been made between impairments or functional limitations and disability (Nagi, 1965; World Health Organization, 1980; Haber, 1990).

The ICD Survey of Disabled Americans

In late 1985, Louis Harris and Associates conducted a telephone survey for the International Center for the Disabled (ICD) and the National Council on the Handicapped to assess the attitudes and experiences of people with disabilities. The survey was designed to reach a representative sample of the population age 16 and over with disabilities, living in households with telephones in all states except Alaska and Hawaii. Individuals were included if they met any one of three criteria: (1) having a health condition that prevented full participation in work, school, or other activities; (2) having a physical disability, a seeing, hearing, or speaking impairment, an emotional or mental disability, or a learning disorder; or (3) reporting that one considered oneself disabled or that others would consider one disabled. In addition to questions on the nature and severity of their disability, the survey asked respondents about the impact of disability on their social and working lives, barriers to entering the mainstream, disability benefits, and other matters. The survey's methodology permitted an estimate of the prevalence of disability in the United States (Louis Harris and Associates, 1986).

Survey of Income and Program Participation (SIPP)

Conducted by the Census Bureau since 1983, the SIPP is an ongoing panel study of the economic well-being of U.S. households. In 1984, during the third round of interviews with its first panel, SIPP collected data on the extent of disability in the civilian noninstitutionalized population. These data include information on: (1) functional limitations; (2) work limitations; and (3) receipt of Social Security or veterans disability benefits (U.S. Department of Health and Human Services, 1989d).

For adults, the degree of functional limitation was based on ability to perform activities of daily living (ADLs),[1] three of the standard instrumental activities of daily living (IADLs)[2] (Katz, 1983), and six other sensory and physical functions. Individuals needing assistance with ADLs were the most severely limited, followed by those needing assistance with IADLs. A broader category of limitation—a "substantial" limitation—included all of those needing assistance with ADLs or IADLs plus people who were unable to perform one or more of the sensory or physical functions, or who had difficulty with two or more of those functions. For children, functional limitation was based on the presence of either a physical condition that limits the ability to walk, run, or play, or a mental or emotional condition that limits the ability to learn or do school work. These limitations in children were considered equivalent to "substantial" limitations in adults. Questions on work limitations were asked of persons ages 16-72. Unlike the NHIS, limitations due to acute conditions were not excluded. The data on receipt of disability benefits cover the noninstitutional resident population ages 18-64.

National Long-Term Care Surveys (NLTCS)

In 1982 and again in 1984, the Health Care Financing Administration conducted surveys of the Medicare-eligible population aged 65 and over to assess the characteristics of persons with chronic disabilities. Both surveys defined disability as a current or expected limitation of 90 days or more in the ability to perform one or more ADLs or IADLs. For the 1982 survey, interviews were conducted only with people living in the community; residents of nursing homes were excluded (Manton, 1989; Macken, 1986). The 1984 survey reinterviewed survivors from the first study, including those who had moved into nursing homes, and conducted first-time interviews with new respondents (Manton, 1989).

Supplement on Aging (SOA) and Longitudinal Study of Aging (LSOA)

Each year the NHIS supplements its core questionnaire with additional questions on special topics. In 1984 the special topic portion of the NHIS, the Supplement on Aging (SOA), addressed the health status and living arrangements of people aged 55 and older. The SOA collected detailed data on subjects that included the respondents' ability to perform ADLs and

---

[1]Dressing, undressing, eating, personal hygiene, getting in/out of bed, and getting around inside the house.

[2]Preparing own meals, doing light housework, and getting around outside the house.

IADLs, the presence of specific health impairments, and the respondents' work histories and disability benefits. The SOA also served as the baseline of a longitudinal study, the Longitudinal Study of Aging (LSOA), intended to study the impact of changes in functional status and living arrangements on institutionalization. The LSOA used three forms of follow-up: the National Death Index was used to locate those SOA respondents who died; Medicare files were used to determine hospital use and costs for respondents who were 65 or older at the time of the SOA interview; and surviving respondents who were 70 or older at the time of the SOA were reinterviewed in 1986 and 1988 (National Center for Health Statistics, 1987b).

PREVALENCE OF DISABILITY

Based on the 1988 NHIS, 33.1 million people, or 13.7 percent of the civilian noninstitutionalized population, have some degree of "activity limitation" due to chronic conditions. When one takes into account the estimated 2.2 million people with disabilities who live in institutional facilities such as nursing homes or residential facilities for the mentally retarded or mentally ill (U.S. Department of Health and Human Services, 1989d), the total number of Americans with disabilities is about 35 million. To describe the composition of this population, we begin with data on activity limitation from the NHIS and then use data from other sources to provide different perspectives.

NHIS Activity Limitation Data

The 33.1 million noninstitutionalized people with activity limitations fall into three groups of roughly equal size. Some 10.3 million (4.3 percent of the population) experience limitations that do not interfere with their major life activities. Another 13.1 million (5.4 percent of the population) are limited in amount or kind of major activities that they can carry out. The remaining 9.7 million (4.0 percent of the population) are unable to carry on the major activity for someone their age (National Center for Health Statistics, 1989a).

The combined prevalence of all three levels of activity limitation increases substantially with age, as shown in Figure 2-1. In 1988, the prevalence of any activity limitation increased from 2.2 percent of children under age 5 to 37.6 percent of adults age 70 or older.

The severity of limitation also increases with age, as Figure 2-1 shows. Among people with activity limitations, an increasing proportion in each age group up to age 70 is unable to carry out their major activities (the most severely affected group). After age 70, however, the proportion unable to carry on their major activities decreases, corresponding to the shift in the

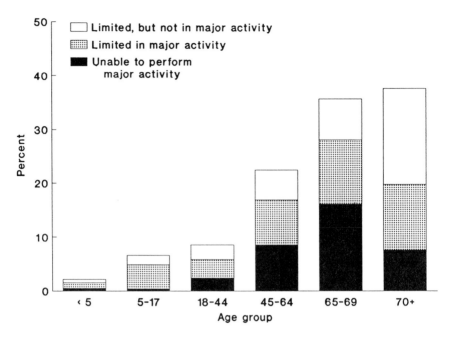

FIGURE 2-1   Prevalence of activity limitation due to chronic conditions by degree of limitation and age, 1988. Source: National Center for Health Statistics, 1989a.

definition of major activity from work to activities of daily living. Another factor in this pattern is that older people are more likely to reside in nursing homes and similar institutional facilities. Because nursing home residents tend to have more severe activity limitations, adding in the institutionalized population would amplify the trend toward increasing severity of disability with age.

Adjusting for the differences in their age distribution, women have slightly lower prevalence rates of activity limitation than men: 12.9 percent vs. 13.2 percent, respectively (National Center for Health Statistics, 1990a). Because women outnumber men in the population and because they have an older age distribution, however, women account for more than 53 percent of the people with activity limitations. Above age 70, women make up 62 percent of the population with activity limitations (National Center for Health Statistics, 1989a).

Blacks experience a higher prevalence of activity limitation than whites— 16.3 percent for blacks vs. 12.8 percent for whites—when differences in age distributions are taken into account. Furthermore, blacks are likely to experience a greater degree of activity limitation: the proportion unable to carry out their major activities is substantially higher for blacks (6.6 percent) than for whites (3.5 percent) (National Center for Health Statistics, 1990a).

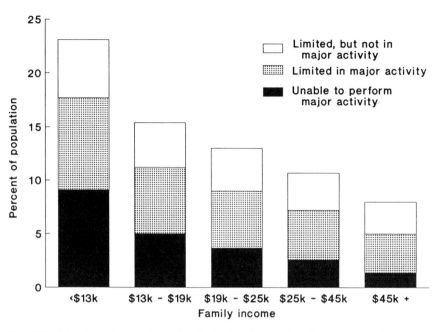

FIGURE 2-2   Prevalence of activity limitation due to chronic conditions, by degree of limitation and family income, 1988.   Source: National Center for Health Statistics, 1990a.

Activity limitation is substantially more prevalent among people with lower family incomes, as Figure 2-2 shows.   The prevalence of activity limitation decreases from 23.2 percent for people with incomes below $13,000 to 8.1 percent for people with annual family incomes above $45,000.   The differential is larger for the most severe activity limitations: the proportion of people unable to carry out their major activities decreases from 9.1 percent in the lowest income group to 1.4 percent in the highest income group. Because the institutionalized population tends to have low incomes, adding this group to the NHIS sample would further amplify this differential (National Center for Health Statistics, 1990a).

It should be pointed out that the cause of these differentials is not clear. To some extent, people with lower socioeconomic status probably experience more disability just as they experience more injuries, higher mortality rates, less access to health care, and generally poorer health.   On the other hand, some people have lower incomes because their disabling conditions restrict their ability to work. Cross-sectional survey data cannot provide any insight into the relative importance of these two very different explanations for the relationship between income and activity limitation.

In general, people with activity limitations are substantially older and poorer than those without limitations. With regard to age, 32 percent of people with activity limitation are over 65, compared with 9 percent of people without limitations. Only 10 percent of the population with activity limitations are under 18, compared with 29 percent of people without limitation. Furthermore, 22 percent of the population with activity limitations—compared with 10 percent of people without limitation—have incomes under $10,000, and 18 percent—compared with 33 percent—have incomes over $35,000.

Other Perspectives

The NHIS data (National Center for Health Statistics, 1989a) also provide perspectives on aspects of disability beyond activity limitation. For instance, respondents were restricted in activity for an average of 14.7 days in 1988 because of acute and chronic conditions, including an average of 6.3 bed-disability days. Furthermore, 39.1 percent of the respondents rated their own health as "excellent," 27.8 percent as "very good," and 23.2 percent as "good." Only 9.9 percent rated their health as "fair" or "poor." This is smaller than the proportion—13.7 percent—that experience any activity limitation. As with activity limitation, the proportion of people who rate their health as fair or poor increases with age, decreases with income, and is higher for blacks than for whites.

As discussed below, a variety of other surveys and data systems generate estimates of the prevalence of disability. Tables 2-1, 2-2, and 2-3 present some of the measures available from the NHIS and other sources. The target population is usually the civilian noninstitutionalized population, but each study uses different criteria for identifying "disability." Without exception, however, people with disabilities tend to be older, to have less education, and to be poorer than the general population.

The ICD survey led to an estimate that about 27 million people, 15 percent of the population age 16 and over, had some disability. Broken down by age in Table 2-1, the prevalence rates are similar to those from the NHIS for the population under age 65. For people 65 and over, however, the NHIS rate is about a third higher. Even though the ICD criteria for disability could be expected to include more people than the NHIS, use of only telephone interviews may have tended to exclude older people with disabilities.

Among those included in the ICD survey, 8 percent reported that they experienced no limitation in their activities, and 50 percent did not consider themselves disabled even though they met at least one of the survey's "disability" criteria. However, 46 percent said that they were prevented completely from working, going to school, or keeping house. Two-thirds of the people under age 65 were not working, and two-thirds of the people who were not working reported wanting to work.

TABLE 2-1 Alternative Estimates of Functional and Activity Limitation by Age: United States

Survey	Under 18	18-44	45-64	65 and Over
Numbers (in thousands)				
Activity limitation				
National Health Interview				
Survey (1985)	3,221	8,391	10,405	10,709
ICD-Louis Harris (1985)	—	8,800[a]	10,200	8,000
Functional limitation				
Survey of Income and				
Program Participation (1984)	2,326	11,139[b]	10,541[c]	15,466
Percent of population group				
Activity limitation				
National Health Interview				
Survey (1985)	5.1	8.4	23.4	39.6
ICD-Louis Harris (1985)	—	8.2[a]	22.7	28.0
Functional limitation				
Survey of Income and				
Program Participation (1984)	3.7	10.1[b]	31.9[c]	58.7

Notes: Definition of disability differs for each survey. *National Health Interview Survey*: Unable to carry out major activity; limited in amount or kind of major activity; or limited, but not in major activity. *International Center for the Disabled—Louis Harris Survey*: Prevented from full participation in work, school, or other activities; having a physical disability, seeing, hearing, or speaking impairment, an emotional or mental disability, or a learning disorder; or considering oneself disabled or considered disabled by others. *Survey of Income and Program Participation*: For adults, needs assistance with ADLs or IADLS; inability or difficulty in at least one function. For children, having a physical condition that limits the ability to walk, run, or play, or a mental or emotional condition that limits the ability to learn or do school work.

[a]Ages 16-44.
[b]Ages 18-49.
[c]Ages 50-64.

SOURCES: National Center for Health Statistics, 1986; Louis Harris and Associates, Inc., 1986; calculated from Rice and LaPlante, 1988a; U.S. Department of Health and Human Services, 1989d.

The relationships among a number of different measures of disability are illustrated in Figure 2-3, from the 1984 SIPP. Each box represents a segment of the population (in thousands) meeting a particular combination of conditions. For example, in the bottom right corner 956,000 people are age 65 to 72 and have a work limitation but report no limitations in func-

DISABILITY IN AMERICA

TABLE 2-2   Alternative Estimates of Work Limitation Among Persons Ages 18 to 64: United States

Survey	Any Work Limit	Unable to Work
Numbers (in thousands)		
National Health Interview Survey (1983-85)	14,347	7,785
Survey of Income and Program Participation (1984)	17,950	8,025
Current Population Survey (1985)^a	13,336	6,893
Disability benefit recipients (1984)	4,400	—
Percent of population group		
National Health Interview Survey (1983-85)	10.1	5.5
Survey of Income and Program Participation (1984)	12.5	5.6
Current Population Survey (1985)^a	8.8	4.5
Disability benefit recipients (1984)	3.1	—

Notes: *Disability Benefit Recipients*: Social Security Disability Insurance, Supplemental Security Income, or Veterans Administration benefits.

^{a}Ages 16-64.

SOURCES: LaPlante, 1988; U.S. Department of Health and Human Services, 1989d; calculated from Haber, 1990, and U.S. Bureau of the Census, 1988.

tioning.   On the basis of functional limitations, the SIPP estimated that 39.5 million people, 17 percent of the noninstitutionalized population, had some degree of disability.   (In Figure 2-3, this number is the sum of all numbers in boxes labeled "limitations in functioning," i.e., 2,326 + 9,677 + 8,422 + 3,443 + 118 + 11,310 + 4,157).   Another example is work limitations, where the number of persons in the population ages 18-64 with any work limitation totals 17.95 million people (i.e., 8,442 + 3,443 + 549 + 5,515).

Table 2-1 shows that the SIPP produced a lower estimate of disability among children than the NHIS.   Some of the difference may be due to different types of questions.   The SIPP asks a general question on whether any children have limitations, and only with a positive response does it go on to ask which children, up to a total of three.   The NHIS includes an individualized inquiry on the presence of activity limitation for each child in the household.   For younger adults, the two surveys produce comparable results.   At older ages, however, the SIPP shows much higher rates of disability than the NHIS.   For people 65 and over, the SIPP rate is half again as high as the NHIS rate.   The more extensive questions in the SIPP on the ability to perform specific functions may provide a greater opportunity for respondents to identify limitations.

The SIPP produces estimates of the prevalence of work limitation somewhat higher than those of the NHIS, 18.0 million vs. 14.4 million. Part of this difference may be due to the exclusion of acute conditions as causes of work disability in the NHIS. About 6.4 million of the people with work limitations in the SIPP report no functional limitations, however. Individuals with mental or emotional conditions that limit their ability to work may not have any difficulty with the physical activities that SIPP uses to define functional limitation (U.S. Department of Health and Human Services, 1989d).

TABLE 2-3 Alternative Estimates of Degrees of Functional Limitation Among Persons Age 65 and Over: United States

Survey	Degree of Limitation		
	More	Less	Any
Numbers (in thousands)			
National Health Interview Survey[a] (1983-1985)			
ADL/IADL	1,507	2,862	4,369
Survey of Income and Program			
Participation[b] (1984)	1,683	2,799	4,482
Long-Term Care Survey[c] (1982)	3,384	1,690	5,074
Long-Term Care Survey[c] (1984)	3,500	1,965	5,465
Percent of population group			
National Health Interview Survey[a] (1983-1985)			
ADL/IADL	5.7	10.8	16.5
Survey of Income and Program			
Participation[b] (1984)	6.4	10.6	17.0
Long-Term Care Survey[c] (1982)	12.7	6.4	19.1
Long-Term Care Survey[c] (1984)	12.9	7.2	20.1

Note: ADL = activities of daily living; IADL = instrumental activities of daily living. The activities related to a specific degree of limitation vary among the surveys. "Any" limitation is the sum of the two separate degrees of limitation.

[a]*National Health Interview Survey:* Major Activity: More = unable to carry out major activity; Less = limited in amount or kind of major activity. ADL/IADL: More = needing assistance in any ADL; Less = needing assistance only in IADLs.

[b]*Survey of Income and Program Participation:* More = needs assistance with ADLs; Less = needs assistance only with IADLs.

[c]*Long-Term Care Surveys:* More = any limitations in ADLs; Less = limitations only in IADLs.

SOURCES: Calculated from LaPlante, 1988; U.S. Department of Health and Human Services, 1989; Macken, 1986; Manton, 1989.

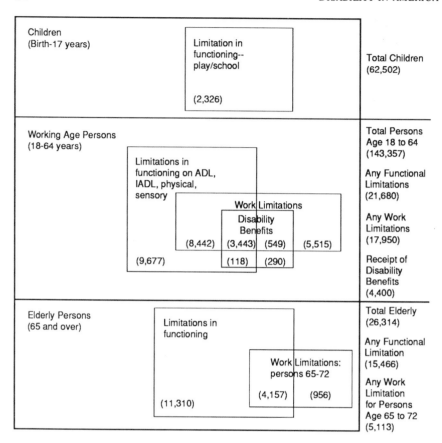

FIGURE 2-3   Illustration of conceptual relationships between disability measures in SIPP (population counts in thousands).   Source: U.S. Department of Health and Human Services, 1989d.

The SIPP also provides estimates of persons receiving disability benefits from Social Security Disability Insurance, Supplemental Security Income, or the Veterans Administration.   Among people ages 18-64, only 4.4 million are receiving benefits.   The NHIS and the SIPP found three to four times as many people with some health condition or impairment that limited their ability to work, but specific eligibility requirements for these benefit programs will exclude many people.

Most efforts to measure disability among people age 65 and over make use of questions on the ability to perform ADLs and IADLs.   Even when surveys seem to use similar approaches to identifying limitations, the results vary.   Table 2-3 shows roughly similar estimates for any limitation in ADLs and IADLs in the noninstitutionalized population ranging from 16.5

percent in the NHIS to 20.1 percent in the 1984 National Long-Term Care Survey (NLTCS). When these estimates are broken down by degree of limitation, however, the two NLTCS surveys show a level of ADL limitations twice that of either the NHIS or SIPP.

Because the size of the population at age 65 and over is growing rapidly, even relatively small differences in the estimates from different surveys can translate into important differences in expected health care and insurance costs. The Interagency Forum on Aging-Related Statistics has made a detailed review of the sources of the variations among 11 national surveys conducted during the mid-1980s (Wiener et al., 1990). They identified several contributing factors, including differences in the lists and groupings of ADLs, in how limitations in these activities were established, in sampling frames, and in the use of proxy respondents.

TRENDS IN THE PREVALENCE OF DISABILITY

The number of people reporting any activity limitation in the NHIS increased from 24 million in 1970 to 33 million in 1988, as shown in Figure 2-4. The increase was greatest between 1970 and 1981, but the trend has been relatively unchanged since then. The proportion of the population with activity limitations has increased less rapidly over the same period, however, changing from 11.8 to 13.7 percent. As Figure 2-4 shows, adjusting for the changing age distribution of the population makes very little difference. The trends in the prevalence of limitation in major activity (not shown) are very similar to those for any limitation.

These trends need to be interpreted with caution because of changes that occurred in the NHIS between 1981 and 1983.[3] At that time, the definition of "major activity" for people age 70 and above was changed from work or keeping house to the ability to carry on the activities of daily living. A second change allowed for all people ages 18-69 to report on limitations in their ability to work. Previously, women who did not work because of chronic conditions were not classified as limited in their major activity if they were able to keep house. A further change altered age ranges for specific major activities. The youngest group was changed from under age 6 to under age 5, and the school-age population shifted from ages 6-16 to ages 5-17 (National Center for Health Statistics, 1990b). With these various changes the proportion of people with any limitation in their major activity dropped correspondingly from 10.9 to 9.9 percent between 1981 and 1983. There was, however, essentially no change in the prevalence of any activity limitation: the proportion decreased from 14.4 to 14.3 percent.

---

[3]A complete set of activity limitation questions was not asked in 1982, and a decision was made not to tabulate the results on the topic that year.

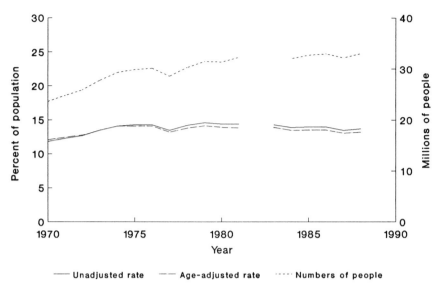

—— Unadjusted rate   — — Age-adjusted rate   ·········· Numbers of people

FIGURE 2-4   Trends in prevalence and numbers of people with any activity limitation. Source: National Center for Health Statistics, 1970-1988.

A more detailed picture of trends in prevalence emerges when the age-specific rates in Figures 2-5 and 2-6 are examined. Prevalence rates are relatively flat for most age groups over the entire period, but there is some increase in the prevalence of activity limitation in the early 1970s, especially for those age 45-64. The changes of definition clearly show up between 1981 and 1983 in Figure 2-6 as an increase in the proportion of children with limitation in major activity and a decrease in the proportion of people 65 and over with limitation in major activity. The differences are especially evident in the figures for people 65 and over with limitations in major activity, as one would expect. The steady overall prevalence of any limitation reflects the balancing of a substantial decrease in prevalence among people over 65 against a smaller proportional increase (in a larger population) among people under age 18.

Colvez and Blanchet (1981) note the increased prevalence of activity limitation in the NHIS data (between 1966 and 1976) and discuss a number of possible explanations. Because the increase is concentrated in men age 45-64 who report that they are unable to work, Wilson and Drury (1984) suggest that the increasing availability of health-related retirement benefits during that period, and perhaps decreasing stigma attached to "disability," could explain a large part of the increase in activity limitation during that period. They also suggest that increased access to health care (especially screening for hypertension and other asymptomatic chronic diseases) could result in physician-ordered activity reduction and improved awareness of

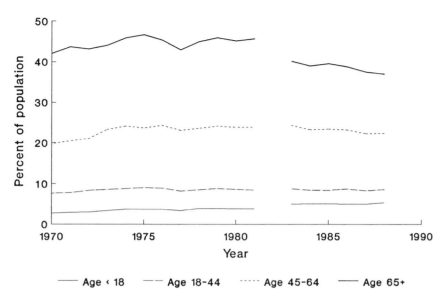

FIGURE 2-5   Trends in prevalence of any activity limitation, by age group. Source: National Center for Health Statistics, 1970-1988.

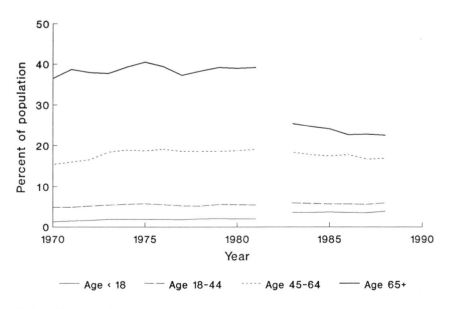

FIGURE 2-6   Trends in prevalence of limitation in major activity, by age group Source: National Center for Health Statistics, 1970-1988.

chronic conditions, thus contributing to the apparent increase in disability without any change in the population's health status. Wolfe and Haveman (1990), in their analysis of trends in work disability from 1962 to 1984, suggest that less stringent eligibility criteria for public disability assistance programs, together with increased willingness to report work limitations, may have acted to increase disability rates through the early 1970s. Subsequent tightening of eligibility criteria appear to have helped reduce the work disability rates from their 1970s peak.

Verbrugge (1984) compares this increase in disability to the decrease in mortality during the same period. After analyzing the possible explanations for these two apparently divergent trends on a disease-specific basis, she concludes that an emphasis on secondary prevention—early detection of chronic disease and intervention to slow its progress—is a major part of the explanation. Based on this analysis, she predicts that health statistics will continue to show increasing morbidity through the turn of the century. Whether this trend continues depends on the success of primary prevention programs to halt the incidence of disease in the future (Verbrugge, 1984).

Other analysts have concentrated on future changes in the prevalence of disability that can be expected due to demographic changes. Assuming that age- and sex-specific disability prevalence rates remain constant, Manton (1989) has estimated that the elderly population with chronic disabling conditions (living in the community and in institutions) could grow by 31 percent to 7.2 million between 1985 and 2000. This compares with a projected 20 percent increase in the nondisabled population. Manton also projects that the most severely disabled population (those with five to six ADL impairments) and the population in institutions could grow even faster. These trends are expected to continue well into the twenty-first century as the baby boom generation ages. In 2060, for instance, the number of people aged 65 or older with chronic disabling conditions could exceed 15 million (Manton, 1989). Schneider and Guralnik (1990) project similar increases in the number of older people requiring nursing home services and experiencing disabling conditions such as dementia and hip fractures.

CONDITIONS LEADING TO DISABILITY

A wide variety of chronic conditions are responsible for activity limitation in the United States. Looking at the single "main cause" of activity limitation as reported by respondents in the NHIS, orthopedic impairments account for 16.0 percent of activity limitations, arthritis for 12.3 percent, heart disease for 11.5 percent. The left half of Table 2-4 gives the 15 single

TABLE 2-4 Percentage of Persons with Activity Limitation Reporting Specified Causes of Limitation, All Ages: United States, 1983-1985

Main Cause	%	All Causes	%
Orthopedic impairments	16.0	Orthopedic impairments	21.5
Arthritis	12.3	Arthritis	18.8
Heart disease	11.5	Heart disease	17.1
Visual impairments	4.4	Hypertension	10.8
Intervertebral disk disorders	4.4	Visual impairments	8.9
Asthma	4.3	Diabetes	6.5
Nervous disorders	4.0	Mental disorders	5.6
Mental disorders	3.9	Asthma	5.5
Hypertension	3.8	Intervertebral disk disorders	5.2
Mental retardation	2.9	Nervous disorders	4.9
Diabetes	2.7	Hearing impairments	4.3
Hearing impairments	2.5	Mental retardation	3.2
Emphysema	2.0	Emphysema	3.1
Cerebrovascular disease	1.9	Cerebrovascular disease	2.9
Osteomyelitis/bone disorders	1.1	Abdominal hernia	1.8

Notes: Nervous disorders include epilepsy, multiple sclerosis, Parkinson's disease, and other selected nervous disorders. Mental disorders include schizophrenia and other psychoses, neuroses, personality disorders, other mental illness, alcohol and drug dependency, senility, and special learning disorders (mental deficiency is not included). Content of other condition categories is described in LaPlante, 1988.

SOURCE: National Health Interview Survey; adapted from LaPlante, 1989b.

conditions most commonly cited by the respondents in 1983-1985 as the main cause of their activity limitations (LaPlante, 1989b).

Because there are many different kinds of conditions that can lead to activity limitation, grouping related conditions helps one to discern the relationship among them. Constrained by the available tabulations (LaPlante, 1988), the committee grouped the conditions as follows (the figures in parentheses are the proportion of people with limitations whose main cause of limitation is in that category):

- mobility limitations (38 percent)
- chronic diseases, namely respiratory, circulatory, cancer, and diabetes (32 percent)
- sensory limitations (8 percent)
- intellectual limitations, including mental retardation (7 percent)
- other (15 percent).

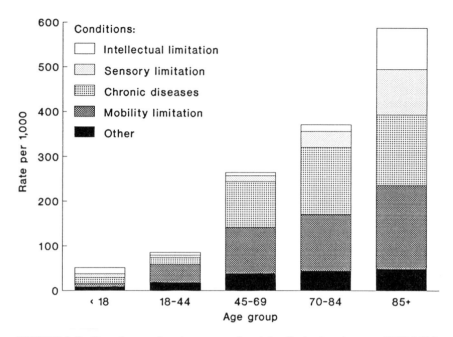

FIGURE 2-7   Prevalence of main causes of activity limitation, by age, 1983-1985.
Source: Calculated from LaPlante, 1988.

Figure 2-7 displays the age-specific prevalence rates for any activity
limitation designated according to these five groups of causes. Figure 2-8
shows the proportion of activity limitation in each age group ascribed to
each of these groups of conditions.

Figures 2-7 and 2-8 show that the main causes of activity limitation vary
markedly with age.   In children under 18, intellectual limitations (two-
thirds of which are mental retardation and one-third mental illness) account
for 27 percent and chronic diseases (two-thirds of which are asthma) account for 26 percent of all activity limitations. Sensory limitations, especially visual and hearing, also account for a relatively high fraction (16
percent), followed by mobility limitations (14 percent).

Above age 18 mobility impairments become more prevalent and are the
leading major cause of activity limitation for all adult age groups.   The
prevalence of activity limitation caused mainly by mobility impairments
increases from 40.5 per 1,000 at ages 18-44 to 188.4 per 1,000 at ages 85
and above. The components of this group change by age, however. For
ages 18-44, back/spine injuries dominate at 48 percent, followed by orthopedic impairments at 29 percent. Arthritis accounts for 11 percent of the

mobility impairments in this age group. For older ages, arthritis becomes increasingly important; its share of the mobility limitation impairments rises from 40 percent at ages 45-69 to 58 percent at ages 85 and above. These increasing percentages are applied to an increasing base of people with mobility limitations, so the prevalence of people with limitations caused mainly by arthritis increases more than 20-fold from 4.6 per 1,000 at ages 18-44 to 109.3 per 1,000 at ages 85 and older.

The importance of chronic diseases (circulatory, respiratory, cancer, diabetes, etc.) as conditions causing activity limitation also increases with age. Taken together, the prevalence of limitation with a main cause in this group increases 10-fold from 15.5 per 1,000 at ages 18-44 to 156.2 per 1,000 at ages 85 and above. Diseases of the heart and circulatory system are the major contributors to this category, increasing from two-thirds of the category at ages 45-69 to three-fourths over age 85.

Verbrugge and colleagues (1989) note that the aggregate measures cited here are actually a function of two components: a condition's prevalence, and whether the condition becomes a disability. These aggregate measures are appropriate measures of public health impact. When comparing the causes of disability, however, it can be helpful to look at each condition's

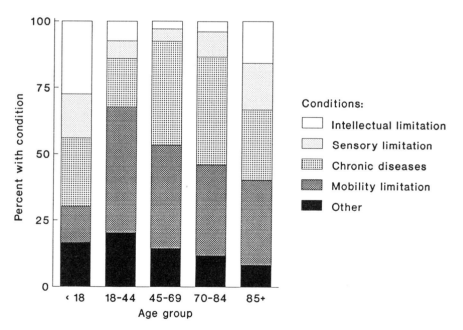

FIGURE 2-8   Percentage distribution of main causes of activity limitation, by age, 1983-1985. Source: Calculated from LaPlante, 1988.

"disability impact"—the probability or level of disability among people with a given condition.[4] Using data from the 1984 Supplement on Aging, Verbrugge and colleagues find a negative relationship between the frequency of a condition and its disability impact. LaPlante (1988) finds a similar relationship in 1983-1985 NHIS data.

The foregoing analyses are based on only the "main" causes of the respondents' activity limitations. Many people who report activity limitations list more than one condition contributing to their limitations. Because there are so many possible combinations of conditions and relatively few people with any particular combination in any survey, analyses of the effect of multiple conditions on disability are limited.

The right half of Table 2-4 shows the prevalence of the 15 most commonly cited conditions responsible for activity limitations, regardless of whether the condition was listed as the main cause. This list is generally similar to the list of main causes. The most notable difference is that hypertension and diabetes move up from ranks 9 and 11 to ranks 4 and 6, respectively, as their prevalence more than doubles. This suggests that a more comprehensive listing of all of the contributing conditions would put more emphasis on chronic diseases than the analysis here of only main causes.

Verbrugge and colleagues have found that as the number of chronic conditions affecting an individual increases, "disability" increases rapidly. This is true when disability is measured in terms of physical or role limitations or by ADL/IADL measures. Only in rare instances, however, is there a synergism between conditions that produce more disability than the two alone would suggest (Verbrugge et al., 1989).

Grouping NHIS data from 1969-1971 and 1979-1981, Rice and LaPlante (1988a) found that the number of chronic conditions reported by those who are limited in their activities increases with age, and that the degree of limitation increases with the number of conditions. The researchers also found that, within every age group and limitation category, the number of conditions has increased over time. It is possible, however, that some of this increase reflects increasing awareness of conditions—perhaps due to improved access to medical care and screening opportunities—rather than a true increase in chronic conditions.

Because they are derived from a single survey, these data on the causes of activity limitation all refer to a cross-section of the population. The "causes"

---

[4]This is not the probability that a given condition will eventually cause activity limitation. It is simply the ratio of the number of people with limitation caused by a condition to the total number of people with that condition. A cohort rather than a period perspective is needed to calculate the proportion of people with a condition who will ever experience an activity limitation caused by that condition. Incomplete reporting on nondisabling conditions, comorbidities, competing causes, and so on also needs to be taken into account.

listed are actually chronic conditions that may have had very different under-lying causes earlier in life. Blindness, for instance, could be a congenital condition or the result of a developmental problem; it could also be due to an injury or a disease such as diabetes. The NHIS data cannot distinguish between these very different possibilities. Furthermore, disability is a dynamic process in which illness and injuries that occur in one life stage have serious implications for the quality of life in later stages. The life table calculations below are a first step toward putting disability in a life course perspective.

LIFE TABLE PERSPECTIVE

Just as one can calculate the average length of life in a population exposed to certain mortality rates, one can also calculate the total number of years a member of this population would spend with various levels of activity limitation. Ideally, this calculation would be carried out using age-specific transition rates among the various categories of activity limitation, just as age-specific mortality rates are used to describe transitions from life to death in ordinary life tables (Rogers, R.G., et al., 1989). Because the necessary transition data are not available for activity limitation, the committee has adopted a hybrid approach (Sullivan, 1971; McKinlay et al., 1989). First, standard life table methods were used to calculate the number of years of life experienced by a cohort in various age groups according to the 1987 U.S. life table (National Center for Health Statistics, 1990c). Second, within each age group for which LaPlante (1988) has tabulated the NHIS activity limitation data, a calculation was made of the number of years lived with various kinds of activity limitations. Based on these results, the committee then calculated the life expectancy without disability and in the various activity-limited states.[5] Because the NHIS figures refer to only the noninstitutionalized population, the committee's calculations underestimate time with activity limitations.

Given current age patterns of activity limitation, an average of 12.8 years out of the current life expectancy at birth of 75.0 years would be spent with some degree of activity limitation. As shown in Figure 2-9, an average of 6.9 of the 16.9 years remaining at age 65 would be spent with some activity limitation. At age 75, the remaining 10.7 years would be expected to include 4.6 with some activity limitation. This analysis suggests that, if current patterns of mortality and activity limitation continue, the 3.8 million children born in 1987 can expect to experience a collective total of 49

---

[5]Specifically, the committee partitioned $_nL_x$ values from the 1987 life table according to the proportions of people with different kinds of activity limitations in the relevant age groups from the NHIS. Just as life expectancy at age x (e_x) would be calculated by summing the $_nL_x$ for age x and above, the life expectancy with a particular kind of activity limitation was calculated by summing the appropriate components of $_nL_x$.

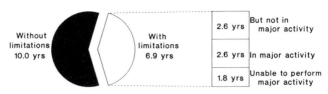

At age 65: 16.9 years

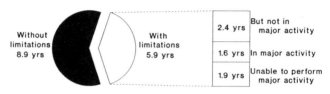

Men at age 65: 14.8 years

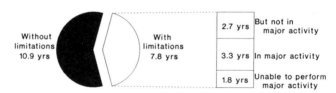

Women at age 65: 18.7 years

FIGURE 2-9 Expected years of life with activity limitation at age 65, by sex, 1987. Source: LaPlante, 1988; National Center for Health Statistics, 1990c.

million disability years. Together, the roughly 2 million Americans who turn 65 each year can expect to experience more than 12 million disability years out of the 33.8 million years of life ahead of them.

As Figure 2-10 further shows, of the 12.8 years of activity limitation expected at birth, the population would average 3.6 years of being unable to carry out a major activity, 5.3 years with a limitation in major activity, and 4.0 years with some other activity limitation. At age 65, the expected years of activity limitation would consist of 1.8 years of being unable to carry out a major activity, 2.6 years with some limitation in major activity, and 2.6 years with a less severe limitation. The expected distribution at age 75 is similar to that at age 65.

Separate calculations for men and women reveal that, while women can expect at birth to live 6.9 years longer than men, both will spend a similar proportion of their lifetimes with some form of activity limitation (see Figure 2-10). At birth women can expect to experience 14.1 years of activity limitation

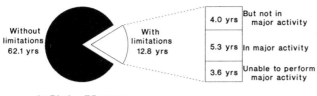

At Birth: 75 years

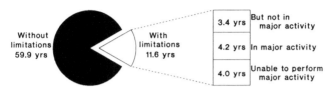

Men at birth: 71.5 years

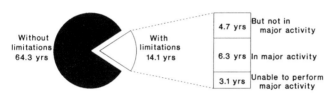

Women at birth: 78.4 years

FIGURE 2-10 Expected years of life with activity limitation at birth, by sex. Source: LaPlante, 1988; National Center for Health Statistics, 1990c

out of a total of 78.4 years. Men can expect 11.6 years out of 71.5. The degree of limitation appears to be more severe in men. For about one-third of their expected years of activity limitation, 4.0 years, men are unable to perform their major activity. Women expect only 3.1 years with this degree of limitation, less than a quarter of the years with activity limitation.

These patterns are similar at age 65. Activity limitation accounts for 40 percent of the expected 14.8 years of additional life for men and 42 percent of the 18.7 years expected for women. Inability to perform major activities continues to account for more limitation for men than for women. For men, however, the largest share of activity limitation, 2.4 years, or 41 percent, is in activities other than their major activity. Limitations in the amount and kind of major activity account for the largest share of women's years of limitation—3.3 years, or 42 percent. By age 75, however, women can expect a greater period of activity limitation than men in both absolute and relative terms: 47 percent of the years of life remaining for women vs. 42 percent for men.

Repeating the life table calculations for earlier years makes it possible to estimate the relative impact of changes in mortality and disability. Use of 1970 mortality (National Center for Health Statistics, 1974) and NHIS data (National Center for Health Statistics, 1972, 1986) shows that while life expectancy at birth increased 4.1 years from 70.9 to 75.0, the number of years with activity limitations increased by 2.4 years from 10.4 to 12.8 years. Thus more than half of the increase in life expectancy in the 1970s and 1980s was lived with some degree of activity limitation. Years of limitation in major activity increased by 2.8 years during this period, implying that there was a decrease in years with less severe limitation. During the same period, life expectancy at age 65 increased by 1.7 years, but less than half of this increase—0.5 years—was time with activity limitation. Taken together, these results show that the increase in activity limitation between 1970 and 1987 was concentrated in people under age 65 who were restricted in their major activities. This is consistent with the trend analysis discussed earlier.

A striking contrast emerges from this overall pattern when men and women are studied separately. For men, expectation of life at birth increased by 4.4 years from 1970 to 1987, and almost two-thirds of that increase, 2.8 years, was in life *without* activity limitations. Women, however, added only 3.6 additional years of life and nearly all of it, 3.3 years, was in life *with* limitations. The changes at older ages were more divergent. For men at age 65, the gain in years of life without limitation, 1.8 years, was greater by 0.1 year than the overall gain in expected years of life. By contrast, women at age 75 can expect 1.5 more years of life with limitations, 0.2 year more than the overall gain during the period.

This apparent worsening of the disability status of women probably reflects at least two factors not directly related to changes in health status. One is the 1982 change in how the NHIS assessed limitation in major activity. Prior to that time, women ages 17-64 who reported that they were able to keep house were not questioned about limitations in their ability to work outside the home. Thus limitation comparable to that experienced by men was missed. The second factor is the increasing number of women between 1970 and the mid-1980s who would define work as their major activity and, therefore, be at risk of limitations in their ability to perform that activity.

Crimmins, Saito, and Ingegneri (1989) have carried out similar calculations comparing 1970 and 1980 data, making use of information available for those years on the institutionalized population and more detailed age, race, and sex categories. Qualitatively, their results are similar to those in this section. Crimmins and colleagues add that, although whites had substantially longer life expectancies than blacks, blacks can expect more years of activity limitation. Furthermore, although life expectancy increased more

TABLE 2-5 Years of Expected Life with Activity Limitations Due to Specified Conditions at Birth, at Age 65, and at Age 75: United States, 1987

Condition	Years at Birth	Years at Age 65	Years at Age 75
All conditions	12.8	6.3	4.6
Mobility limitations	4.7	2.2	1.6
Intellectual impairments	0.9	0.4	0.4
Sensory impairments	1.0	0.6	0.6
Chronic diseases	4.3	2.3	1.6
Other conditions or impairments	1.8	0.7	0.5

SOURCE: Calculated from National Center for Health Statistics, 1990c, and LaPlante, 1988.

for blacks than for whites between 1970 and 1980, the expected number of activity-limited years also increased more for blacks. The researchers also note that, although the United States, Canada, and France had similar total life expectancies around 1980, Canadians and the French could expect 2 to 5 additional years free of activity limitation.

The life table perspective can also be used to determine the average impact of the conditions that are reported as the main cause of activity limitation. Table 2-5 shows the number of years of activity limitation expected at birth and at ages 65 and 75 that would be attributed to mobility limitations, intellectual impairments, sensory impairments, chronic disease, and other kinds of conditions and impairments. Mobility limitations and chronic diseases account for about 70 percent of the years of activity limitation expected at birth and at older ages. At birth, mobility limitations are a slightly more prominent cause of activity limitation than are chronic diseases (4.7 vs. 4.3 years, respectively), but at age 65 chronic diseases are slightly more prominent than are mobility limitations (2.3 vs. 2.2 years).

The conditions that lead to activity limitation differ substantially in the age at which they occur, and hence in the number of years that people live with disabilities associated with them. Disability that begins early in life is most commonly associated with developmental disabilities and mobility limitations caused by injuries. Disability that begins later in life is more commonly associated with chronic diseases and mobility limitations due to arthritis. The relative impact of different disabling conditions on the health of the public is clearly of interest in setting prevention priorities. Although the available data do not allow one to calculate the impact of different underlying causes, the life table analysis presented here can provide a rough approximation of the relative impact of disabilities acquired early and late in life. For this analysis the committee defined "early in life" as occurring before age 45 and "late in life" as after age 45.[6] The results of this calculation are that about 6.1 of the 12.8 years of activity limitation expected at birth—slightly less than half—are due to conditions that had their onset before age 45. Thus, although conditions acquired early in life lead to more years of disability per case, the number of individuals who acquire disabilities after age 45 is much greater. Comparing the two in a life course perspective suggests that, in the aggregate, more years of disability are experienced by people acquiring limitations later in life (after age 45). Thus, despite the length of time that people live with developmental disabilities and mobility limitations due to injuries at early ages, more disability years are experienced by people whose disability appears later in life (after age 45), primarily because of chronic diseases and mobility limitation due to arthritis.

The analyses in this section are based on a hybrid analytical approach that mixes current-status activity limitation data with dynamic mortality data. Rogers and colleagues have developed a more sophisticated approach to this issue that makes use of data on transitions into and out of disability, and from one degree of disability to another. Their approach allows them to go beyond general statistics for the population as a whole to estimates of the expected time with different degrees of disability for people who have (or do not have) a disability at a particular age (Rogers, R.G., et al., 1989; Rogers, A., et al., 1989). The method they developed, however, requires data from a panel study of individuals surveyed at two points in time.

---

[6]The committee estimated the relative impact of activity limitations occurring before and after age 45 as follows. Age 45 was chosen as a break point because the calculations required use of an age break available in the tabulated NHIS data. All limitations experienced by people under age 45 clearly were initiated before that age, so every activity-limited year experienced before age 45 was counted in the first category. Next, an assumption was made that X percent of the population in every age group above 45 experiences activity limitations due to conditions arising before age 45, where X is the prevalence of activity limitations in the 18-44 age group. These activity-limited years were added to the number experienced before age 45. The difference between the total number of years with activity limitation and the number attributed to conditions with early onset gives the activity-limited years associated with conditions that were acquired after age 45.

This calculation requires two assumptions that are clearly not correct, but which partially counteract one another. First, X—the proportion of the population acquiring an activity limitation before age 45—was estimated by the proportion of the 18-44 age group with a limitation. This is clearly an underestimate because the 18-44 age group includes people who have not yet had a chance to acquire the conditions they might expect to have acquired by age 45. Second, an assumption was made that X percent of the population at every age over 45 has a limitation acquired before age 45. This would only be true if mortality rates were the same for people with and without activity limitations. Because people with activity limitations are likely to have higher mortality rates, the true fraction is likely to be less than X, tending to offset the error caused by the first assumption.

Because disability data of this type for the general population are lacking, the method has only been applied to data on older adults. To make their estimates, Rogers and colleagues used data on ADLs reported by individuals interviewed in both the 1984 Supplement on Aging of the NHIS and the 1986 Longitudinal Study of Aging (LSOA), and they defined "dependence" as requiring assistance with seven ADLs. The researchers found that individuals who were independent at age 70 could expect to live 13.4 years on average and had a life expectancy of 3.4 years in a dependent state (25 percent of their life expectancy). Individuals who were dependent at age 70 had a total life expectancy of 12.5 years and a dependent life expectancy of 6.1 years (49 percent). Rogers and his colleagues also found differences in the active life expectancies of men and women. Among those independent at age 70, men had a lower life expectancy than women (11.3 vs. 15.4 years) but a proportionally shorter dependent life expectancy (18 percent vs. 29 percent of total life expectancy). The same pattern held among people who were dependent at age 70. Men had a 9.9-year life expectancy, 40 percent of which was in a dependent state, and women had a 14.5-year life expectancy, 53 percent of which was in a dependent state (Rogers, R.G., et al., 1989).

ECONOMIC COST OF DISABILITY

Disability imposes an enormous economic cost on society. It is costly to the nation in terms of the medical resources used for care, treatment, and rehabilitation; in reduced or lost productivity; and in premature death. For example, persons with disabilities use more medical care services than those without them. In 1979, 15 percent of the noninstitutionalized population that was limited in activity due to chronic conditions made 29 percent of the visits to physicians and accounted for 40 percent of the hospitalizations. Persons with activity limitations made 9.5 physician visits per person, compared with about 3.9 visits for persons with no activity limitation (National Center for Health Statistics, 1981a). Those unable to carry on their major activities made 11.9 visits per person per year. The hospitalization rate for those with activity limitations is almost four times that for people with no activity limitations: 38.3 discharges per 100 persons compared with 9.8 per 100, respectively.

Not surprisingly, older persons with chronic and disabling conditions are high utilizers of medical resources. The elderly with activity limitation had 8.7 visits to physicians per year, in contrast with 4.3 visits for persons with no activity limitation. They had 41.2 hospitalizations per 100 elderly persons per year, in contrast with 14.8 hospitalizations per 100 people with no limitation of activity. The 46 percent of elderly people who were limited in activity because of a chronic condition accounted for 63 percent of physician contacts, 71 percent of hospitalizations, and 82 percent of all the days that older people spent in bed because of health conditions (National Center for Health Statistics, 1981a). Among the 1.5 million nursing home residents in 1985, more than four-fifths (82.1 percent) were reported by their next of kin at the time of admission as being dependent in one or more activities of daily living. More than half (50.5 percent) were dependent in four or more ADLs (National Center for Health Statistics, 1989b).

In addition, current medical service, social services, and entitlement programs for persons with disabling conditions are not well coordinated at the national and state levels and offer uncertain benefits with regard to restoring persons with disabling conditions to their highest levels of functioning. Assessments of the effectiveness of these programs are largely unsatisfactory because the evaluations usually measure traditional medical outcomes (physiological and biochemical results) rather than quality of life.

Health services research is needed for the development and application of improved methodologies to measure the effectiveness of the health and social service systems on maintaining those persons with disabling conditions at maximal functional capacity and quality of life.

Several estimates of the high economic costs of disability in the United States are now available. Chirikos (1989) estimates aggregate economic disability losses at $176.8 billion in 1980, as shown in Table 2-6. Included are:

1. net consumption attributable to disability, that is, the difference in medical care utilization and costs before and after the disabling condition occurred. This amounts to $90.6 billion, 51 percent of the total, and includes expenditures for hospital, medical, and institutional care of people with disabilities, paid household work, and non-health-care spending;

2. primary market time, or the value of reduced productivity on the part of persons with chronic disability, valued at $68.4 billion, or 39 percent of the total; and

3. secondary market time, or the value of productivity losses for members of the households of persons with disabilities, valued at $17.7 billion, or 10 percent of the total.

Disability losses for males were significantly higher than for females— $115 billion and $62 billion, respectively. Losses for the working population were estimated at $112 billion; losses for dependents were estimated at $65 billion.

Berkowitz and Greene (1989) used a different approach for estimating the cost of disability. They estimated disability expenditures in 1986 for the

TABLE 2-6 Disability Losses (in millions of dollars) for the Population
Aged 18-64 Years, by Sex and Age, 1980

Age Group	Total	Males	Females
Total	$176,778	$115,140	$61,638
Working population	111,605	82,680	28,925
15-24	6,726	4,198	2,528
25-44	32,117	23,102	9,015
45-64	72,762	55,380	17,382
Dependents	65,173	32,460	32,713
Under 15	4,206	2,630	1,576
65-74	29,858	18,408	11,450
75 and over	31,109	11,422	19,687

SOURCE: Adapted from Chirikos, 1989.

population aged 18 to 64 years to be $169.4 billion, comprising three types
of expenditures:

1. transfer payments (transfer of funds from one payer to another in
which no new goods or services are produced) amounted to $87.3 billion;
included are social insurance programs, individual and employer programs,
and income support;

2. medical care expenditures, which amounted to $79.3 billion in 1986;
included are expenditures under public programs (Medicare, Medicaid, Department of Defense, Veterans Administration, and Workers' Compensation) and private insurance; and

3. direct service expenditures, which amounted to $2.8 billion; included
are expenditures for rehabilitative services, veterans services, services offered to persons with specific impairments, general federal programs, and
employment assistance programs (Table 2-7).

Berkowitz and Greene (1989) also present disability expenditure trend
data. Disability expenditures rose almost ninefold, from $19.3 billion in
1970 to $169.4 billion in 1986; as a percentage of GNP, disability expendi-
tures rose from 1.9 percent in 1970 to 4 percent in 1986 (Figure 2-11). In
per capita terms, expenditures rose from $167 to $1,136 during this 16-year
period. The largest growth was between 1970 and 1975, when real disability
expenditures (adjusted for rising prices) rose 13 percent annually. The
second half of the 1970s showed a slowing rate of increase in disability
expenditures; the 1980s was a period of contraction in government spending, resulting in an average rate of real growth of 5 percent per year. Berkowitz
and Greene conclude the following: "These fluctuations in disability expenditures are not matched by corresponding fluctuations in injuries or dis-

TABLE 2-7 Disability Expenditures by Type of Expenditure, 1986

Type of Expenditure	Amount (millions)	Percent Distribution
Total	$169,407	100.0
Transfer payments	87,319	51.6
Social insurance (OASDI[a])	22,474	13.3
Individual and employer-provided insurance	10,840	6.4
Indemnity	44,987	26.6
Income support	9,018	5.3
Medical care expenditures	79,315	46.8
Medicare	8,828	5.2
Department of Defense	108	0.0
Private health insurance	46,043	27.2
Veterans medical care	3,732	2.2
Workers' compensation	4,540	2.7
Medicaid	15,588	9.2
Medical vocational rehabilitation	349	0.2
St. Elizabeth's Hospital	127	0.1
Direct service expenditures	2,773	1.6
Rehabilitative services	1,654	1.0
Veterans	423	0.2
Services to persons with specific impairments	183	0.1
Social services (Title XX)	355	0.2
Employment assistance programs	158	0.1

[a]OASDI = Old Age, Survivors, and Disability Insurance.

SOURCE: Berkowitz and Greene, 1989.

eases. These changes then must be accounted for by demographic changes, changes in social and economic conditions, changes in public perception of disability, and the way that the benefit laws are administered."

Newacheck and McManus (1988) analyzed data from the 1980 National Medical Care Utilization and Expenditure Survey to obtain data on the use, charges, and financing of medical care for children (under 21 years of age) with disabilities. Total charges for medical care services for children and youth with disabilities, defined as those limited in activity, amounted to $2.4 billion in 1980 and $3.9 billion in 1986 dollars. On a per capita basis, medical expenditures in 1980 amounted to $760 per person limited in activity, almost three times the amount spent by those without limitations. The 4 percent of children and youth who were limited in their activities accounted for 11 percent of total health care expenditures for the under-21 population.

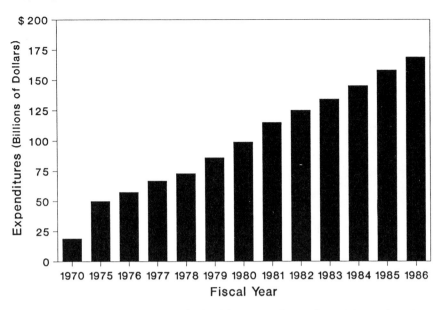

FIGURE 2-11   Estimated value of disability expenditures for 1970 and for 1975-1986. Expenditures in 1986 were more than $169.4 billion. Source: Berkowitz and Greene, 1989.

Rice and LaPlante (1988a) also analyzed the 1980 National Medical Care Utilization and Expenditure Survey, focusing on the costs of chronic comorbidity (i.e., more than one condition existing at the same time) for all ages. They estimated that total expenditures for medical care for persons limited in activity amounted to $63 billion in 1980, more than two-fifths of the total medical care expenditures for noninstitutionalized persons (Table 2-8). Persons limited in activity due to one condition incurred medical expenditures of $49.4 billion; for those with two or more conditions, expenditures amounted to $13.6 billion. Sixteen percent of the total noninstitutionalized population with a limiting chronic condition incurred 41 percent of total medical care expenditures (Figure 2-12). On a per capita basis, medical spending amounted to $1,620 per person for those individuals limited by one condition and $2,456 for those persons limited by two or more conditions, compared with $486 for those not limited in activity (Table 2-8). The distribution by age showed that per capita spending for medical care increases with age for those with and without disability. However, there are higher relative differentials in per capita spending between those with limiting conditions and those with none for the under-65 population.

Rice and LaPlante (1988b) inflated the 1980 costs of disability to 1987 dollars by the increase in per capita national health expenditures over the 7-

TABLE 2-8 Total and Per Capita Medical Expenditures in the Noninstitutionalized Population of People With and Without Disability, by Number of Limiting Conditions and Age, 1980

Age and Sex	All Persons		Persons Without Disabilities		Persons With Disabilities			
					One Condition		Two or More Conditions	
	Amount (millions)	Per Person	Amount (millions)	Per Person	Amount (millions)	Per Person	Amount (millions)	Per Person
All ages	$153,863	$691	$90,856	$486	$49,369	$1,620	$13,638	$2,456
Under 65	112,330	568	74,552	433	31,554	1,424	6,223	1,886
Under 19	21,705	319	19,468	300	2,202	734	35[a]	267[a]
19-44	50,911	591	36,543	482	12,925	1,371	1,444	1,637
45-64	39,713	911	18,542	588	16,427	1,687	4,744	2,075
65 and over	41,533	1,650	16,303	1,116	17,815	2,144	7,415	3,290

[a]Indicates that the relative standard error exceeds 30 percent.

SOURCE: Rice and LaPlante, 1988a. Reprinted with permission.

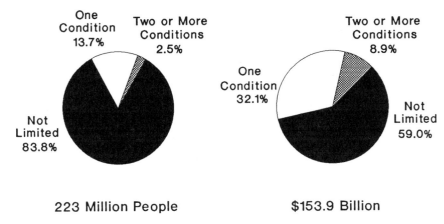

223 Million People $153.9 Billion

FIGURE 2-12   Distribution of population and medical care expenditures by number of limiting conditions, 1980. Source: Rice and LaPlante, 1988b. Reprinted with permission.

year period and estimated that the medical care costs of disability totaled $117.6 billion in 1987. For those limited by one condition, medical care costs amounted to $92.2 billion; the remaining $25.4 billion are for those with two or more limiting chronic conditions. These cost estimates do not include losses in productivity due to disability (indirect costs), nor do they include transfer payments.

Although the above estimates of the costs of disability vary because of the different methodologies employed, it is clear that disability imposes a large economic cost on the public and private sectors of our society. The data show that the economic cost of multiple chronic conditions causing activity limitations is significant and high, a result that is not very surprising because the probability of disability and medical care use is greater for persons with multiple or comorbid conditions regardless of other factors. Thus targeting measures to prevent or reduce disability and its high economic toll is clearly in the nation's interest and should be given high priority.

CONCLUSION

Disability statistics rely on a wide variety of measures. The general-purpose NHIS data rely primarily on activity limitation as a measure of disability. Other data systems, designed for different purposes, use different measures: work disability, disability compensation, ability to perform particular tasks, and so on. The result is a patchwork of data that reflect the complexity of the concept of disability. Unfortunately, for technical reasons, it is often difficult to compare data from different sources.

Furthermore, unresolved conceptual difficulties in measuring disability can make it difficult to compare and comprehend the implications of existing data. Some clinical measures of functional status, for instance, which were developed to follow individual patients in the course of treatment, are too detailed and require too much medical expertise and/or equipment to be used in a broad-based population survey (Guralnik et al., 1989a). Some issues are difficult to measure through respondents. For instance there can be confusion between one's ability to carry out a specific task and whether one gets assistance in carrying it out (Wilson and Drury, 1984).

Just as role expectations influence whether a functional limitation becomes a disability (Nagi, 1965), statistical measures of functional limitation can be affected by what people expect or are expected to be able to do. For instance, if health promotion messages convince an older woman that she should walk more often, a mild case of arthritis that did not limit her activity before could interfere with walking on some days. Despite a probable improvement in health status, she would legitimately then be counted by the NHIS among those with activity limitations. A similar effect explains part of the apparent increase in disability in the 1970s among middle-aged men. Improved chronic disease screening, increased opportunities for disability compensation, and changing societal norms about early retirement allowed many men to enter medical treatment and to retire earlier than had been possible, probably increasing their health prospects and quality of life. In the official statistics, however, it appears that disability has increased (Wilson and Drury, 1984).

Given these limitations, it is clear that comprehensive measures of health status and quality of life are needed to understand the full complexity of disability and the factors leading up to it. Such measures have been developed, but they have been applied primarily in clinical studies. Research on their extension to population-based surveys is underway (Erickson et al., 1989).

As was apparent in the life table analyses, there are very few data extant on transitions in the disabling process. Although one can estimate on a cross-sectional basis the relationship between chronic conditions and activity limitation in the NHIS, and between different measures of activity limitation and disability in the SIPP, it is not possible to say much about the transitions from particular chronic conditions to particular functional limitations to different types of disability, for example, work disability. To develop efficient prevention programs it is critical to know the likelihood and rate of a large number of these transitions and their associated risk factors.

Finally, it is apparent that the available data focus on the chronic health conditions, not on the underlying processes and events that lead to these conditions and ultimately to disability. For instance, intentional and unintentional injuries are a major cause of the mobility limitations that are so prevalent in young adults, but no data are available to directly tie particular kinds of injuries—motor vehicle accidents or firearm injuries, for instance—to functional limitations or disabilities. This kind of information is clearly needed to develop effective programs for the prevention of disability.

In summary, taking into account all of the data discussed above, it is clear that the number of persons with disabilities depends on the definition of disability. Combining the number of noninstitutionalized people with any activity limitation estimated in the NHIS and the population of all ages in nursing homes, it appears that 35 million people live with disabling conditions. SIPP data point to about 46 million people with some type of work or functional limitation. With definitions focused only on inability to work or to carry out other major activities, or on receipt of disability benefits, the number of people with disabilities is substantially smaller. By any definition, however, people with disabling conditions, on average, are older and have lower incomes than others.

Because disability has many dimensions, different measurement concepts are necessary. Data are needed on (1) the clinical conditions that lead to functional limitations, (2) the impact of these limitations on the activities that individuals are able to carry out, and (3) the social and economic impacts these individuals experience because of functional limitations. Each of these aspects of disability can legitimately be measured in different ways, and because social programs are tied to some measures of disability, different definitions to match eligibility requirements are necessary. Although it would be extremely costly and technically difficult for any single data system to deal with all of these concepts and measurement systems simultaneously, it is important that attention be paid to improving the quantity, quality, comprehensiveness, and relevance of data on disability in the United States for consumers and for setting policy.

3

A Model for Disability and Disability Prevention

A common understanding of such terms as injury, impairment, handicap, functional limitation, and disability is essential to building effective, coherent prevention programs. Several frameworks have been advanced to describe disability-related concepts, but none has been universally adopted. The lack of a uniformly accepted conceptual foundation is an obstacle to epidemiological research and surveillance and to other elements critical to effective disability prevention programs. This chapter describes a conceptual framework of disability that is derived primarily from the works of Saad Nagi (1965; Appendix A, this volume) and the World Health Organization (1980). The framework is used as the basis upon which to build a model of the interacting influences involved in a stagelike disabling process that can lead to disability and that includes risk factors and quality of life.

CONCEPTUAL FRAMEWORK

There are two major conceptual frameworks in the field of disability: the International Classification of Impairments, Disabilities, and Handicaps (ICIDH), and the "functional limitation," or Nagi, framework, which is not accompanied by a classification system. The ICIDH is a trial supplement to the World Health Organization's International Classification of Diseases; it has stimulated extensive discussions of disability concepts, received both positive and negative reviews in the literature, and is used widely around the world. Several European countries including France and the Netherlands have adopted the ICIDH and use it extensively in administrative systems and clinical settings. As a classification system that has received broad international sponsorship the ICIDH deserves considerable attention, and the WHO is to be commended for its efforts in developing a system that has met with such success. As has been pointed out in the literature, however, the ICIDH is neither a classification of persons nor a research tool. The original intent of the ICIDH was to provide a framework to organize information about the consequences of disease (Haber, 1990). As such, the ICIDH has been considered by some as an intrusion of the medical profession into the social aspects of life—as a "medicalization of disablement" (Badley, 1987). The WHO is planning a revision of the ICIDH in the near future, however, which will provide opportunities for significant improvements.

Both frameworks (i.e., the ICIDH and the Nagi) have four basic concepts. In the ICIDH the four concepts are disease, impairment, disability, and handicap. In the Nagi framework the four concepts are pathology, impairment, functional limitation, and disability. Several authors have compared the two frameworks, and most have noted similarities, particularly between Nagi's concept of pathology and ICIDH's concept of disease and between the two frameworks' characterizations of impairment (Nagi, Appendix A, this volume; Duckworth, 1984; Frey, 1984; Granger, 1984; Haber, 1990).

The more important distinctions between the Nagi framework and the ICIDH occur in the last two conceptual categories and go beyond simple terminology. The ICIDH concept of disability seems to correspond to Nagi's concept of functional limitation, or "activities of daily living" (as used in the National Health Interview Survey), and the ICIDH concept of handicap (which subsumes role limitations) seems to correspond to Nagi's concept of disability. Both frameworks recognize that whether a person performs a socially expected activity depends not simply on the characteristics of the person, but also on the larger context of social and physical environments. Conceptual clarity, however, seems to be a problem with some of the classifications in the ICIDH. As Haber (1990) points out, for example, some of the classifications in the ICIDH are confusing, such as classifying certain social role limitations (e.g., family role, occupational role) under "behavior disabilities," instead of "occupation handicaps" or "social integration handicaps." Another example (Haber, 1990) is the distinction between "orientation handicaps" and disabilities associated with self-awareness, postural, or environmental problems.

In considering the options for a conceptual framework, the committee was faced with the fact that the ICIDH includes the term *handicap* in its classification. Traditionally, *handicap* has meant limitations in performance, placing an individual at a disadvantage. Handicap sometimes has been used to imply an absolute limitation that does not require for its actualization any interaction with external social circumstances. In recent years, the term has fallen into disuse in the United States, primarily as a result of a feeling on the part of people with disabling conditions that handicap is a negative term.

Although the term handicap is used often as a synonym for disability in American legislation, at least three federal agencies have changed their names to use the term *disability* instead of *handicap*: the former National Council on the Handicapped became the National Council on Disability in January 1989, the National Institute of Handicapped Research was redesignated the National Institute on Disability and Rehabilitation Research in 1986, and the President's Committee on Employment of the Handicapped was renamed the President's Committee on Employment of People with Disabilities in 1988. Mostly out of deference to those who feel that handicap is a denigrating term when used to describe a person, this committee decided not to use it. Yet the shadow of handicap as a commonly used term hovers behind the concept of "quality of life" and has the effect of reducing quality of life even though impairment, functional limitation, and even disability do not necessarily do so. Much as the term "cripple" has gone out of style, "handicap" seems to be approaching obsolescence, at least among people with disabilities in the United States.

The committee concurs with those who have noted internal inconsistencies and lack of clarity in the ICIDH concepts of disability and handicap (Nagi, Appendix A, this volume; Haber, 1990). It notes the opportunity and calls attention to the need for its pending revision, prefers not to use the term *handicap* in this context, and offers an alternative framework that does not focus on the consequences of disease. The committee's alternative framework draws on the widespread acceptance and success of the ICIDH and the conceptual clarity and terminology of the Nagi framework, and then adds risk factors and quality of life into a model of the disabling process. The committee found this framework and model to be useful in understanding and describing the relationships that exist among and between components of the disabling process as well as in identifying strategic points for preventive intervention. It is hoped that this will be considered as a viable alternative in the revisions of the WHO/ICIDH.

The conceptual framework used in this report is composed of four related but distinct stages: pathology, impairment, functional limitation, and disability. In the course of a chronic disorder, one stage can progress to the next. But depending on the circumstances, progressively greater loss of function need not occur, and the progression can be halted or reversed. Thus disability prevention efforts can be directed at any of the three stages that precede disability, as well as at the disability stage itself, where efforts can focus on reversal of disability, restoration of function, or prevention of complications (secondary conditions) that can greatly exacerbate existing limitations and lead to new ones. The four stages of the framework are summarized in Figure 3-1 and are briefly discussed below. A more detailed discussion and description of Nagi's concepts and terminology, vis-à-vis the alternative approach developed by the WHO (1980), appear in Appendix A. A recent editorial by Mervyn Susser (1990) adds considerable insight into the historical development of related concepts.

PATHOLOGY →	IMPAIRMENT →	FUNCTIONAL LIMITATION →	DISABILITY
Interruption or interference of normal bodily processes or structures	Loss and/or abnormality of mental, emotional, physiological, or anatomical structure or function; includes all losses or abnormalities, not just those attributable to active pathology; also includes pain	Restriction or lack of ability to perform an action or activity in the manner or within the range considered normal that results from impairment	Inability or limitation in performing socially defined activities and roles expected of individuals within a social and physical environment
Level of reference			
Cells and tissues	Organs and organ systems	Organism— action or activity performance (consistent with the purpose or function of the organ or organ system)	Society— task performance within the social and cultural context
Example			
Denervated muscle in arm due to trauma	Atrophy of muscle	Cannot pull with arm	Change of job; can no longer swim recreationally

FIGURE 3-1 An overview of the concepts of pathology, impairment, functional limitation, and disability.

Pathology

Pathology refers to cellular and tissue and changes caused by disease, infection, trauma, congenital conditions, or other agents. Much pathology is a reflection of the mobilization of the body's defenses against abnormalities. In the case of acute diseases, destruction of the normal cell architecture may result in particular manifestations (some combination of signs and symptoms) that aid identification of the underlying cause, or etiology. Many chronic diseases have multiple or uncertain etiologies. High serum cholesterol, hypertension, and smoking, for example, all increase the risk of heart disease, but not all people with these traits develop heart disease.

Predisposing factors that can lead to pathology are called risk factors. In the committee's model, risk factors can be biological, lifestyle and behavioral, or environmental (physical or social). Risk factors are discussed in greater detail later in the chapter.

Impairment

Impairment is defined as a discrete loss or abnormality of mental, physiological, or biochemical function. Impairment includes losses caused by all forms of pathology. A specific impairment might have different etiologies and different types of pathology. All pathologies, however, are accompanied by impairments (Figure 3-2).

Impairments include anomalies, defects, or losses and relate to the specific functioning of an organ or organ system but not to the organism as a whole. Examples of impairments are absence or displacement of body parts, reduced blood flow, mechanical problems of joints, paralysis, stiffness, and numbness. The severity of impairment varies by condition, by the tissues and organs affected, and by the extent to which tissues and organs are damaged. For example, the human immunodeficiency virus (HIV) attacks T-cells, compromising the immunity of the infected person. Compromised immune function is but one impairment associated with HIV exposure. Depending on the extent of immune system suppression, several other conditions and impairments may occur. In contrast, other diseases such as arthritis are more specific in terms of the type and location of impairments they cause.

Functional Limitation

Functional limitation is the term proposed by Nagi to describe effects manifested in the performance or performance capacity of the person as a whole. An example of a functional limitation is the inability to lift a 25-pound box and carry it 25 feet. This type of limitation may be caused by impairment of any one of several body systems, including reduction of pulmonary function (emphysema), denervation of muscle tissue (amyotrophic lateral sclerosis), or restriction in range of joint motion (arthritis).

All functional limitations result from impairments, but not all impairments lead to functional limitation (Figure 3-2). Several factors other than the nature and degree of impairment affect functional performance. For example, of two individuals with the same level of pulmonary function, one may be able to complete an activity such as walking upstairs, whereas the other cannot. Only the latter individual has a functional limitation as a result of this particular impairment. Such variation may be related to the capacities of the individual's other body systems (e.g., cardiovascular fitness, muscular strength, or pain tolerance).

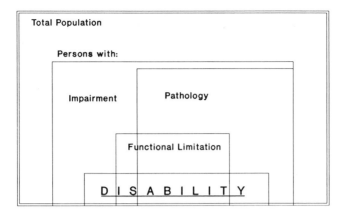

FIGURE 3-2 According to the Nagi framework, all pathology is associated with impairment, but not all impairments lead to functional limitations. Similarly, all functional limitation and disability is associated with impairment, but not all functional limitations lead to disability. Disability can also exist in the absence of functional limitation (e.g., disfigurement). (This diagram serves to illustrate the conceptual relationship among the categories in Nagi's framework; the sizes of the boxes do not reflect the relative size of that category in the U.S. population.)

Disability

Disability is the expression of a physical or mental limitation in a social context—the gap between a person's capabilities and the demands of the environment. People with such functional limitations are not inherently disabled, that is, incapable of carrying out their personal, familial, and social responsibilities. It is the interaction of their physical or mental limitations with social and environmental factors that determines whether they have a disability. Most disability is thus preventable, which not only will significantly improve the quality of life for millions of Americans but also could save many billions of dollars in costs resulting from dependence, lost productivity, and medical care.

Pathology, impairment, and functional limitation all involve different levels of organismic function. *Disability*, however, refers to social rather than organismic function. According to Nagi (Appendix A, this volume):

[Disability is a] limitation in performing socially defined roles and tasks expected of an individual within a sociocultural and physical environment. These roles and tasks are organized in spheres of life activities such as those of the family or other interpersonal relations; work, employment, and other economic pursuits; and education, recreation, and self-care. Not all impairments or functional limitations precipitate disability, and similar patterns of disability may result from different types of impairments and limitations in function. Furthermore, identical types of impairments and similar functional limitations may result in different patterns of disability. Several other factors contribute to shaping the dimensions and severity of disability. These include (a) the individual's definition of the situation and reactions, which at times compound the limitations; (b) the definition of the situation by others, and their reactions and expectations—especially those who are significant in the lives of the person with the disabling condition (e.g., family members, friends and associates, employers and co-workers, and organizations and professions that provide services and benefits); and (c) characteristics of the environment and the degree to which it is free from, or encumbered with, physical and sociocultural barriers.

Thus one way in which disability differs from pathology, impairment, and functional limitation is in the role of factors external to the individual. Disability is defined by the attributes and interactions of the individual and the environment, whereas the preceding stages are defined solely by characteristics of the individual. For example, whether a person with an impairment is able to work depends not only on the nature and severity of his or her impairment and resulting functional limitation but also on such factors as the state of the economy, characteristics of the workplace, availability of transportation, and the individual's particular work skills and training. Whether a person with a functional limitation lives independently may be determined by supportive social contacts and the architectural features of his or her home.

Pathology, impairment, and functional limitation can be determined by examination and testing of the individual, but disability is a relational attribute—the interaction of an individual's functional limitation with the demands of expected tasks and roles and with the environmental conditions under which roles and tasks are to be performed. Referring to specific pathologies or impairments as disabilities ignores the interactive nature of the process that can lead to disability.

To understand disability as it is defined here, one must also understand the concepts of roles and tasks, and how they relate to each other. The concept of task is best understood in relation to the concept of role. Simply put, roles—such as being a teacher, researcher, parent, or civic leader—are organized according to how individuals participate in a social system (Parsons, 1958). Tasks are specific physical and mental actions through which an individual (not a subsystem of an individual, which would be at the impairment level) interacts with the physical and social world and performs his or her roles. One task does not define a role; roles are made up of many tasks, which are modifiable and somewhat interchangeable.

Finally, although disability can be prevented by improving the functional capacity of the individual—the traditional aim of rehabilitation—this is not the only nor perhaps even the most effective method. Disability can be prevented by changing societal attitudes that now restrict employment opportunities for persons with functional limitations, by modifying the buildings in which such people work, or by providing accessible modes of transportation (all of which are components of the Americans with Disabilities Act). Disability can be prevented by building living quarters, parks, and other facilities with fewer obstacles restricting access and use by persons with functional limitations. The opportunity to prevent disability by manipulating characteristics external to the individual greatly expands the traditional medical notions of disability and the consequent approaches to treatment and services, and reflects more of a public health approach.

Personally and socially expected activities can be accomplished by changing the means to the ends. Capacities are the means; expected activities are the ends. One reason why impairments and functional limitations do not necessarily lead to disability is that individuals with a given impairment may overcome specific functional limitations by compensating with other functional capacities to avoid disability. Installing ramps in buildings, for example, enables people with mobility limitations to perform activities that would otherwise be denied to them.

In summary, disability begins with physical or mental health conditions that limit the performance of individuals in personally, socially, and culturally expected roles. The limitation may be total, rendering an activity unperformable, or it may be partial, restricting the amount or kind of an activity a person can perform. Although conceptually distinct, disability is often confused with disease and impairment. For example, specific diagnostic conditions and impairments, such as mental retardation, cerebral palsy, or multiple sclerosis, are erroneously referred to as disabilities. But depending on various factors, these conditions may or may not lead to disability (although the risk of disability is high for each of the examples given). Moreover, the scope and severity of limitation that follows even the most physiologically damaging disorders—those that pose the greatest risk of physical disability—vary among individuals, including those with the same condition.

MODEL OF DISABILITY

Building on the conceptual frameworks of Nagi and the WHO, and placing disability within the appropriate context of health and social issues, the committee developed a model for disability. The model, shown in Figure 3-3, depicts the interactive effects of biological, environmental (physical and social), and lifestyle and behavioral risk factors that influence each stage of the disabling process; the relationship of the disabling process to quality of life; and the stages of the disabling process that often precede disability. Each component of the model (i.e., risk factors, quality of life, and the disabling process) is discussed below.

Risk Factors

Risk factors are biological, environmental (social and physical), and lifestyle or behavioral characteristics that are causally associated with health-related conditions (Lalonde, 1974; Last, 1988). They can be identified by comparing the frequency of a condition's occurrence, such as disability, in a group having some specific trait with the frequency of the same condition in another group without that trait. Identifying such factors can be a first step toward identifying a mechanism of action, and then developing preventive interventions. For example, workers in a factory where there is high exposure to dust may have higher rates of respiratory disease than other factory workers. In this case, exposure to dust-borne hazardous particles may be identified as a cause, the mode of biological action elucidated, and appropriate preventive measures identified.

Some risk factors are implicated in a variety of chronic diseases, resulting in what has been termed general susceptibility (Syme and Berkman, 1976). Socioeconomic status is important among these risk factors. Epidemiologists have also called attention to changes in the nature and distribution of disease as nations develop economically and standards of living change accordingly (Omran, 1979). Such changes have engendered debate on the relative importance of lifestyle, sanitation, nutrition, and public health in the changing incidence and prevalence of chronic diseases.

Similarly, there are many risk factors and causal routes associated with disability. Marge (1988) lists the following 16 causes of disabling conditions:

- Genetic disorders
- Acute and chronic illness
- Violence
- Lack of physical fitness
- Tobacco use
- Educational deficiency
- Familial-cultural deleterious beliefs
- Inaccessibility to adequate health care

- Perinatal complications
- Unintentional and intentional injuries
- Environmental quality problems
- Alcohol and drug abuse
- Nutritional disorders
- Deleterious child-rearing practices
- Unsanitary living conditions
- Stress

Whether through injury, disease, personal-choice behaviors, genetic traits, or some other causal mechanism, multiple risk factors of various types can converge to predispose an individual to the disabling process, as shown in Figure 3-3. In addition, risk factors interact at the different stages of the disabling process (note the circles between the stages that represent the

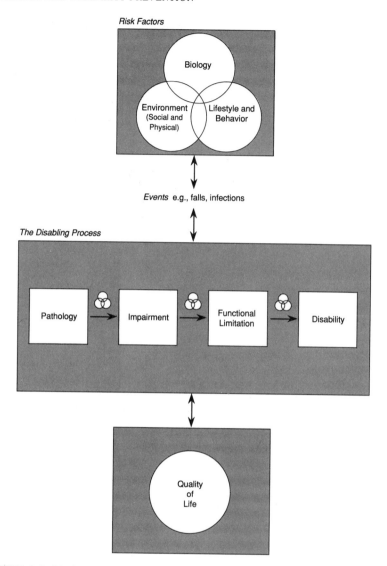

FIGURE 3-3 Model of disability showing the interaction among the disabling process, quality of life, and risk factors. Three types of risk factors are included:
biological (e.g., Rh type); environmental (e.g., lead paint [physical environment],
access to care [social environment]); and lifestyle and behavior (e.g., tobacco consumption). Bidirectional arrows indicate the potential for "feedback." The potential
for additional risk factors to affect the progression toward disability is shown between
the stages of the model. These additional risk factors might include diagnosis, treatment,
therapy, adequacy of rehabilitation, age of onset, financial resources, expectations,
and environmental barriers, depending on the stage of the model.

various risk factors), and these are often different risk factors than those that precipitate the initial condition. In addition, risk factors exist internally (e.g., through individual choices) and externally (e.g., through the physical and social environment).

The disability research and service communities have not yet adopted a systematic, comprehensive conceptual model for understanding risk factors for disability. This committee, however, believes that the model described in this report, incorporating three risk factor categories—biological, environmental (physical and social), and lifestyle and behavioral—will help move the disability research and service communities closer to a more unified understanding of disability and disability prevention. Although many disability risks cannot be neatly categorized, and many occur at the intersection of two or three categories, this model presents an initial framework for exploring possible points for preventive interventions. The scope of each risk category is discussed briefly below.

Biological Factors

Biological risk factors are those that develop within the body as part of one's basic biology and organic makeup. They include genetic and other inborn or inherited characteristics as well as the metabolic aspects of maturation, growth, aging, and the interactions of the varied and complex systems of the body.

Biological risk factors associated with disabling conditions are often the same as those associated with specific diseases because the disabling condition often results from the disease (e.g., arthritis, diabetes, atherosclerosis). Many biological risk factors are genetic, as in the case of Tay-Sachs disease, a condition that causes progressive retardation, paralysis, blindness, and death by age 3 or 4.

Preventive strategies directed toward decreasing biological risk factors include pharmaceutical prophylaxis and treatment, nutritional modification, exercise, and prenatal care.

Environmental Factors

The defining characteristic of environmental risk factors is that they are health-related risks that exist outside the person and over which the individual has little or no control. There are two types: social and physical. The social-environmental risk factors overlap to some extent with the lifestyle and behavioral risk factors, but are primarily the product of societal structures. The physical-environmental risk factors are primarily the product of the built (i.e., human-made) environment.

The social (i.e., social-environmental) risks for disability are a function of the expectations and opportunities that accompany specific sociocultural environments. Attitudes, assumptions, preferences, and prejudices encountered throughout society help create social-environmental disability risks. For example, in agricultural occupational settings individuals are expected to have certain physical skills, abilities, and characteristics. Because of the physical demands and sociocultural expectations of that environment, the likelihood or risk of a functional limitation becoming a disability is greater than in a cultural setting that assigns less value to these characteristics. Thus job settings can create a social-environmental risk for disability when individuals are required to perform tasks that exceed their physical (or mental) abilities.

Individuals with disabling conditions often report that their independence of action is significantly influenced by the attitudes of those in their environment. These attitudes are reflected both in the way individuals relate to those with disabling conditions and in the public policies that are adopted by society. Paternalism, for example, whereby individuals provide resources but not freedom of choice in the use of those resources, is not uncommon. This practice requires a compliance on the part of those with disabling conditions that affects self-esteem negatively and encourages dependent roles—a result that can contribute to a lack of initiative and independence in social and work situations. It also is not uncommon for persons with disabling conditions to encounter discriminatory attitudes and behavior—for example, being prejudged as unable to assume roles such as worker, spouse, sports participant, or independent resident. It is also not uncommon for those with physically disabling conditions to be treated as though they had mental impairment as well.

Much as social-environmental risk factors stem from sociocultural expectations and opportunities, physical-environmental risk factors have their source in the physical places in which people conduct their daily lives. Like social-environmental risk factors, physical-environmental risk factors also occur in a variety of forms. The risk can occur as a direct result of the physical design of public places or of the individual's workplace or living arrangements. These environments can put an individual at risk for injury or disease, which can trigger a process that leads to disability; they also can place individuals in circumstances in which impairments and functional limitations become disabling. Examples of the former risk include workplaces in which employees are not protected from dangerous machinery, households with slippery floors (or other problems that promote injuries), or exposure to toxicants (e.g., lead paint) and other disease-causing agents. Examples of the latter include inadequate access to the built environment for individuals who use wheelchairs, prostheses, orthosis, or guide or hearing dogs. Inadequate public transportation also can put individuals with impairments or functional limitations at increased risk for disability.

Designing intervention strategies for environmental risks can be difficult. There often is not a clear-cut option between modifying the environment or targeting the intervention to the individual with the disabling condition. In some cases, such as the inaccessibility of public accommodations, a legislative approach—one that requires modification of the environment—is the solution. The recent passage of the landmark Americans with Disabilities Act is an excellent example. Unfortunately, not every environmental risk lends itself to such a solution. In many cases interventions require a careful balance of modifications to the physical and social environments (e.g., altering the workplace and increasing educational efforts) and interventions designed to assist people with disabling conditions in adjusting to the environment (e.g., rehabilitation and retraining). These issues are discussed in more detail in Chapter 7.

Lifestyle and Behavioral Factors

Lifestyle and behavioral risk factors consist of personal decisions and habits that affect one's health and over which one has considerable control. Lifestyles and behaviors that are detrimental to health create self-imposed risks. Research has made it clear that unhealthy lifestyles contribute to mortality and morbidity in affluent, industrialized countries. The Centers for Disease Control has estimated that 50 percent of the deaths attributed to the 10 leading causes of mortality can be directly related to "lifestyles." Foremost among these behavioral risk factors, according to Hamburg (1984), are smoking, excessive alcohol intake, illicit drug use, poor dietary habits, insufficient exercise, reckless driving, noncompliance with medication regimens, and maladaptive responses to stressful experience. As Hamburg notes, "A new awareness has dawned: much of disease and disability is related to human behavior, and therefore the role of behavior in keeping people healthy must be understood scientifically. In this direction lies the possibility of preventing much disease and promoting health. This promising approach affects the well being of people everywhere."

Because Hamburg's list of risk factors was published in 1984, it did not include unsafe sexual behavior as a major contributor to mortality and morbidity. With the AIDS (acquired immune deficiency syndrome) epidemic, however, unsafe sexual behavior must be added to the list of behaviors that contribute to disability and mortality in the United States. Moreover, Hamburg points to cigarette smoking as the most important environmental factor and alcohol abuse as the most serious drug problem in America, but the toll taken by cocaine abuse also now must be taken into account. For example, Hahnemann University Hospital in Philadelphia reports that 40 percent of a consecutive series of 500 mothers who delivered babies and who were insured by Medicaid had evidence of cocaine in urine or blood samples at the time of delivery (M. R. Spence, Department of Obstetrics and Gynecology, Hahnemann University Hospital, personal communication, 1990). Cocaine use during pregnancy and the consequent intrauterine exposure of cocaine to the developing fetal brain increases the risk of reduced learning and socializing abilities and the development of disabling conditions.

Many health-damaging behaviors, such as smoking, overeating, and alcohol and drug abuse, are extremely resistant to permanent change (Matarazzo et al., 1984). It is therefore time- and resource-consuming to try to effect change in these behaviors. Matarazzo and coauthors conclude that public health programs designed to change health-related behaviors should be undertaken only after careful pilot studies. To do otherwise, they warn, is to risk damaging society's willingness to invest fiscal and human resources in prevention. Nonetheless, it is increasingly obvious that successful programs have the potential to yield large returns to individuals and to society.

Belloc (1973) identified seven specific personal health practices that were highly correlated with the physical health of some 7,000 Americans. These health practices included sleeping 7 to 8 hours daily; eating breakfast almost every day; never or rarely eating between meals; currently being at or near a prescribed height-adjusted weight; never smoking cigarettes; moderate or no use of alcohol; and regular physical activity. A correlation was found between long survival and an increase in the number of health-related behaviors adopted. These behaviors also resulted in a decrease in the morbidity associated with many disorders, such as heart disease, lung cancer, and hypertension—illnesses that cost society substantial medical care dollars and losses resulting from forgone productivity.

Health-related behaviors such as those described above greatly influence the onset and progression of disabling conditions. Physical fitness, for example, can affect both the severity of an injury sustained from a fall and the recovery from it. Fitness and exercise are also major factors in maintaining maximal functioning in people with paraplegia, for example, to prevent progression in the disabling process and the development of secondary conditions.

Finally, many risk factors exist at the intersection of the three risk factor categories described above. Personality, for instance, is probably a product of all three—biological, behavioral, and environmental.

Quality of Life

Quality of life generally corresponds to total well-being, encompassing both physical and psychosocial determinants (Wenger et al., 1984). So defined, quality of life closely approximates the World Health Organization's definition of health as a state of complete physical, mental, and social well-being, and not merely the absence of disease or infirmity (WHO, 1947). Components of quality of life include performance of social roles, physical status, emotional status, social interactions, intellectual functioning, economic status, and self-perceived or subjective health status (Wenger et al., 1984; Patrick and Erickson, 1988; Levine and Croog, 1984). Indicators of quality of life have included standard of living, economic status, life satisfaction, quality of housing and the neighborhood in which one lives, self-esteem, and job satisfaction. Quality of life is also clearly the product of broad social forces that influence, for example, education and employment opportunities or that result in differential treatment of groups within the population.

The concept of quality of life subsumes many aspects of personal well-being that are not directly related to health. It is becoming increasingly clear, however, that health is the product of a complex array of factors, many of which fall outside the traditional province of health care. Similarly, the health of the population has commercial, economic, and social importance. Thus, quality of life is assuming greater importance in the practice and evaluation of medicine (Levine, 1987), and its enhancement, in addition to curing disease or improving survival, is becoming an accepted goal of the health care professions. Concerns of health care providers now include, for example, whether a patient's physical state or treatment modality causes depression or dependency, limits role performance, or creates poor perceptions of health. Indeed, functioning and role performance are considered important, if not central, variables in applying the quality of life concept in health assessments.

Quality of life is relevant to all stages of the disabling process, beginning with pathology. Indeed, gradual deterioration in function, as in the case of some chronic diseases, or the sudden occurrence of disability, as in the case of serious injuries, must be viewed in the context of how quality of life is affected. For people facing such circumstances, preventing deterioration in function is tantamount to maintaining their lives at a certain level of quality. In turn, conditions within society greatly affect the health and well-being of these individuals. Those who have functional limitations may not have the opportunity to participate in society if it does not accommodate their limitations. Affected individuals may be healthy in the sense that their residual impairments have stabilized and they are free of pathology, but they are not healthy in a social sense. If the essence of health is, as some have maintained, the ability to perform personally valued activities, then disability is a social definition of ill health.

As depicted in Figure 3-3, quality of life affects and is affected by the outcomes of each stage of the disabling process. Within the disabling process, each stage interacts with an individual's quality of life; it is not an endpoint of the model but rather an integral part. There is no universal threshold—no particular level of impairment or functional limitation—at which people perceive themselves as having lost their personal autonomy and diminished the quality of their lives. Perceptions of personal independence and quality of life, however, are clearly important in determining how individuals respond to challenges at each of the four stages of the disabling process. (A similar theoretical model for health status and quality of life is described by Patrick and Bergner, 1990.)

In addition, social roles are valued differently by individuals and social groups. In the evaluation of disabling conditions, considerable attention is often paid to the socially valued roles, principally work. To the individual, however, other roles and activities may be more important and rewarding than work. Thus, it is important to assess both the objective aspects of quality of life, such as whether a person has changed jobs because of an impairment or health problem, and the subjective aspects, such as the individual's satisfaction with the job.

Quality of life for persons with disabling conditions can be enhanced or at least maintained even if functioning cannot be improved. Modification of the environment, such as the construction of a ramp into a building or the reduction of negative attitudes and stereotypes, can help to improve an individual's quality of life as well as prevent disability by restoring role performance even when functional limitations cannot be redressed.

Improved measures of quality of life are needed for use in assessments of health and disability.

The Disabling Process

At the center of the model is the disabling process. Although it seems to indicate a unidirectional progression from pathology to impairment to functional limitation to disability, and although a stepwise progression often occurs, progression from one stage to another is not always the case. An individual with a disabling condition might skip over components of the model, for example, when the public's attitude toward a disfiguring impairment causes no functional limitation but does impose a disability by affecting social interaction. It is also important to note that the effects of specific stages in the model can be moderated by such interventions as assistive devices. Similarly, environmental modification (e.g., elimination of physical obstacles and barriers) is an important form of disability prevention, as is legislation such as the recently enacted Americans with Disabilities Act—a landmark in antidiscrimination legislation directed toward ensuring the rights of people with disabling conditions.

An important feature of the disabling process is its interaction with risk factors—a feature that is essential to the development of preventive interventions. For example, the outcome of heart disease is not predetermined at the time of diagnosis, and changes in diet, regular exercise, adoption of less stressful work habits, and other health-promoting practices may actually result in improved functioning, even though the underlying condition will persist. In addition, risk factors can interact with so-called protective factors (not shown) to increase or decrease the likelihood of further change in health status. Thus there are "feedback loops" in the disabling process that can hasten, slow, or prevent the progression to disability.

Implicit in the model is the influence of important social and medical variables, such as the timely availability of appropriate medical and rehabilitative care, employment opportunities, and adequate housing. High rates of disability among low socioeconomic groups and low rates of disability among people with advanced educations are but two of many pieces of compelling evidence demonstrating the significant influences of social variables, which generally are not addressed in traditional medical approaches to treating people with disabling conditions.

Thus a variety of personal, societal, and environmental factors can influence the progression of a potentially disabling condition from pathology to disability, the degree of limitation or disability, and the occurrence of secondary conditions. Several of these factors are discussed below.

Health Status

Health status prior to the onset of a potentially disabling condition, as well as after the initiation of the disabling process, can significantly influence the degree of limitation and the ability to avoid the development of secondary conditions. Obesity, for example, can limit the amount of ambulation by an individual with neurological impairment, making that person more susceptible to skin infections or joint and muscle contractures. Skin infections and contractures, in turn, can lead to additional impairment and functional limitation.

Psychological Status

Successful management of potentially disabling conditions and prevention of secondary conditions depends greatly on the psychological status of the individual with the condition. Thus the realization and acceptance of a potentially disabling condition, combined with a focus on adaptation, are necessary components of preventive interventions as they apply to primary and secondary conditions. In addition, an individual's attitudes toward solving problems and functioning independently become important in minimizing both primary and secondary conditions. Also, coping skills as demonstrated prior to the onset of a disabling condition are important to those facing a major disabling event, particularly those skills relating to flexibility in coping with change. Motivation for adaptation is poorly understood but is uniformly seen as necessary for successful rehabilitation.

Socioeconomic Status

Socioeconomic status and the risk of disability are inversely related. In part, this relationship is explained by the income-suppressing effects of disability (Luft, 1978). The same inverse relationship is found, however, between disability risk and level of educational attainment (LaPlante, 1988), which is less sensitive to such income effects. Clearly, there are factors associated with being poor that powerfully increase the risk of pathology and the progression to disability. Differences in personal expectations, demands of the social and living environments, ability to control personal and social circumstances, access to adequate health care, and individual behavior have all been hypothesized to play a role.

Although we know that rates of disability are higher among lower socioeconomic groups, we do not know precisely why. People in low socioeconomic groups are at higher-than-average risk for a variety of chronic diseases and injuries (Susser et al., 1985; Syme and Berkman, 1976), and they are more likely to work in physically demanding occupations that afford little control over the conditions of their jobs and work sites. Moreover, they are less likely than those in higher socioeconomic groups to get the health care they need to avoid impairment and functional limitation. Although health and welfare programs defray expenses and help offset income losses for persons with disabling conditions, they do so only for those with the most severe disabilities. Even for these people, however, some acute and long-term care needs go unaddressed.

Educational Status and Vocational Training

On average, earnings rise in tandem with levels of educational attainment, and higher levels of earnings perhaps are an incentive for returning to work following the onset of disability. Indeed, among the population of people with disabling conditions, those with college-level educations are less likely to be unemployed or underemployed than those with lower levels of educational training. Moreover, education is believed to be correlated with flexibility and adaptability, which are necessary for adjusting to the changes imposed by a potentially disabling condition. Nevertheless, after taking into consideration these obvious factors, the reason why people with higher levels of education have lower levels of disease and disability remains largely unexplained (Sagan, 1987). More knowledge about this topic is important to understanding disability causation and prevention.

Previous job experience also tends to increase the options available to an individual with functional limitations. Experience and training serve as the basis for occupational planning. Those with easily transferable skills are more likely to return to work than those who have narrow job experience and who, because of their functional limitations, cannot return to their previous employment. Thus people who were involved in physically demanding occupations usually are less able to return to their former job than those who were engaged in sedentary, white-collar jobs prior to the initiation of the disabling condition. Another key variable influencing employability is the attitude of the previous employer. Some employers are willing to make major work-site modifications, whereas others are quite rigid in their requirements for conformance to usual job descriptions.

Climate

The opportunity for independent community living and access to work for people with disabling conditions often are influenced by the characteristics of the climate (e.g., typical weather patterns), as well as of the social environment (e.g., social attitudes and programs). Frequent snow and limitations in its removal, for example, can influence the mobility of a physically restricted individual. Another example is the fact that urban areas often have social support programs for persons with major disabling conditions than do relatively isolated rural areas.

Some advocacy groups have noted an apparent migration of individuals with disabling conditions from relatively rural to more urban areas that offer more support and opportunity. At times, those with disabling conditions are able to enhance their independence by moving to an area with a different and less restrictive environment or climate. However, the net effect of such moves is a function of many variables, including the individual's social support system, as well as factors related to the regional environment.

The relationship between risk factors, such as health, education, socioeconomic status, and psychosocial status, and the disabling process needs to be elucidated.

Multiplicity of Conditions and Disabilities

In considering the disabling process, it is important to recognize that persons can have multiple chronic conditions, multiple functional problems, and even multiple disabilities because each role that an individual normally performs produces an opportunity for disability to manifest. Thus an independent disabling condition can develop in a person who already has one. A more likely situation, however, is one in which additional disabling conditions result as a consequence of a primary disabling condition. An example is the disuse syndrome, in which a person with paralysis (primary condition) develops pressure sores (secondary condition). In this example, an impairment (paralysis) causes the development of other conditions (pressure sores) and additional losses of capability. In addition, the risk of progression from impairment to functional limitation to disability will increase if other conditions are present (Guralnik et al., 1989b). Similarly, the risk of progression from functional limitation to disability can be expected to increase in the presence of multiple functional limitations in such a way that a previously low risk of disability is elevated to high probability.

Thus multiple disabling conditions arise in many different ways and may or may not be causally related. If there is neither a direct nor an indirect linkage between conditions, that is, if they are independent, then the two conditions would be expected to occur no more frequently than by chance alone. Analysis of National Health Interview Survey (NHIS) data, however, shows that several combinations of disabling conditions, including hypertension with arthritis and hypertension with heart disease, occur more frequently than would be expected by chance alone. In addition, persons with multiple disabling conditions are more likely to have severe limitations in activity. Thus prevention of secondary conditions is an important aspect of reducing disability and improving the quality of life. (Prevention of secondary conditions is discussed in more detail in Chapter 7.)

THE NEED FOR EPIDEMIOLOGY

Epidemiology is the study of the distributions and determinants of states of health in human populations. Despite the significance of disability as a health and social issue, it has received little attention from the epidemiological community (Nagi, 1976; Appendix A, this volume). Nagi (1976) attributes this seeming lack of interest to the preoccupation of epidemiology with pathology and impairment, the conceptual confusion surrounding the meaning of disability and related terms, and problems in the reliability and validity of available measures. As discussed later in this chapter in relation to the need for surveillance, the available epidemiologic data are mostly prevalence data. Incidence data on disability are more difficult to obtain and are lacking. The purpose of this section is to discuss the need for epidemiologic studies of disability, that is, beyond pathology and impairment. The need applies to all of the elements in the conceptual framework of disability, including risk factors, quality of life factors, pathology, impairment, functional limitation, disability, and levels of functional performance in everyday living.

As noted previously, disability refers to limitations in carrying out activities that people are generally expected to be able to perform (Haber, 1988; Nagi, 1965; Appendix A, this volume). Human activities vary in many ways, including whether they are necessary, the degree to which an individual is expected by others to perform them, and the degree to which the individual desires to perform them. In addition, disease, injury, and congenital and developmental conditions limit human behavior; the distribution of these limitations is not random in human populations; and epidemiological principles can be used to study health-related limitations in human activity and how they might be prevented.

Epidemiologists traditionally study the distribution of disease in a population and attempt to understand the determinants of that distribution. The usefulness of this approach for the study of disability is somewhat limited because the concept of disability does not fit the traditional disease model. For example, a developmental condition, injury, or disease does not necessarily lead to disability. Whether it does depends on many factors, including the level of functional limitation associated with the condition, the activities the person with the condition is expected to perform or may want to do, and features of the living and work environments.

In much traditional epidemiological research, it is necessary only to identify the existence of a disease, condition, or injury. In epidemiological research on disability, however, social and behavioral variables must be taken into consideration. Nonetheless, the same principles that guide epidemiological research on disease are relevant to research on disability. For example, a fundamental premise of epidemiological research is that disease does not occur randomly in the population. Disabilities, like diseases, also are not randomly distributed. In addition, as with diseases, rates of disability vary among population groups. Epidemiological methods can be used to describe these distributions, help identify risk factors, and, in turn, guide development of disability prevention programs. The challenge is to recognize the shortcomings of traditional methods for addressing disability and then develop the tools and data networks necessary to identify the causes of disabilities and their associated risk factors. Gathering this information will require studying social and behavioral variables that were once considered to be outside the domain of epidemiology and even public health.

This task will be speeded by the broader epidemiological perspective that appears to be evolving today in the field of public health. For example, public health interest in AIDS has helped pave the way for a more sophisticated epidemiology of disability by targeting efforts toward the behaviors and events that result in the transmission of the HIV and the onset of AIDS. As the life spans of people with AIDS are prolonged, however, the field of public health will need to direct additional attention to issues of long-term disability management.

Although the relationship between some risk factors and certain disabilities is well understood, much remains unknown. Some needed information can be obtained by organizing and analyzing data that are already available.

But much of the available information on people with disabling conditions has been collected piecemeal by many agencies, each with the aim of meeting its own particular needs. Thus large voids remain that cannot be filled with existing data, and a more comprehensive approach to data collection is needed to develop an adequate knowledge base on the risk of disability.

Standard terminology and conceptual clarity are essential to meaningful discourse, productive research, and effective prevention efforts. As mentioned above, conceptual confusion surrounding the meaning of disability and related terms has hindered epidemiologic research on disability, and an underlying obstacle to data collection and analysis continues to be the lack of a widely accepted, uniformly applied conceptual framework. During the past 10 to 15 years two major options have emerged: the Nagi and the ICIDH model frameworks. The ICIDH has become the de facto international standard, but neither framework is dominant in the United States, and scientific consensus is lacking.

The need for conceptual clarity and uniform terminology in the field of disability prevention is essential and immediate. The model developed by this committee reflects its recommendation for standardized concepts and terminology that can serve as the basis for developing preventive interventions and an epidemiology of disability.

Once a nationally accepted framework is in place, future survey research efforts related to disability should be required to demonstrate that the concepts, terms, and questions used in the survey are anchored within the agreed-upon framework. Such a grounding would increase the probability that the results from one survey could be compared with those of another, thereby improving the utility of survey data.

Data Needs

Disability prevention requires continuing population surveillance. To be effective, such surveillance should be more thorough than the existing patchwork system, be based on an improved understanding of the causes of disabilities and associated risk factors, and reflect greater knowledge of the economic and social consequences of disability, including the effects of disability on quality of life. In short, the paths of the model in Figure 3-3 must be explored and quantified, the mechanisms described, and intervention strategies developed. Questions that must be addressed if we are to set priorities for disability prevention include the following: Do conditions with the highest risks of disability also pose the highest risks of functional limitation and impairment? To what extent do behavioral factors combine with impairment and functional limitation to determine disability outcomes? How does the environment affect disability outcome, and does the effect of the environment depend on the nature of the impairment and functional limitation? The following sections discuss data and research needs that should be addressed to ensure that basic epidemiological elements of effective prevention efforts are in place.

Risk Factors

Research on biological, environmental (physical and social), and behavioral risk factors is one of the cornerstones of epidemiology and, consequently, of health promotion and disease prevention. As the model of the disabling process illustrates, knowledge of risk factors is central to disability prevention. Indeed, a comprehensive understanding of risks is critical to answering three fundamental questions:

* Given exposure to environmental agents or other provocations, why do some persons develop potentially disabling conditions and others do not?
* Given such exposure and the occurrence of pathology or injury, why does one person develop a disability and another does not? That is, what determines the progression toward functional limitation and disability?
* At the aggregate level, why do some population groups have higher rates of disability than others?

At each stage in the disabling process, biological and behavioral characteristics and features of the social and physical environment have determinative effects on individual outcomes. The genetically determined healthy or unhealthy nature of an individual's body systems is not the sole factor in the development of disease or disability. For example, not all people with abnormal glucose levels develop diabetes, and not all diabetics develop functional limitations or disabilities. An epidemiology of disability requires an expanded perspective on risk factors because any specific type of disability can be the product of many different kinds of pathology, impairment, and functional limitations. Moreover, a complex array of variables, many of them outside the bounds of the usually emphasized biological risk factors, can speed, slow, halt, or reverse the stage-to-stage progression to disability. Such variables include the adequacy and availability of social and medical services, socioeconomic status, marital status, job experience, and amount of educational and vocational training.

Research has demonstrated the importance of psychosocial risk factors in disability (Haan et al., 1989), but the findings thus far are largely in the form of leads for further research. Critically important details remain to be identified—for example, the influence of social support, a concept that refers to the quality and breadth of one's relationships with a mate, other family members, friends, and others. Lack of social support has been associated with an increased risk of heart disease, complications of pregnancy and delivery, suicide, and other conditions (Dutton and Levine, 1989; U.S. Department of Health, Education, and Welfare, 1979). An important question is, what underlying biological mechanisms are affected by social support? The answer to the question of underlying biological mechanisms may not emerge if the focus of investigation is limited to only one condition. Perhaps the most productive way to detect the underlying mechanism in this case is to study all health consequences associated with inadequate social support (Haan et al., 1989).

Although the condition-specific approach of epidemiology has increased our understanding of diseases and their prevention, it may lead to overly narrow perspectives on prevention, corresponding to disease classifications (see Table 3-1). An alternative approach would be based on risk factors that predispose an individual to several disease conditions that can lead to disability, such as those shown in Table 3-2. From the viewpoint of public health, a classification scheme that identifies causative features common to several disabling conditions may foster more efficient prevention programs, focusing on risk factors implicated in multiple conditions that predispose an individual to disability. This strategy might offer opportunities to achieve benefits that are larger than the sum of the returns to individual disorder-specific initiatives.

Although epidemiology is essential to disability prevention, very little epidemiological research on risk factors for disability or on disability per se has been done, and few studies have been conducted to identify populations at increased risk of disability. Most relevant data relate to clinical conditions, which correspond most closely to the pathology and impairment stages of the committee's model. Some functional limitation and disability information can be extrapolated from the NHIS data (see Chapter 2), but this methodology does not produce very precise measures. In addition, although potentially disabling conditions are dynamic and can improve as well as deteriorate, existing data systems can neither measure the dynamics of disability progression nor identify risk factors that accelerate progression from impairment to functional limitation to disability.

More specific epidemiological data are needed on the incidence and prevalence of functional limitation and disability and their attendant risk factors. Populations at higher risk for disability need to be identified and their risk factors assessed to develop interventions to prevent disability. Longitudinal studies are needed to help define the dynamic nature of impairment, functional limitation, and disability and to describe the natural history of chronic conditions and aging in terms of these functional outcomes.

TABLE 3-1   Major Causes of Death and Associated Risk Factors, United States, 1977

Cause	Percentage of All Deaths	Risk Factors
Heart disease	37.8	Smoking, hypertension, elevated serum cholesterol, diet, lack of exercise, diabetes, stress, family history
Malignant neoplasms	20.4	Smoking, work-site carcinogens, environmental carcinogens, alcohol, diet
Stroke	9.6	Hypertension, smoking, elevated serum cholesterol, stress
Non-vehicular injuries	2.8	Alcohol, drug abuse, smoking (fires), product design, handgun availability
Influenza and pneumonia	2.7	Smoking, vaccination status
Motor vehicle crashes	2.6	Alcohol, no seat belts, speed, roadway design, vehicle engineering
Diabetes	1.7	Obesity
Cirrhosis of the liver	1.6	Alcohol abuse
Arteriosclerosis	1.5	Elevated serum cholesterol
Suicide	1.5	Stress, alcohol and drug abuse, gun availability

SOURCE: Matarazzo, 1984. Reprinted with permission.

The Need for Surveillance

The changing demographic profile of the U.S. population and the associated patterns of disability risk demonstrate the necessity of continued surveillance of the incidence and prevalence of chronic physical and mental health conditions, injury, and disability. Some research indicates that the risk of disability has been increasing for all population age cohorts, although there is considerable debate about the reasons for this trend. There has also been a noticeable increase in work disability rates (Chirikos, 1989). In addition, the aging of the population may bring increased risks of disability.

Existing national data sets that track the prevalence of chronic conditions over time are useful for disability surveillance. The lack of data on incidence rates, however, is a serious void in disability surveillance and an impediment to fundamental understanding of the disabling process. Incidence data provide a measure of the rate at which a population develops a chronic condition, impairment, functional limitation, or disability and thereby yield estimates of the probability or risk of these events. Most existing data, however, provide information only on prevalence, not incidence. Prevalence is the net result of changes in incidence and the duration of time a person has a condition. Duration is determined by rates of recovery and mortality. When one compares population groups, only incidence data provide a clear picture of how risks differ among populations. Prevalence data, on the other hand, reflect not only these risks but also differences in rates of recovery and mortality. Thus populations with equal risks of developing

TABLE 3-2 Risk Factors in Chronic Disease and Disability

Risk Factor	Some Related Conditions
Smoking	Lung cancer
	Emphysema
	Bronchitis
	Other respiratory diseases
	Coronary artery disease
	Burns (especially home fires)
Alcohol abuse	Injuries sustained in motor vehicle accidents,especially head injuries and pedestrian injuries
	Cirrhosis
	Fetal alcohol syndrome
Lack of prenatal care	Mental retardation
	Cerebral palsy
	Congenital heart abnormalities (via rubella)
	Various congenital anomalies (e.g., through failure to control blood sugar in pregnant diabetic women)
	Other developmental disabilities
Socioeconomic status	Low birthweight
	Injury
	Coronary heart disease
	Lung cancer
	Osteoarthritis
	Death
	Diabetes mellitus
	Cervical cancer

disability may differ in prevalence because of differences in access to medical and rehabilitative care. Information on incidence is therefore critical to understanding the causes of disability. Data on duration, however, are useful to gauge rates of recovery and mortality. Only when incidence and duration are known can one understand what causes disability and what determines its course. Collecting data on the incidence and duration of pathology, impairment, and functional limitation as well as secondary conditions is an important component of the disability surveillance effort that is needed.

Although the NHIS includes some disability-related questions, it is quite limited in scope because it is a general-purpose survey of the health of the nation and not designed to investigate efficiently the causes and risks of disability. To conduct such an investigation requires a comprehensive longitudinal survey that could address each path of the model displayed in Figure 3-3, particularly the biological, lifestyle and behavioral, and physical and social environmental factors influencing transitions from pathology to impairment and on to functional limitation and disability.

A longitudinal survey of disability is needed to assist in determining the causes and rate of transition between pathology, impairment, functional limitation, and disability. The survey should make use of data linkages to existing agency data sets on need, use, and costs of services; be responsive as a policy development resource tool; and evaluate the causal relationship between socioeconomic status and disability. The development and implementation of this survey should be a collaborative effort involving the U.S. Census Bureau, the Centers for Disease Control, the National Center for Health Statistics, the National Institute on Disability and Rehabilitation Research, the National Institute on Aging, the Health Care Financing Administration, the Social Security Administration (SSA), and other relevant agencies.

Before conducting a new survey, however, consideration should be given to the utility of longitudinal analysis of existing data sources such as the SSA 1971-1974 disability survey, the Boston University project of the Framingham Study, the SSA 1969-1970 Retirement History Survey, the Census Bureau's SIPP, and the Department of Labor manpower mobility surveys.

The Need for Priorities

In terms of goals and implementation, disability prevention is usually thought to mean *primary* prevention—averting the onset of a potentially disabling pathology or an impairment that leads to a disability (see section on primary prevention that follows). The model set forth in this chapter, however, underscores the fact that well after the onset of a potentially disabling condition, multiple points of intervention exist at which to prevent disability or diminish its severity. Although this model can help lead to many new opportunities for prevention, it does not specify what priorities to place on the possible points of intervention. Priority setting must include an analysis of epidemiological data pertaining to the causes and natural history of various disabling conditions.

As noted in Chapter 2, some of the less prevalent potentially disabling conditions (e.g., spinal cord injury) have a high risk of disability, whereas some of the more prevalent conditions (e.g., arthritis) have a fairly low risk of disability. The inverse relationship between the prevalence of a condition and the risk of disability presents an enormous challenge in forging prevention strategies. Primary prevention strategies are normally targeted to higher-than-average risk groups in the general population, even though the overall risk of acquiring a disabling condition is very small. Secondary prevention strategies are targeted to those who have already acquired a condition but may not be experiencing its disabling effects. Neither course of action may be necessarily efficient or cost-effective.

The committee considered several competing and overlapping principles and criteria on which priorities for prevention could be based. These included the following:

- prevalence of specific conditions that can cause disability;
- number of persons who are likely to experience some degree of limitation or disability associated with a particular condition;
- severity of disabling conditions and their probable impact on the individual, the family, and society;
- the number of expected disability years (not merely the prevalence of a condition or its limitations); and
- how the prevalence and severity of selected conditions are likely to grow in future years.

As discussed in the recent National Research Council report on disability statistics (NRC, 1990), a study is needed in which a combination of the above-mentioned principles and criteria is used to conduct an objective analysis that will lead to alternative indexes of disability risk and public health impact. These indexes can then be used to set priorities for prevention efforts among all conditions.

A disability index or group of indexes is needed to help establish priorities for disability prevention among conditions and to gauge and monitor the magnitude of disability as a public health issue. This index or group of indexes should include measures of independence, productive life expectancy (both paid and unpaid), and quality of life.

In the absence of such an index, the committee is reluctant to recommend prevention strategies that favor one disabling condition over another. However, in succeeding chapters the committee cites some of the needs and issues related to several categories of individual disabling conditions. Major gaps exist in the data and knowledge about risk factors associated with disability. One reason for these gaps is that most disability-related data are oriented toward clinical categories or impairments. Such categories may have clinical utility for addressing the treatment needs of persons with specific impairments, but they are not useful in fostering an epidemiology based on risk factors such as those related to the social and physical environment.

As discussed earlier (under the section on risk factors), the committee believes that specific conditions may not always be the most appropriate or effective means for setting priorities or identifying targets for the development of preventive intervention strategies. An alternative method for consideration is to focus on risk factors or causes that are generic to the etiology of several disabling conditions. Some examples include smoking, alcohol abuse, drug abuse, socioeconomic status, and lack of prenatal care (see Table 3-2). These risk factors are already associated with many of the nation's leading health problems. Less understood is their relationship to disability.

Cause-oriented disability data need to be considered possible alternatives in the development of approaches to identifying priorities in disability prevention.

APPLYING TRADITIONAL PREVENTION STRATEGIES TO DISABILITY

The standard public health model delineates three categories of prevention efforts—primary, secondary, and tertiary—each one focusing on distinct stages in the natural history of diseases. This same model is applicable to the prevention of disability. And, as is true for all prevention programs, epidemiological data and analyses are the cornerstones of effective planning and evaluation. Thus the quality and quantity of the available epidemiological data, as discussed in the previous section, will be critical to the development of effective intervention strategies. Here, the committee briefly summarizes the primary, secondary, and tertiary approaches to prevention and how they might be applied to disability (see Patrick and Peach [1989] for additional information). Prevention efforts that are specific to various disabling conditions are discussed in more detail in succeeding chapters.

Primary Prevention

Primary prevention focuses on healthy persons, seeking to avoid the onset of pathological processes by reducing susceptibility, controlling exposure to disease-causing agents, and eliminating or at least minimizing behaviors and environmental factors that increase the risk of illness, injury, or disability. Interventions include (1) health promotion and education, which are largely tailored to fostering adoption of healthy lifestyles; (2) health protection, such as measures designed to improve air quality or food safety; and (3) preventive health services, such as immunization or counseling.

Most public health efforts fall into the category of primary prevention. Unfortunately, and incorrectly, people with potentially disabling conditions often are not recognized as a target population for primary prevention efforts, despite the fact that having a potentially disabling condition frequently increases the need for good health promotion and disease prevention practices. With respect to disability, primary prevention usually means preventing the initiation of a potentially disabling condition such as spinal cord injury. However, having a disabling condition does not preclude the need for other primary prevention activities such as exercise and immunization. Primary prevention of disabling conditions is a focus of attention in this report, but additional emphasis is focused on people who already have potentially disabling conditions, i.e., secondary and tertiary prevention.

Health-promoting practices, appropriate medical care, and other measures that help ensure good health and a reasonable quality of life are as important to people with disabling conditions as they are to people without them. Similarly, they are as important to the elderly as they are to the young. It is never too late to benefit from quitting smoking, adopting good dietary practices, or engaging in regular exercise, as illustrated in the report on the benefits of smoking cessation for those with coronary heart disease who are over 55 years of age (Hermanson et al., 1988). These and other health-promoting measures pay health dividends to all. Indeed, health promotion directed toward older adults has great potential for impact because the benefits of healthy behaviors may be achieved relatively quickly. Given that the prevalence of chronic diseases rises sharply in this age group and that this segment of the population is growing rapidly, the societal benefits of health promotion and disability prevention during later life may be great (Institute of Medicine, 1990a).

Moreover, the purpose of health promotion is not simply to extend life but also to improve the quality of life and to extend active life free of disability (Fries, 1988; Katz et al., 1983). Health promotion is applicable to all age groups and although the messages might change for different ages, the major themes with respect to exercise, diet, substance abuse, and injury prevention are often the same. Reinforcing messages in the community, at schools, at the workplace, and in the doctor's office provides the social context that can facilitate behavior change. Health promotion for children should help establish lifelong habits for maintaining health. For adults, the emphasis should be on modifying risk factors related to disease and disability and maintaining healthy behaviors (Institute of Medicine, 1990a; Keil et al., 1989; Pinsky et al., 1985).

Secondary Prevention

Secondary prevention activities include early detection and treatment of persons with early or asymptomatic disease, reduction in risk factors, vocational and educational counseling, and social interventions. Common approaches include periodic screening of high-risk individuals and subsequent treatment of the pathology. Secondary prevention can in many cases cure a specific pathology, but in other cases secondary prevention merely slows the progression of a pathology toward becoming a clinical condition. People with chronic diseases and those with disabling conditions can benefit significantly from secondary prevention efforts, and, as noted earlier, much of this report focuses on secondary and tertiary prevention.

Not all diseases and disabling conditions, however, can be prevented. Examples include conditions that are strongly related to the process of aging (Fries and Crapo, 1981). Aging-related conditions include arteriosclerosis, non-insulin-dependent diabetes, cancer, osteoarthritis, emphysema, and cirrhosis, as well as numerous other conditions that are less prevalent. Prevention measures are applied differently to aging-related conditions because individuals are seldom observed to be totally free of pathogenic changes. Plaque deposits in arteries, for example, can be found in most individuals, even at very young ages. Fries and Crapo (1981) argue, therefore, that it is better to think of controlling (or eliminating) risk factors to affect the progression of these conditions rather than to prevent the onset of the underlying pathological process. They maintain that primary prevention of aging-related conditions is not possible because such conditions are a part of aging and occur in all individuals. However, the rate at which such universal conditions progress can be reduced so that clinically significant symptoms can be avoided or delayed.

Thus prevention of many aging-related conditions begins with secondary prevention that aims to reduce the progression of these universal pathological processes. In some instances, although the condition may not disappear, secondary prevention is considered successful if from the standpoint of the affected individual the symptoms are not noticeable and do not require clinical treatment. In such cases the condition in essence has been prevented. What are often considered to be primary prevention activities, such as not smoking, are often secondary interventions for many aging-related, and potentially disabling, conditions because the condition has already been initiated.

Tertiary Prevention

Tertiary prevention strategies concentrate on arresting the progression of a condition and on preventing or limiting additional impairment, functional limitation, and disability. These strategies can be directed toward the person, his or her environment, or society as a whole. Rehabilitation efforts, which attempt to restore function and the capacity to perform one's roles, are in the domain of tertiary prevention. Rehabilitation can address not only the individual with a functional limitation or disability but also elements of the physical and social environments that preclude participation in the activities of society by people with disabling conditions. Modifying or eliminating social and physical obstacles to personal autonomy and societal participation present opportunities for prevention strategies that are not often enough accepted into the traditional province of public health. Measures designed to foster independent living and help ensure a reasonable quality of life should clearly be major elements of disability prevention policies and strategies.

Tertiary prevention, as well as secondary prevention, has not received as much emphasis in public health as the health-promoting, disease-preventing measures of primary prevention. However, the fact that more than 35 million people already have some type of disabling condition underscores the need to develop and implement secondary and tertiary prevention strategies that are directed toward people with disabling conditions, and that will reduce the risks of additional limitation and prevent disability and secondary conditions. With the aging of the population there is growing interest in the prevention of age-related chronic disease and disability and the secondary and tertiary strategies that are designed to prevent them (Patrick and Peach, 1989).

Given the dynamics of the disabling process and the variety of interacting risk factors, primary, secondary, and tertiary preventive measures will often be required in concert. To take AIDS as an example, primary prevention is needed in the form of educating individuals about high-risk behaviors. Testing for exposure to HIV, especially in high-risk populations, and treatment to postpone the progression of the disease to AIDS or the characteristic set of symptoms known as AIDS-related complex (ARC) constitute secondary prevention. Tertiary prevention includes rehabilitation programs and social services that seek to reduce the effects of AIDS or ARC so that affected people can perform desired roles and live independently.

Another example is people who use wheelchairs and therefore have increased risk of developing pressure sores. Preventive intervention strategies would include passive restraints that prevent spinal cord injury in automobile crashes (primary prevention), modifying wheelchairs or teaching the individual who uses the wheelchair how to relieve pressure to reduce the likelihood of pressure sores (secondary prevention), and treating the sores to prevent infection and promote healing (tertiary prevention). In this, as in other cases, there are many opportunities to interrupt the disabling process and the progression toward disability.

Finally, although tertiary prevention might be where most prevention of disability itself occurs, primary and secondary strategies are essential elements of disability prevention because they intervene in the disabling process to reduce the likelihood of progression of predisposing conditions toward disability. Thus the public health and medical aspects of disability prevention are important, but should not overshadow or undercut the essential understanding of the social context of disability, as described throughout this report. Given the existence of predisposing functional limitations, the predominant means of disability prevention and amelioration are often social and economic.

4

Prevention of
Developmental Disabilities

The term *developmental disabilities* was introduced in the late 1960s to describe clinical disorders and diseases that cause disability, begin early in life, and require supportive services. This generic term covers a broad spectrum of impairments, ranging from mild to serious, and includes conditions characterized by mental retardation, cerebral palsy, epilepsy, and serious sensory impairment, as well as other childhood chronic illnesses associated with significant developmental delay.

In 1970 the term was given a narrower legal definition in Public Law 91-517 for the purposes of public planning and policy. This definition was subsequently altered and given its current form in the Developmental Disabilities Act of 1984 (P.L. 98-527). Here, Developmental Disabilities (using uppercase letters) were legally defined solely as severe, chronic conditions attributable to a mental or physical impairment, manifest before age 22, and likely to continue indefinitely, resulting in substantial limitations in a prescribed set of activities and requiring special interdisciplinary care. This restrictive definition generally has been interpreted to include only the most serious conditions.

This chapter will address developmental disabilities in the broader sense of the term, focusing on clinical disorders and diseases that can cause developmental delay. The concepts of prevention discussed here apply to all chronic health conditions that potentially can cause disability in childhood.

PUBLIC HEALTH SIGNIFICANCE

The scope of developmental disabilities is broad. An estimated 2 million to 4 million persons of all ages have such disabilities. The upper estimate is derived from the 1.7 percent prevalence rate in a study by Wistar and Vernon

(1986). The lower estimate is based on national survey data by LaPlante (1989a) and Sirrocco (1987). The two most common developmental disabilities, mental retardation and cerebral palsy, rank first and fifth as chronic conditions causing major activity limitation among persons of all ages (Table 4-1) (LaPlante, 1989a) and rank ninth and eighth, respectively, as conditions that create a need for assistance in carrying out basic life activities.

Disability years, a measure introduced by Houk and Thacker (1989), represents the number of years people survive with disabilities and thus provides an estimate of the public health impact of disability. By this measure, developmental and other childhood disabilities accounted for 35 percent of all disability years in 1986 (Table 4-2). This highlights the importance of preventing childhood disabilities, because significant gains in this area will have a "multiplier effect," substantially decreasing the number of disability years.

The national costs of caring for children with developmental disabilities are substantial. Data from the 1980 National Medical Care Utilization and Expenditure Survey (NMCUES) indicate that children who experience limitations in normal activities use more medical services than other children, resulting in significantly higher health costs for this group (Newacheck and McManus, 1988).

Of an estimated total of $40.5 billion spent on health care for all children under the age of 21 in 1988 (based on updated 1980 National Medical Care Utilization and Expenditure Survey data), approximately $4.4 billion was spent on children with chronic disabling conditions. Thus an average of $1,406 was spent on each child with a chronic disabling condition, compared with an average of $487 for other children. Four percent of those under the age of 21 accounted for nearly 11 percent of total health care expenditures for that population (Newacheck and McManus, 1988). However, these cost figures underestimate the individual and total charges because of the significant changes in medical care costs and out-of-pocket expenditures since 1980.

A 1986 study of state, local, and federal government expenditures on institutionalization, income maintenance, and special education revealed combined spending of $16.5 billion in 1984, a 23 percent increase over 1979. These figures represent $7.28 billion in federal expenditures, $6.08 billion in state expenditures, and $3.12 billion in local expenditures (Braddock and Hemp, 1986).

The following section provides a descriptive epidemiology of developmental disability.

Epidemiology of Developmental Disabilities

Clinical disorders and diseases associated with developmental disability can be categorized by time of onset as follows: hereditary disorders, early

TABLE 4-1 Conditions with the Highest Risk of Disability, All Ages: United States, 1983-1986

Chronic Conditions	Number of Conditions (thousands)	Percent Causing Activity Limitation	Rank	Percent Causing Major Activity Limitation	Rank	Percent Causing Need for Help in Basic Life Activities	Rank
Mental retardation	1,202	84.1	1	80.0	1	19.9	9
Absence of leg(s)	289	83.3	2	73.1	2	39.0	2
Lung or bronchial cancer	200	74.8	3	63.5	3	34.5	4
Multiple sclerosis	171	70.6	4	63.3	4	40.7	1
Cerebral palsy	274	69.7	5	62.2	5	22.8	8
Blind in both eyes	396	64.5	6	58.8	6	38.1	3
Partial paralysis in extremity	578	59.6	7	47.2	7	27.5	5
Other orthopedic impairments	316	58.7	8	46.2	8	14.3[a]	12
Complete paralysis in extremity	617	52.7	9	45.5	9	26.1	6
Rheumatoid arthritis	1,223	51.0	10	39.4	12	14.9	11
Intervertebral disk disorders	3,987	48.7	11	38.2	14	5.3	—
Paralysis in other sites (complete/partial)	247	47.8	12	43.7	10	14.1[a]	13
Other heart disease/disorders[b]	4,708	46.9	13	35.1	15	13.6	14
Cancer of digestive sites	228	45.3	14	40.3	11	15.9[a]	10
Emphysema	2,074	43.6	15	29.8	—	9.6	15
Absence of arm(s)/hand(s)	84	43.1	—	39.0	13	4.1[a]	—
Cerebrovascular disease	2,599	38.2	—	33.3	—	22.9	7

[a]Figure has low statistical reliability or precision (relative standard error exceeds 30 percent).

[b]Heart failure (9.8 percent); valve disorders (15.3 percent); congenital disorders (15.0 percent); all other and ill-defined heart conditions (59.9 percent).

SOURCE: LaPlante, 1989b. Reprinted with permission.

TABLE 4-2 Estimated Effect of Disability in the United States, in Terms of "Disability Years"

Age of Onset	Number of Persons (millions)	Percent of Persons with Disability	Survival (years)	Years of Disability Number (millions)	Percent
Birth-15 years	5.6	20	50	280	35
16-34 years	7.0	25	40	280	35
35-54 years	6.4	23	25	161	20
55 years and older	8.7	31	10	87	10

SOURCE: Houk and Thacker, 1989.

alterations of embryonic development, late pregnancy or perinatal conditions, acquired childhood conditions, and conditions of unknown etiology. Table 4-3 presents these categories of origin, associated causes or pathologies, and some examples of conditions and their estimated prevalences in the United States. This is a slightly modified scheme from that of Crocker (1989) in that there is no category for environmental problems and behavioral syndromes; these have been primarily subsumed under the acquired childhood condition category. The following sections present general descriptions of these categories and some examples.

Hereditary Disorders

Some conditions originate prior to conception in the genotype of the parents. These conditions often have multiple somatic effects, but variation in expression is common as a result of single-gene interactions with other genic and environmental forces. The underlying causes or pathologies of these conditions are metabolic disorders, single-gene abnormalities, chromosome abnormalities, and polygenic familial syndromes.

Fragile X Syndrome Fragile X syndrome, a hereditary disorder caused by a chromosomal abnormality, is a common cause of mental retardation among males (Friedman and Howard-Peebles, 1986). Estimates of fragile X prevalence in males range from 0.5 to 0.9 per 1,000 (Blomquist et al., 1983; Froster-Iskenius et al., 1983; Herbst and Miller, 1980; Sutherland, 1982). Diagnosis is made by laboratory identification of the characteristic fragile site on the X chromosome or by inference from the pedigrees of affected family members.

TABLE 4-3 Category of Origin, Associated Cause/Pathology, and Examples (with Prevalence Estimates) for Developmental Disabilities

Category of Origin	Cause/Pathology	Examples[a] (prevalence per 1,000)
Hereditary	Metabolic disorders	Tay-Sachs disease (>0.01)[1] Phenylketonuria (0.08)[2] Maternal phenylketonuria (0.08)[3] Congenital hypothyroidism (0.33)[1] Hurler syndrome (0.01)[2]
	Other single-gene abnormalities	Neurofibromatosis (0.02)[2] Tuberous sclerosis (0.6)[4] Muscular dystrophy (0.02 - 0.10)[4]
	Chromosomal abnormalities	Fragile X syndrome (0.7)[4]
Early alterations of embryonic development	Chromosomal changes	Down syndrome (1.0)[1]
	Intrauterine toxicity	Fetal alcohol syndrome (1.4)[1] Lead exposure toxicity
	Intrauterine infection	Congenital rubella syndrome (<0.1)[2] Congenital cytomegalovirus infections (3.0)[2] Congenital syphilis (0.2)[2]
	Structural malformations	Absence of or shortened limbs (0.5)[1] Hydrocephalus (1.8)[1] Microcephalus (0.5)[1] Spina bifida (0.4)[1]
Late pregnancy or perinatal conditions	Premature birth	Very low birthweight, < 1,500 grams (12)[1] Central nervous system hemorrhage (6)[5] Retrolental fibroplasia (0.07)[2]
	Perinatal hypoxia	5-minute Apgar < 4 (6)[1]
	Infection	Perinatally acquired human immunodeficiency virus infection (0.4)[2]
Acquired childhood conditions	Postnatal infection	Bacterial meningitis (0.8)[2] Measles encephalopathy (<0.1)[4]

TABLE 4-3 *Continued*

Category of Origin	Cause/Pathology	Examples[a] (prevalence per 1,000)
	Childhood injury	Spinal cord injury $(0.04)^6$ $(0.4)^7$ Traumatic brain injury $(2.2)^4$ Near drowning $(1.0)^4$
	Environmental toxicity	Lead encephalopathy $(>0.1)^4$ Low-lead toxicity (not available)^4
	Psychosocial disadvantage	Mental retardation of deprivational causes $(3-5)^4$
Unknown		Autism $(0.4)^4$ Cerebral palsy $(2-4)^4$ Epilepsy $(3.5)^4$ Mental retardation of unknown cause $(3-5)^4$ Learning disorders $(50-100)^4$

[a]Superscript numbers indicate the age group used in determining the prevalence estimates, as follows: 1, at birth; 2, early childhood; 3, of all births; 4, childhood; 5, newborn period; 6, age 10; and 7, age 20.

SOURCE: Adapted from Crocker, 1989.

Early Alterations of Embryonic Development

Circumstances in early gestation can affect mitosis and embryogenesis. Generally, the resulting conditions are relatively stable after birth. The underlying causes or pathologies of these conditions are chromosomal changes, intrauterine toxicity, intrauterine infection, and structural malformation.

Fetal Alcohol Syndrome Fetal alcohol syndrome (FAS) is a condition caused by intrauterine toxicity. FAS is diagnosed when infants have characteristic dysmorphic features and when a history of maternal alcohol use in early pregnancy is determined. Infants with FAS have prenatal onset growth deficiency, facial abnormalities, and mental retardation. Congenital malformations, especially microcephaly, are common (Goodman and Gorlin, 1983; Smith, 1976). The national prevalence of FAS is estimated to be 1.4 per 1,000 live births. FAS rates among blacks are as much as six times higher than those for whites; among Native Americans the prevalence is 30 times greater (Chavez et al., 1988).

FAS is only one of a number of adverse outcomes associated with alcohol use in pregnancy. Mental retardation, in the absence of FAS, and learning disorders are other disabling conditions that become apparent in the school-age years (Streissguth et al., 1989). The cause of mental retardation and learning disorders in children of women who use alcohol during pregnancy is often not clear. More study is needed to determine the contribution of maternal use of illicit drugs (especially cocaine)—often associated with heavy alcohol use—in the etiology of central nervous system impairment. Children of parents who use alcohol and illicit drugs have an increased risk for child abuse or neglect (Orme and Rimmer, 1981), which can also cause central nervous system impairment. Additional work is needed in the area of postnatal parental behavior that increases the vulnerability of this group of children.

Down Syndrome   Children with Down syndrome, a condition caused by chromosomal changes, have a characteristic facies and almost always have mental retardation (Cicchetti and Sroufe, 1976; Dahle and McCollister, 1986). The presence of a third chromosome 21 is diagnostic for the condition. The risk of Down syndrome increases with the age of the mother from rates of less than 1 per 1,000 pregnancies among women in their twenties, to more than 10 in 1,000 among women over 40 years old (Hook and Lindsjo, 1978). In the United States today, the prevalence of the condition is 1 per 1,000 live births (Centers for Disease Control, 1988b), a decrease from the prevalence rates of more than 2 per 1,000 observed in earlier decades. Eighty-seven percent of children with Down syndrome survive to at least age 5 years; most deaths are due to heart malformations (Masaki et al., 1981). Persons with Down syndrome are at risk for developing hypothyroidism (Cutler et al., 1986) and instability of the neck (Van Dyke and Gahagan, 1988), as well as Alzheimer disease (Miniszek, 1983) for those living into their forties.

Late Pregnancy or Perinatal Conditions

During gestation and after morphogenesis, fetuses undergo a relatively long period of growth and development. If this growth period ends prematurely, the result is small, low-birthweight babies with increased vulnerabilities. The underlying causes of these conditions are prematurity, perinatal hypoxia, and infection.

Perinatally Acquired Human Immunodeficiency Virus Infection   Data from the Centers for Disease Control (CDC) national serosurveys suggest an HIV seroprevalence rate of 1.5 per 1,000 among women delivering liveborn babies in the United States. Approximately one-third of these pregnancies result in HIV infection of the infant as well. Thus, in 1990, between 1,500 and 2,000 infants (0.5 per 1,000 live births) are expected to develop perinatally acquired HIV infection.

The clinical course of HIV infection in children is varied. Belman and colleagues (1985) report that 90 percent of infants with HIV infection had central nervous system involvement including developmental delay, loss of developmental milestones, microcephaly, and encephalopathy.

Acquired Childhood Conditions

Many postnatal hazards can modify the body's development during childhood and do damage, from which varying degrees of recovery are possible. The underlying causes of these conditions are postnatal infection, childhood injury, environmental toxicity, and psychosocial disadvantage.

Traumatic Brain Injury   It has been estimated that 2.2 per 1,000 children (birth through 19 years) each year have traumatic brain injury (Centers for Disease Control, 1990a). Approximately 40 per 1,000 persons sustain a traumatic brain injury in the first 19 years of life (based on annual age-specific rates). The major consequence of traumatic brain injury is death. Other outcomes such as intellectual, motor, and emotional/behavioral impairment have not been adequately studied. Existing data suggest that loss of consciousness and motor and sensory impairments are usually only short-term sequelae, but intellectual limitation, especially loss of memory and concentration, is an important long-term complication (Bruce, 1983; Klonoff et al., 1977; Lange-Cosack et al., 1979). It has also been reported that about a third of children who remained unconscious for more than one week had IQ scores less than 70. Some children, however, have long-term intellectual limitation/mental retardation after comas lasting only three to four days (Heiskanen and Kaste, 1974). However, Haas and colleagues (1987) report that 50 percent of persons with head injury had a record of poor academic performance before their injury.

Lead Toxicity   Lead toxicity, an acquired childhood condition caused by environmental lead exposure, is the most common environmental disease of young children. Lead is a toxicant that affects every system in the body and is particularly harmful to the developing brain and nervous system. It has been estimated that in 1984, more than 3 million U.S. children (ages 6 months to 5 years) had lead levels high enough to cause clinical or subclinical effects (U.S. Department of Health and Human Services, 1988a). Children in the inner cities, who are already disadvantaged by poor nutrition and other factors, are particularly vulnerable.

Recent prospective studies have shown that adverse effects on the fetus and child probably begin at blood lead levels of 15 micrograms per deciliter (µg/dl) and below. These effects include decreases in IQ (Grant and Davis, 1989), delays in reaching developmental milestones (Bellinger et al., 1987; Vimpani et al., 1989), decreases in birthweight (Bornschein et al., 1989) and in postnatal stature (Schwartz et al., 1986), and shorter gestation (McMichael et al., 1986). There may be no threshold for some of the adverse effects of lead.

Conditions of Unknown Origin

There are a significant number of developmental disabilities for which the etiology remains obscure. These conditions include epilepsy, autism, and much cerebral palsy and mental retardation.

Cerebral Palsy Cerebral palsy (CP) is a group of disorders in which a disease of the brain causes impairment of motor function (Ingram, 1984). Although mobility limitation is the most common result of CP, coexisting mental retardation also occurs in about half of all cases (McDonald and Valmassey, 1987). In a review of CP prevalence studies in industrialized countries, Paneth and Kiely (1984) estimate that 2 per 1,000 school-aged children require services. About half of all occurrences of CP are associated with underlying prenatal conditions such as intrauterine infection, perinatal anoxia and maternal metabolic disease, and postnatal events such as trauma, infection, toxic exposure, and vascular problems. In the other half of CP cases, no underlying health problem can be identified.

There is a common misconception that most CP results from perinatal hypoxia. Blair and Stanley (1988) have shown that perinatal hypoxia was a possible cause of CP in less that 10 percent of children with the disorder.

Learning Disorders Learning disorders occur in persons who do not have mental retardation and include conditions such as hyperactivity and attention deficit disorder, along with specific "disabilities" of reading, writing, and mathematics. These learning disorders are usually not recognized until the child is academically challenged in school. A prevalence range of 50 to 100 per 1,000 children was found in studies reviewed in a 1987 report (U.S. Interagency Committee on Learning Disabilities, 1987). A few factors, such as very low birthweight (Calame et al., 1986; Nickel et al., 1982), fetal alcohol effects (Streissguth et al., 1989), low-lead-exposure syndrome (Needleman et al., 1990), and neurofibromatosis (Stine and Adams, 1989), are known to be associated with learning disorders, but in most cases the underlying cause is unknown.

There is both a need and a high potential for the prevention of developmental disabilities. The most readily preventable conditions include fetal alcohol syndrome, lead toxicity, many premature births, intrauterine and postnatal infection, and disabling conditions related to psychosocial disadvantage. Although more research is needed to improve interventions, current knowledge is adequate to warrant the expansion of existing prevention programs.

Employing the New Model

The terms *impairment, functional limitation, disability,* and *handicap* are commonly used to describe developmental disabilities. But their use has not been consistent, leading to some conceptual confusion. The committee's model of the disabling process (Figure 3-3) provides a new perspective for assessing and evaluating developmental disability. The model is useful in identifying similarities between developmental disabilities and other disabling conditions and in improving understanding of developmental disabilities as nonstatic disabling conditions. As a result, this model should facilitate the development of preventive interventions.

The clinical conditions described above correspond generally to the first two stages of the model of the disabling process, that is, pathology and impairment. Thus the prevalence of developmental disability does not equal the prevalence of functional limitation and disability according to the committee's model; other measures are needed to describe the prevalence of functional limitation and disability.

Functional limitations associated with developmental disabilities can be described as occurring in three categories: *intellectual limitation/mental retardation, mobility limitations,* and *sensory and communication limitations.* (Note that the committee's definition of functional limitation differs from that used in the Apt Associates report that provided terminology for federal legislation on developmental disabilities.) Examples of measurements that can be used for these categories of functional limitation appear below. It is important to note that functional limitations in childhood are caused not only by Developmental Disabilities but also by other potentially disabling conditions such as congenital heart defects, asthma, cystic fibrosis, and sickle cell anemia.

As described earlier, disability is the expression of a functional limitation in a social context, that is, a limitation in performing socially defined roles and tasks. Disability estimates can be made using activity limitation data (as measured by the National Health Interview Survey) and school-related limitation data (as measured by the use of special education services).

Functional Limitations

As noted above, developmental disabilities cause three major types of functional limitation: intellectual limitation/mental retardation, mobility limitation, and sensory and communication limitation. Some of the disabling conditions that can cause these functional limitations are discussed below. Monitoring their prevalence, in relation to the categories of origin, should be useful in developing intervention strategies and evaluating their effectiveness.

Intellectual Limitation/Mental Retardation   Mental retardation (MR) is often divided into two categories: serious MR (IQ of less than 50) and mild MR (IQ 50 to 70). Serious MR is more likely than mild MR to be associated with discernible pathology. Susser and colleagues (1985) cite a range of reported prevalence for serious MR between 2.9 and 3.5 per 1,000 children. In the studies they examined, about 35 percent of the serious MR was associated with chromosomal changes, between 15 and 20 percent with late pregnancy or perinatal conditions, and between 15 and 25 percent of unknown causes (Figure 4-1).

Children reared in psychosocially disadvantaged family settings are at greater risk for MR (Butler et al., 1984; Broman et al., 1987; Shonkoff, 1982), but the relationship between socioecomonic risk and mental retardation is complex and not well understood. Subtle neurological abnormalities and minor obstetrical risk factors (Zigler and Cascione, 1984) are thought not to be sufficient cause (Breitmayer and Ramey, 1986).

Comprehensive day care programs have been developed in response to observed differences between homes with and without psychosocial disadvantage (Ramey and Campbell, 1984). A 13-point improvement in IQ scores of low-birthweight children has been reported in a recent trial of such programs (Infant Health and Development Program, 1990).

Mobility Limitation   The prevalence of mobility limitation among children under 18 years of age was 1.5 per 1,000 (LaPlante, 1989b). Walker and colleagues (1988) studied the underlying health conditions of children using crutches and wheelchairs and reported that 43 percent have cerebral palsy, 12 percent have spina bifida, and 8 percent have muscular dystrophy (Figure 4-1). Prevalence estimates for these disorders are 2 per 1,000 for cerebral palsy (Kudrjavcev et al., 1983), 0.4 per 1,000 for spina bifida (Centers for Disease Control, 1988b), and between 0.02 and 0.1 per 1,000 for muscular dystrophy (Gardner-Medwin and Sharples, 1989; Tangsrud and Halvorsen, 1989).

Sensory and Communication Limitation   A range of prevalence between 0.93 and 2.3 per 1,000 has been reported for childhood hearing impairments

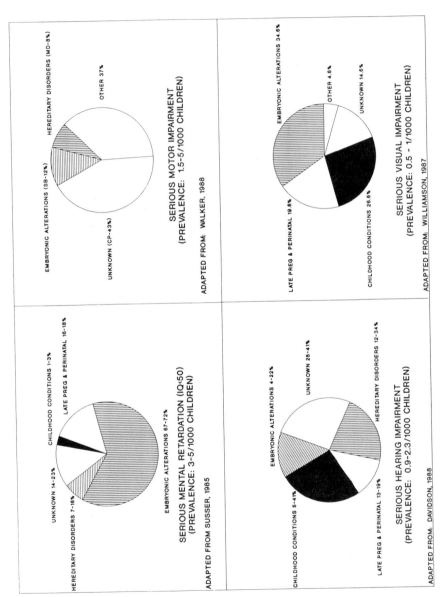

FIGURE 4-1 Proportions of serious mental retardation, visual, hearing, and motor impairments associated with

(Figure 4-1) (Davidson et al., 1988). Hereditary and other prenatal causes accounted for between 31 and 52 percent of all hearing limitation; late pregnancy and perinatal causes for between 13 and 19 percent; and postnatal causes for between 5 and 41 percent. The underlying disorder (cause/pathology) was unknown in between 25 and 41 percent of the subjects.

In a population-based study of infants and toddlers, Williamson and colleagues reported that 1 child per 1,000 under age three had a severe vision impairment that could not be corrected (Figure 4-1) (Williamson et al., 1987). Twenty-five percent of these cases were attributable to prenatal disorders, 20 percent to late pregnancy/perinatal conditions, and 25 percent to postnatal infection or injury. The cause was unknown in 15 percent of the cases.

Multiple Impairments and Functional Limitations A person who has a serious impairment that causes functional limitation in one area may have additional impairments causing other functional limitations. For example, a child with mental retardation may also have mobility limitations caused by cerebral palsy. About two-thirds of all children with developmental disabilities have more than one clinical disorder. Of children with mental retardation, 10 percent have cerebral palsy (and mobility limitation), 3 percent have serious hearing impairment, 1 percent have visual loss, and 40 percent have emotional or behavioral disorders (Accardo and Capute, 1979). Children with more serious mental retardation are more likely to have additional functional limitations.

Disability

At least two survey indicators are useful in determining childhood disability: activity limitation (measured in the National Health Interview Survey) and use of special education services (measured by public education agencies). Based on the 1983-1985 National Health Interview Surveys, 40.2 children per 1,000 aged 5 through 17 were limited in their major activities (LaPlante, 1988). The prevalence of children who needed help to carry out activities of daily living (ADL) was 3.3 per 1,000. Of the 15 per 1,000 children aged 5 through 17 who were found to have mental retardation, 90 percent (13 per 1,000) were limited in their major activity (school), and 6 percent (0.9 per 1,000) needed help in ADLs. Of the 2.4 per 1,000 children who had cerebral palsy, 74 percent (1.8 per 1,000) had activity limitations, and 13 percent (0.3 per 1,000) needed help in ADLs. Children with mental retardation and cerebral palsy accounted for 26 and 10 percent, respectively, of all children needing help in ADLs.

The prevalence of children aged 3 through 21 who received special educational services in 1987-1988 was 66 per 1,000 (U.S. Department of

Education, 1989b). Forty-seven percent of these children were categorized as learning disabled, a prevalence of 31 per 1,000 children. Fourteen percent were labeled mentally retarded, a prevalence of 9.6 per 1,000 children.

Secondary Conditions

When more than one potentially disabling condition is present in the same individual, it is important to determine whether the conditions had different origins or whether one led to the other. This distinction has important implications for prevention. If one condition, such as mobility limitation, is an antecedent to another, such as decubitus ulcers, then elucidating the causal mechanism can help to identify effective interventions to prevent development of the secondary condition. In children with cerebral palsy and mobility limitations, for example, muscle contractures that further limit mobility are secondary conditions and can be prevented. Data are limited, however, on secondary conditions, and it is often difficult to differentiate between dependent and independent conditions. The Centers for Disease Control (CDC) is attempting to identify and classify preventable secondary conditions associated with cerebral palsy. Five types have been tentatively identified: neuromusculoskeletal, health maintenance, psychosocial, communication, and quality of life (see Table 4-4) (M. Pavin, Centers for Disease Control, personal communication, 1990).

An improved understanding of the relationships that exist between clinical conditions and the model for the disabling process is needed to facilitate the development and evaluation of improved intervention strategies. Prevalence data on functional limitations and disabilities need to be evaluated in relation to the categories of origin of developmental disability, the progression in the disabling process, and the interactions with risk factors and quality of life. Research should include assessments of risks associated with socioeconomic and psychosocial disadvantage, the effectiveness of habilitative services, and the identification of secondary conditions.

APPROACHES TO PREVENTION

The development of successful prevention strategies in recent decades is illustrated by the history of the prevention of kernicterus and cerebral palsy from Rh hemolytic disease. Prior to the Second World War, there was virtually no understanding of the cause of the hemolytic anemia and severe jaundice that produced some cases of cerebral palsy. Progress in understanding blood types during the war led to the discovery that the hemolytic anemia was caused by a genetic incompatibility between the mother and the

TABLE 4-4 Secondary Conditions, Their Associated Risk Factors, and Interventions in Persons with Cerebral Palsy

Secondary Condition	Risk Factors	Recommended Interventions
Neuromusculoskeletal		
Deformities of hip, knee, spine	Poor positioning	Range of motion exercises; positioning; wheelchair type
Falls	Deconditioning	Treatment selection that recognizes short- and long-term consequences
Health maintenance		
Respiratory problems	Dysphagia	Food selection; oral/swallowing therapy
Skin breakdown	Compromised skin integrity	Nutrition, positioning
Psychosocial		
Low self-esteem, depression	Inadequate modes of communication; limited community integration	Augmentive communication devices; access and training; peer interaction at all ages
Limited communication	Unintelligible expressive language	Speech and language skills therapy; use of augmentive communication devices; access and training
Quality of life— limited integration, independence, and productivity	Lack of employment opportunities; lack of community access (e.g., inadequate transportation and architectural barriers)	Supported employment; community education policy; legislation and regulation

fetus. Subsequently, exchange transfusions after birth became a common procedure to prevent toxic brain effects that caused cerebral palsy.

The late 1960s and early 1970s saw further advances in the prevention of hemolytic anemia that resulted from several factors: an understanding of the biology of blood types, the development and use of an Rh immune globulin, and a change in reproductive patterns (women began to have fewer babies). The condition is now virtually eliminated. Thus the battle against this genetically caused developmental disability has progressed from treating a condition to prevent the impairment to preventing the underlying pathology.

Many types of interventions reduce the incidence of potentially disabling conditions among infants and children. As seen in Table 4-5, genetic interventions are the prime method when the underlying condition is a hereditary disorder. Immunization and avoidance of prenatal toxic exposures are important measures to prevent early alterations in embryonic development. Programs that reduce the rate of prematurity prevent some disabling conditions associated with the perinatal category of origins. Medical care, injury control, and family support services are examples of interventions to reduce disabling conditions associated with acquired childhood conditions. The types of interventions are ranked in three categories according to their effectiveness: those proven to be effective (such as immunizations to prevent congenital rubella); those showing promise (such as prenatal care to prevent prematurity); and those requiring further research (such as periconceptional multivitamin supplementation).

Effective secondary preventive strategies include corrective surgery for congenital anomalies, newborn metabolic screening, early detection of serious hearing impairment, and habilitation to reduce limitations in communication. Tertiary prevention includes habilitation, peer support, and prevention of secondary conditions in persons with existing disabilities.

Preventive interventions can be grouped into four general categories: health care, education, environmental control and adaptive assistance, and peer support. Some examples of each of these categories are presented below.

Health Care Interventions

Health care before pregnancy (preconception care) can ameliorate disease, improve risk status, and help prepare a family for childbearing (Institute of Medicine, 1988c). The components of preconception care include health promotion activities and interventions to reduce risk. Such care for women with known medical conditions may prevent anomalies or illnesses in the newborn. A discussion of other health care interventions follows.

Prenatal and Well-Child Care

Preventive interventions have been developed for normal health care practices in pregnancy, during the prenatal and perinatal periods, and during childhood. Recommendations on the content of such programs, including specific risk assessment and health promotion activities, have been developed by the Institute of Medicine (1985) and the U.S. Public Health Service (1989), among others. Risk assessment is done by evaluating an individual's medical history and conducting a physical examination. Pertinent elements of history, such as prematurity in a previous pregnancy or genetic disease in a family member, can be indications for special care. During the physical examination, blood pressure, weight gain, and pelvimetry findings can also signal the need for intervention.

TABLE 4-5 Known Risk Factors and Types of Interventions That Reduce the Incidence and Severity of Certain Conditions

Condition	Risk Factor	Type of Intervention
HEREDITARY DISORDERS		
Metabolic disorders		
Maternal phenylketonuria	Maternal diet	Program to inform young women with phenylketonuria of preventive diet[a]
Hurler syndrome	Family history Laboratory marker	Genetic interventions[b]
Tay-Sachs disease	Family history Laboratory marker Ashkenazi Jews	Genetic interventions[b] Screening and pregnancy planning[b]
Other single-gene abnormalities		
Muscular dystrophy	Family history Laboratory marker	Genetic interventions[a]
Cystic fibrosis	Family history Laboratory marker	Genetic interventions[a]
Sickle cell anemia	Family history Laboratory marker	Genetic interventions[b]
Hemophilia	Family history Laboratory marker	Genetic interventions[b]
Chromosomal abnormalities		
Fragile X syndrome	Family history Laboratory marker	Genetic interventions[a] Population screening and pregnancy planning[c]
EARLY ALTERATIONS OF EMBRYONIC DEVELOPMENT		
Chromosomal changes		
Down syndrome	Maternal age Laboratory markers	Genetic interventions[b]
Toxic exposure syndromes		
Fetal alcohol syndrome	Maternal alcohol use	Parenting supports[a] Child placement[a] Family planning[a] Addiction treatment programs[a]
Kernicterus	Rh hemolytic disease	Rh immune globulin[b]

TABLE 4-5 *Continued*

Condition	Risk Factor	Type of Intervention
Accutane embryopathy	Maternal exposure	Labeling and patient information[a] Counseling[a]
Intrauterine infection		
Congenital rubella syndromes	Rubella exposure	Immunization[b]
Congenital syphilis	Maternal infection	Prenatal detection and maternal treatment[b]
Congenital malformations		
All types	Maternal diabetes	Prenatal medical management[a]
Spina bifida	Family history Laboratory marker	Genetic interventions[b]
	No maternal vitamin use	Periconceptional vitamin supplementation[c]

LATE PREGNANCY AND PERINATAL CONDITIONS

Premature birth	Lack of prenatal care	Prenatal care[a]
	Adolescent pregnancy	Adolescent pregnancy prevention programs[a]
Perinatal hypoxia	High-risk pregnancy	Prenatal care[a] Tertiary perinatal care[a]
Infection		
Perinatally acquired		
HIV infection	Maternal infection	Counseling[b]
Congenital herpes	Maternal infection	Family planning[a] Cesarean delivery[a]

ACQUIRED CHILDHOOD CONDITIONS

Postnatal infection		
Bacterial meningitis	HFlu immunity	Immunization[a]
Poliomyelitis	Immune status	Immunization[b]
Measles encephalopathy	Immune status	Immunization[b]
Mumps encephalopathy	Immune status	Immunization[b]
Childhood injury		
Unintentional head trauma and spinal cord injury	Seat belts and child safety seats	Child safety seat legislation[b]

TABLE 4-5 *Continued*

Condition	Risk Factor	Type of Intervention
		Child safety seat programs[a]
	Motorcycle helmets	Helmet legislation[b]
	Bicycle helmets	Bicycle helmet programs[a]
	Unsafe diving	Health education[a]
	Playground hazards	Surface modification[b]
Child abuse (physical)	Family history of violence	
	Impoverished family environment	See deprivational syndromes below
	Parental alcohol and drug addiction	Addiction treatment programs[a]
	Adolescent parents	Adolescent pregnancy prevention programs[a]
	Childhood disability for all above risks	Respite care[a]
Near drowning	Unsupervised swimming	Health education[a]
	Unfenced home pools	Local ordinances[a]
	No caretaker CPR skills	CPR training programs[a]
Burns	Hot water temperature	Health education[a] Local ordinances[a]
Environmental toxicity		
Lead exposure toxicity	Environmental lead in paint, dust, and air	Abatement in housing[a] Low-lead gasolines[a] Lead-free paints[a] Protection in workplace[b]
Deprivational syndromes	Impoverished family environment	Head Start[b] Comprehensive day care[a] Food supplementation for women and children[a] Housing programs[a] Social services[a]

[a]Interventions that are promising and should be implemented, but that should also be monitored closely and evaluated.
[b]Interventions that have been proven effective and that should be implemented and monitored.
[c]Interventions that require further research.

Guidelines on preventive measures in labor and delivery procedures, infection control in nurseries, and other areas have been issued by the American Academy of Pediatrics and the American College of Obstetricians and Gynecologists (Frigoletto and Little, 1988). A recent report by the U.S. Preventive Services Task Force (U.S. Department of Health and Human Services, 1989a) also includes sections on care during the prenatal period, at birth, and during childhood.

> *There is a need to increase the use of preventive measures in prenatal care and well-child care. This could be accomplished by increasing public awareness of the need for family planning and prenatal care and by ensuring that every child who has, or is at risk of developing, a developmental disability has access to continuous, comprehensive preventive and acute health services.*

Genetic Interventions

Major advances in genetic screening during the past 20 years have allowed families and physicians to recognize hereditary and other genetic disorders at very early stages, thereby facilitating preventive and treatment decisions for patients earlier in the course of the condition. During the next decade, genetic interventions are likely to play a major role in reducing the incidence and severity of developmental disabilities.

Genetic screening has reduced the birth incidence of Down syndrome, other chromosomal aberrations, and inborn errors of metabolism such as Tay-Sachs disease. The success of these interventions highlights the responsibility of health care providers to counsel potential parents about test results and discuss with them a range of possible options. Some tests can give a definitive diagnosis for a disease, whereas others, such as maternal serum alpha-fetoprotein screening, can give only an indication of risk. Clinicians must be able to provide sufficient detail about risk and therapy to provide couples with a range of reproductive options. In certain circumstances, the availability of pregnancy termination may be an important option to some parents. It is important to note, however, that this option in health care delivery does not prevent the occurrence of disabling conditions—only their birth incidence.

Continued success with genetic technology opens the way for rapid gains in carrier screening for hundreds of genetic diseases known to cause developmental disabilities, and probably for the many genetic diseases that are yet to be discovered as causes of developmental disabilities. Understanding the genetic basis for these diseases may one day lead to primary prevention or true cures through gene therapy.

Newborn screening for metabolic conditions also shows promising developments for secondary prevention. For example, genetic technology is currently used to identify children who will develop mental retardation upon exposure to phenylalanine. The next decade is likely to see a growing list of conditions that are caused by susceptibility of the rare individual to common environmental exposures. Interventions will be developed to provide early identification and appropriate avoidance of exposures.

Genetic interventions, as part of preconception counseling and prenatal care, can play a major role in reducing the birth incidence of disabling conditions. Genetic screening and counseling, with associated services, should be accessible to all who choose to use them. Using sensitivity and care, physicians should discuss all possible interventions with prospective parents.

Multidisciplinary Care

A 1987 report by the U.S. surgeon general emphasized that health care for children with disabling conditions should be delivered in a family-centered, community-based system. The Association for the Care of Children's Health and the Maternal and Child Health Bureau have developed specific recommendations to ensure that health care delivery is flexible, accessible, and responsive to family needs (Shelton et al., 1987). Moreover, parents should be involved in all health care decision making, and physical therapists, speech therapists, orthopedic surgeons, and other involved health professionals should coordinate the delivery of care.

State systems of services for children with, or at risk of developing, chronic and disabling conditions must be expanded to provide adequate multidisciplinary care for the prevention of developmental disabilities and associated secondary conditions.

Education

Head Start and Comprehensive Day Care

Head Start programs are designed to provide educational opportunities to three- and four-year-old children from low-income families (Barnett, 1985; Lazar et al., 1982). Children in Head Start programs are better prepared for school, demonstrate less need for special education, and have less chance of being retained in a grade. Success in school was associated with lower rates of delinquency, teenage pregnancy, and welfare usage, and with higher rates of high school completion and employment.

Comprehensive day care programs for disadvantaged children younger than age three also show promise. The Infant Health and Development Program

(1990) reported that such programs improved the developmental outcomes of low-birthweight and premature infants. Infants from one to three years old who were assigned to the intervention, which included attending a child development center five days a week, showed improved IQ scores.

Positive effects from these programs are possible if they are adequately funded and staffed with well-trained, competent teachers (U.S. Department of Health and Human Services, 1985; Schweinhart and Weikart, 1986).

Head Start and comprehensive day care programs have been shown to be effective interventions in reducing the incidence of school failure. Early educational interventions should continue to be implemented but should be evaluated further.

Community Educational Priorities

Communities can promote prevention in a broad variety of settings, such as clinics in public schools. Community leaders also have successfully used public school curricula, newspapers and other media, churches, and the business sector to promote information in priority areas. Health promotion and disease prevention education should be an integral part of the curriculum in public schools and should include the rationale for preventive measures such as immunization and newborn metabolic screening.

Recent efforts to evaluate the effectiveness of school-based health education will enhance the quality of the prevention science base (Kolbe, 1986), and the National Cancer Institute's program to assess the impact of school curricula on student health behavior provides a useful model for evaluating prevention in the developmental disabilities area. In addition, several of the Health Objectives for the Year 2000 (U.S. Department of Health and Human Services, 1990) focus on increasing instruction in specific prevention activities. Many of these objectives are relevant to developmental disabilities prevention.

The effectiveness of school-based programs in health education should be reviewed and improved as necessary to educate children about prevention including the prevention of disability.

Access to Public Education

Landmark 1975 legislation (P.L. 94-142) mandated the education of children with disabilities in the least restrictive environments and required the provision of special education services to make school completion possible. Although there is considerable variability in placement policies among school districts, on average, 27 percent of "students with handicaps" were placed in regular classrooms in 1986-1987 (U.S. Department of Education, 1989b). Special resource rooms were provided for another 43 percent, 25 percent were placed in separate classes, and 4 percent were placed in separate schools. Less than 2 percent of special educational services were provided in homes, hospitals, residential facilities, or correctional facilities.

Sixty percent of "handicapped students" aged 16 to 21 graduated with a diploma or certificate. Twenty-five percent dropped out. The highest drop-out rates were reported among the "emotionally disturbed" (42 percent) and the "learning disabled" (26 percent) (U.S. Department of Education, 1989a).

In 1986, amendments to the 1975 legislation (P.L. 99-457) encouraged states to identify children with disabling conditions as early as possible and provide early intervention services (Smith, 1976; DeGraw et al., 1988). States are now discussing how to implement these programs.

Environmental Interventions

Environmental Control

Environmental control programs are designed to protect children from exposure to toxicants such as lead and asbestos. With respect to lead, prevention strategies focus on efforts to identify major environmental sources of lead exposure (such as house paint, automobile emissions, and water) and to identify children with elevated blood levels of lead (Centers for Disease Control, 1985). Federal, state, and local regulations are directed at keeping environmental exposures at safe levels.

Childhood lead exposure is an important cause of preventable developmental disability, and screening programs in high-risk areas should be expanded. Surveillance also should be established to monitor childhood lead poisoning more closely, and governmental health, housing, and environmental agencies should work together to increase the removal of lead paint and dust in high-risk areas.

Accessibility and Adaptation

Methods of adaptive assistance that reduce secondary conditions are evolving, including personal care attendants, respite care, and a vast array of assistive technology. Communication devices, feeder plates, computers, and electric wheelchairs are among the most widely used assistive technologies, but devices also can be customized for individuals with unique needs. The impact of some environmental obstacles, such as curbs and buildings, has been lessened, but many obstacles remain, including inadequate transportation in rural areas.

Environmental modification and adaptive assistance are essential components of a prevention program focused on developmental disability.

Peer Support Groups

Organizations such as local Parent to Parent groups, Associations of Retarded Citizens groups, United Cerebral Palsy Associations, and Independent Living Centers provide community-based peer support for individuals with disabling conditions and their families. These groups provide an invaluable resource for emotional support and information. For example, support groups are the major source of referrals to professionals who specialize in care for persons with disabling conditions, and to systems of health care reimbursement. In addition, support groups are excellent sources of advice on career alternatives, training, and job opportunities.

Peer support groups also play a major advocacy role. Through the concerted efforts of several such groups, legislation has been adopted to improve access to public buildings and transportation. These groups also have been instrumental in developing many state-based disability prevention programs.

Persons with disabling conditions, their families, personal attendants, and advocates need improved access to information and training in disability prevention. In particular, there is a need for enhanced disability advocacy, information, and support in many rural communities where physical distances limit group interactions.

OPPORTUNITIES AND NEEDS

Current efforts in the prevention of developmental disabilities as described above provide numerous opportunities. There is much room for improvement, however. Some of the opportunities and needs that have been identified are described below, organized into five categories: organization and coordination, surveillance and epidemiology, research, access to care and preventive services, and professional education.

Organization and Coordination

The vast array of disability-related activities in both the public and private sectors is evidence in itself of the need for coordination. There are numerous examples of duplicate and underutilized services. Efforts are under way at national and state levels to better coordinate prevention programs. Some of these are briefly described below.

National Coordination

National Council on Disability   The National Council on Disability is a presidentially appointed council that has made prevention of disability one of its highest priorities. Its efforts include promoting the development of a national disabilities prevention plan. In addition, the council has worked with the Office of Disease Prevention and Health Promotion to cosponsor a federal task force to coordinate disability prevention planning.

The National Coalition for the Prevention of Mental Retardation   The National Coalition for the Prevention of Mental Retardation comprises representatives from the President's Committee on Mental Retardation, the American Academy of Pediatrics, the American Association on Mental Retardation, the Association for Retarded Citizens of the United States, and the American Association of University Affiliated Programs. This group meets regularly to discuss major activities in the area of developmental disabilities prevention.

The Office of Disease Prevention and Health Promotion   In coordinating the development of the Health Objectives for the Year 2000 (U.S. Department of Health and Human Services, 1990), the Office of Disease Prevention and Health Promotion has promoted objectives that address disability prevention. These objectives will prescribe measurable improvements in health status, risk factor reduction, health education, and preventive services related to the prevention of disabilities.

State-based Coordination

States that accept planning money under federal legislation (P.L. 99-457) must establish interagency coordinating councils. Under the direction of a state agency (usually the department of education or health), representatives of state government divisions dealing with childhood disability interventions must meet regularly to discuss the design of intended service programs.

A new systematic approach to the prevention of developmental disabilities has been launched under recent federal legislation (P.L. 100-102). This approach involves cooperative agreements between the CDC and the respective states to develop coordinated state disability prevention programs. A major goal of this effort is to develop a scientific data base on incidence, prevalence, and relative effectiveness of intervention strategies.

The many disability-related activities in the public (federal, state, and local levels) and private sectors need to be coordinated with additional emphasis on prevention.

Surveillance and Epidemiology

The creation of effective preventive measures requires an informed analysis of data on the types and prevalences of disabling conditions and their underlying conditions. Surveillance data on younger children can be used to estimate their potential needs in subsequent years. Surveillance data also provide the basis for epidemiologic research to evaluate preventive measures and to discover more causes of developmental disabilities. Analysis of community- and state-based surveillance data can provide the basis for etiologic research (Thacker and Berkelman, 1988). The systematic collection of surveillance data should always be examined with the goal of spreading knowledge about the availability of health services. Several sources of nationally published data are described below to illustrate the variety of available data and the need to coordinate data collection and analysis.

Centers for Disease Control

CDC has an established program in epidemiologic research and birth defects surveillance and is building on this experience to study other developmental disabilities such as mental retardation and cerebral palsy. The birth defects surveillance program has two elements: the Metropolitan Atlanta Congenital Defects Program (MACDP), and the national Birth Defects Monitoring Program (BDMP). Developmental disabilities are being studied in the Metropolitan Atlanta Developmental Disability Study (MADDS).

Metropolitan Atlanta Congenital Defects Program   MACDP is a population-based active surveillance program in metropolitan Atlanta designed to provide reliable prevalence estimates of several hundred types of birth defects. Because many prevention programs and environmental agents that exist in Atlanta are also found throughout the country, this program has served as a source of data for national policy decisions.

Reports based on MACDP data have shown no increased risks for birth defects associated with maternal Bendectin exposure (Cordero et al., 1981) or with paternal opportunity for exposure to Agent Orange (Erickson et al., 1984). Another study showed that women who took multivitamin supplements prior to pregnancy were only half as likely as unsupplemented women to have an infant with spina bifida (Mulinare et al., 1988).

Birth Defects Monitoring Program   The BDMP provides a national perspective on birth defects, using hospital discharge diagnoses from large numbers of hospitals. Comparison of BDMP birth defect rates with those obtained from MACDP is helpful in interpreting national findings and monitoring trends over time. Patterns discerned from these data include decreasing trends of anencephaly and spina bifida (Edmonds and Windham, 1985) and increasing trends in renal agenesis and ventricular septal defect (Centers for Disease Control, 1988b). These and other data gained from birth defects surveillance programs potentially can be used to inform eligible families of the availability of clinical services. Iowa and Colorado are investigating the feasibility of using surveillance data to refer families to early intervention programs.

Metropolitan Atlanta Developmental Disabilities Study Birth defects are a major component of developmental disabilities and are easier to ascertain on a population basis than are non-birth defect developmental disabilities. Surveillance methods are now being developed in this more difficult area. MADDS is a prevalence survey of five developmental disabilities (mental retardation, cerebral palsy, severe hearing and vision impairments, and seizure disorders) in metropolitan Atlanta. In addition, cases and controls are being studied to search for causes.

There is a need for a national surveillance system to monitor the incidence and prevalence of developmental disabilities. The CDC surveillance systems for birth defects and developmental disabilities represent an important base from which to develop this capacity.

National Center for Health Statistics

In addition to its birth defects and developmental disabilities surveillance efforts, the CDC has several other programs for collecting information on health status. These programs, directed by the National Center for Health Statistics (NCHS), which also compiles vital statistics data, can be a rich source of information on disability. The most important of the NCHS surveillance efforts are the National Health Interview Survey (NHIS), the 1980 National Medical Care Utilization and Expenditure Survey (NMCUES), the National Maternal and Infant Health Survey, and the National Health and Nutrition Examination Surveys (NHANES).

National Health Interview Survey The NHIS has been conducted annually since 1957, with approximately 50,000 households providing information in a personal interview. A core questionnaire solicits data on perceived health status, limitation of activity, disability days, the incidence of acute conditions, prevalence of selected chronic conditions, and health care utilization. Conditions such as mental retardation, cerebral palsy and sensory impairment are included in the core data, but no information on underlying clinical disorders is gathered. A Child Health Supplement to the NHIS, added in 1981 and 1988, solicits information on childhood conditions.

1980 National Medical Care Utilization and Expenditure Survey NMCUES was a 1980 study that collected data on disability, health status, acute and chronic conditions, use of health services, and source of expenditures from 17,000 noninstitutionalized civilians. NMCUES was replicated, in part, by the 1987 National Medical Care Expenditures Survey conducted by the National Center for Health Services Research.

National Maternal and Infant Health Survey   Ten thousand mothers of live-born babies were interviewed in this 1988 survey. A longitudinal follow-up study of this group is planned in 1990. This study will help establish expected distributions of health status measures, but the sample size will not allow adequate statistical description of individual developmental disabilities.

National Health and Nutrition Examination Surveys   Data on hearing, vision, and intelligence were collected in three cycles of NHANES studies begining in 1971, providing another source of normal descriptive data. The samples studied in NHANES I, NHANES II, and Hispanic HANES were approximately 20,000 (1971-1974), 20,000 (1976-1980), and 12,000 (1982-1984), respectively.

National Institutes of Health

National Institute of Child Health and Human Development   NICHD, part of the National Institutes of Health (NIH), has supported research on the genetic and environmental causes of mental retardation, autism, epilepsy, and cerebral palsy (National Institutes of Health, 1989). NICHD-funded investigators in 12 mental retardation research centers carry out biomedical and behavioral studies of these issues. Biomedical research has focused on applications of new genetic approaches to investigate a variety of developmental disabilities. NICHD Mental Retardation Research Centers have also provided a setting for longitudinal studies of environmental and social factors, along with research on secondary conditions and quality of life issues. NICHD also houses the new National Center for Medical Rehabilitation Research (seee Chapter 8).

National Institute of Neurological Disorders and Stroke   Another branch of NIH, NINDS funds biomedical research on brain development during infancy and childhood and on disorders that influence cognition, learning, behavior, and performance (NIH, 1989). NINDS-supported investigators study conditions that damage the central nervous system early in life and contribute to mental retardation.

Bureau of Maternal and Child Health and Resources Development

To complement their health service delivery program, the Health Resource Services Administration's BMCHRD administers a grant program for research (BMCHRD, 1989). These grants support a broad spectrum of studies, ranging from descriptive epidemiology to evaluation of major preventive interventions. Evaluation of interventions to reduce the incidence and severity of secondary conditions is also a priority in the BMCHRD research program.

Department of Education

National Institute on Disability and Rehabilitation Research The NIDRR administers two grant programs: one to support research and training centers, and a second to promote individual research. The research and training centers, which are principally university based, recently have focused on the identification and treatment of secondary conditions. The NIDRR is also promoting the development of assistive technology and is cofunding (with the National Institute of Mental Health) a study of service systems used by children with emotional disorders.

Office of Special Education Programs The U.S. Department of Education supports research activities on the effectiveness of special education and publishes annual data on the use of special educational services. The State/Federal Evaluations Studies Program funds studies of the effectiveness of programs implemented under the Education of the Handicapped Act.

The Department of Education publishes special education statistics in an annual report to Congress. Use of services is categorized by type of impairment (e.g., mental retardation, learning disorders, hearing and visual impairment). National data are difficult to interpret because case definitions may vary greatly among local school districts.

State- and Local-level Data Bases

Disability data are collected at the state and local level by a number of health and education agencies. Some states have begun interagency collaboration to share data to improve planning and inform families of available services. For the most part, however, data are used only within the agency that collected them.

There is a great potential for increasing the applications of these data for both service and research purposes. More complete discussions of these varied data sets are provided by Gortmaker and Walker (1984) and by Crocker (1986) in his widely used unpublished article, "Data Collection for the Evaluation of Mental Retardation Prevention Activities: The Fateful Forty-three."

Birth and death records are usually maintained by the state health agency. The number of annual births, by state and region, is often used with established prevalence rates to calculate the expected number of persons with specific potentially disabling conditions. Such synthetic estimates can provide a basis for evaluating the comprehensiveness of service programs.

State- and local-level data can provide the foundation for epidemiologic research in selected regions. National surveillance for developmental disabilities could benefit from such epidemiologic research.

Other Important Data Bases on Developmental Disabilities

Several other valuable data bases document important aspects of developmental disabilities. These include surveys by the National Center for Health Services Research, the Social Security Administration, the Health Care Financing Administration, and the Bureau of the Census.

Public access data bases are available from the Collaborative Perinatal Study of 50,000 pregnancies in the early 1960s and the Child Health and Development Studies of 20,000 infants in the mid-1970s. Both studies include follow-up data on cognitive and other neurological development of the children studied.

Research

Preventive interventions are directed at reducing risk factors. For developmental disabilities, the interactions of biologic, behavioral, and environmental (social and physical) risk factors in pregnancy and early childhood are of obvious importance. However, because many children with congenital anomalies are born to parents who practice healthy lifestyles, there is a clear need for identifying risk factors that remain unknown.

Maternal use of alcohol during early pregnancy clearly can cause mental retardation. But it is not known why some infants with heavy alcohol exposure during early pregnancy have no discernible impairment. Understanding these differences may provide clues for prevention. The belief that the nutritional status of the mother is an important determinant of infant health provides the basis for the Women, Infants, and Children (WIC) food supplementation programs. More can be learned about how to maximize the impact of this intervention.

Recent studies show that women who use multivitamin supplements prior to conception and throughout early pregnancy have a lower risk of having an infant with spina bifida (Smithells et al., 1983; Mulinare et al., 1988; Milunsky et al., 1989). It is not clear whether this protective effect is attributable to vitamin supplements or to some other maternal behavior. More definitive studies are needed in this important area.

Expanded surveillance and epidemiologic research can greatly improve our ability to prevent developmental disabilities. A national surveillance program is needed to establish the magnitude of the problem, to measure our success in reaching prevention goals, and to determine gaps in prevention stemming from poorly implemented programs or services. Epidemiologic research is also needed to identify the causes of the large proportion of developmental disabilities with unknown origins and to find the basis for the excess of developmental disabilities observed among the socioeconomically disadvantaged.

Improved and expanded surveillance, epidemiology, and applied research is needed as part of a coordinated research program on the prevention of developmental disabilities.

In summary, the goal of these efforts is to prevent developmental disabilities and reduce the incidence and severity of secondary conditions. To reach this goal, effective preventive measures must be implemented. The scientific base of known preventive interventions should be expanded by further evaluating promising strategies and by identifying the preventable risk factors that may underlie disabilities of unknown origin and etiology.

Comprehensive, coordinated services in health care, education, environmental control, and peer support are encouraged at the federal, state, and community levels. In addition, efforts to monitor prevention programs and establish uniform definitions and data collection methods will advance program coordination and accountability.

Access to Care and Preventive Services

The financing of health care and preventive interventions in the United States is complex, involving contributions from public programs, private insurers, and families (Table 4-6). This complicated strategy makes it increasingly difficult for all citizens to have equal access to health care and preventive services.

Inadequate insurance coverage is the single greatest barrier to equal access to health care, according to a Robert Wood Johnson Foundation study (1987). Lack of insurance coverage for preventive care services for women of childbearing age is a particular problem. More than 14 million women in this category (ages 15 to 44) do not have prenatal or other maternity coverage, 9 million are completely uninsured, and 5 million have private insurance coverage that excludes maternity care (Alan Guttmacher Institute, 1987).

The cost of immunizations and other pediatric preventive care is a strong disincentive for uninsured families who might otherwise obtain these services. Nineteen percent of children under 18 (10.6 million) had no insurance coverage in 1986 (Chollet, 1988). Thirty-three percent of all uninsured children had family incomes below the poverty level. In 1987, children under age 21 represented 52 percent of all Medicaid recipients and only 19 percent of expenditures. The average payment per child was $742, compared with $3,362 for adults (U.S. Health Resources and Services Administration, 1989).

TABLE 4-6 Various Normal and Special Care Prevention Activities for Developmental Disabilities and Their Usual Sources of Funding

Type of Care	Usual Source of Funding for Prevention Activities	
	Private Funds (third-party reimbursement)	Public Funds (programs of state, city, and volunteer agencies)
Normal care		
Prior to pregnancy		Family life education Avoidance of teen pregnancy Improved parenting Role of alcohol in pregnancy AIDS education Family planning
Prenatal	Maternal serum alpha-fetoprotein Ultrasound and amniocentesis as needed	[a]Appropriate prenatal care
Perinatal	Hospital delivery	
		[a]Newborn screening PKU, thyroid, etc.
Childhood	A medical "home" for each child Immunization Automobile restraints	Lead screening Developmental screening
Special care		
Prior to pregnancy	Genetic counseling Carrier testing	Family assistance
Prenatal	Prenatal diagnosis as needed	Family assistance
Perinatal	Regional newborn intensive care	
Childhood		[a]Early intervention programs [a]Effective services for child progress family support

[a]Usual sources of funding for these activities are both public and private.

To help redress these inequities, governmental programs have been established to provide preventive services to two groups: persons with disabilities, and families with socioeconomic disadvantage. Because socioeconomic disadvantage is a risk factor for disability, persons may be members of both groups.

Public Programs for Persons with Developmental Disabilities

The major federal programs for persons with developmental disabilities are coordinated by the Administration for Developmental Disabilities (ADD) of the Department of Health and Human Services. ADD supports councils in each state that plan and coordinate services and advocate changes to reduce the disadvantage associated with developmental disabilities. ADD also awards grants to state offices providing legal and administrative assistance to individuals with developmental disabilities. Special project grants are awarded to encourage innovative work that will help integrate persons with disabling conditions into the community. ADD also supports the University Affiliated Programs, which offer clinical evaluation for children and training for providers in the field.

In addition to ADD-sponsored programs, the Medicaid and Supplemental Security Income (SSI) programs provide medical insurance and income assistance for persons with developmental disabilities. Guidelines are expected to be revised soon that will make more children eligible for SSI support.

Several other federal departments offer assistance to persons with developmental disabilities, including the Department of Education (special education and vocational education, among other programs), the Department of Transportation (grants to improve access to public transportation), and the Department of Housing and Urban Development (housing construction loans).

Public Programs for Families with Socioeconomic Disadvantage

Many preventive services programs for families with socioeconomic disadvantage are jointly financed by federal and state funds. At the federal level, the Departments of Health and Human Services, Education, and Agriculture are responsible for directing these programs. Agencies at the state and local levels manage the programs. Table 4-7 contains a partial list of existing programs for the prevention of developmental disability.

Within the Department of Health and Human Services, the Maternal and Child Health Bureau (Health Resources and Services Administration) administers block grants that provide major support for state prenatal care programs, newborn intensive care units, newborn screening, genetic ser-

TABLE 4-7 Partial List of Existing Programs for the Prevention of
Developmental Disabilities

Program	Activity
FEDERAL PROGRAMS	
Maternal and Child Health Bureau (Health Resources and Services Administration)	MCH block grants include major support for states in public prenatal care programs, newborn intensive care units, newborn screening, services for children with special health care needs, etc. Additional elements are provided for genetics programs, AIDS education and prevention, and special projects.
Centers for Disease Control	Disabilities Prevention Program, epidemiologic studies; injury control program, lead poisoning prevention; childhood immunization, school health, AIDS prevention programs
Office of Special Education and Rehabilitative Services	P.L. 94-142, P.L. 99-457, and special projects
Office of Disease Prevention and Health Promotion	Health Objectives for the Year 2000
Office of Human Development Services	Head Start, Administration on Developmental Disabilities
Health Care Financing Administration	Early Periodic Screening, Diagnosis, and Treatment, Medicaid
National Institute of Child Health and Human Development	Studies in causation, pathophysiology, and intervention; Mental Retardation Research Centers
National Institute on Disability and Rehabilitation Research	Studies of interventions to reduce secondary conditions in persons with disabilities; assistive technology research
National Council on Disability	National advocate for federal civil rights legislation for persons with disabilities and for a national disabilities prevention program; introduced concept of prevention of secondary conditions in persons with disabilities
President's Committee on Mental Retardation	Guidelines for state prevention planning, convenes National Coalition on Prevention of Mental Retardation

TABLE 4-7 *Continued*

Program	Activity
STATE PROGRAMS	
Department of Health	Prenatal care clinics, standards of obstetric care, newborn screening, services for children with disabilities, special chronic disease programs, supports for immunization, lead screening and lead poisoning prevention, developmental screening, genetic counseling, family planning, AIDS programs, automobile restraints, education of the public, professional awareness
Departments of Mental Retardation, Developmental Disabilities, and/or Mental Health	Early childhood services, family support, counseling
Department of Social Services	Family support, child protection, respite, foster care, adoption
Departments of Welfare, Public Assistance	Family support, care coordination, Medicaid
Department of Education	Family life curricula, school health services, and early intervention programs
Office for Children	Standards, certification, advocacy
Office for Prevention	Prevention planning, monitoring, collaborative efforts
COMMUNITY PROGRAMS	
City health departments	Immunization, prenatal care, AIDS work, lead programs
Other city agencies	Recreation, youth programs, transportation
Health care centers	Screening, counseling, supports
Neighborhoods	Education, lead poisoning prevention
PRIVATE PROGRAMS	
Voluntary and consumer organizations	Education of public, counseling services, family planning, parent-to-parent services, screening, case-finding, advocacy, pressure on state agencies, and research (March of

TABLE 4-7 *Continued*

Program	Activity
	Dimes, Associations for Retarded Citizens, National Tay-Sachs Allied Diseases Association, National Mucopolysaccharidosis Society, Epilepsy Foundation of America, and United Cerebral Palsy Association)
Professional organizations	Member education, advocacy, studies, standard development, data collection (American Association on Mental Retardation, American Association of University Affiliated Programs, American Academy of Pediatrics, Association of Maternal and Child Health Programs)
University centers	Genetic counseling and services, other services, technical assistance, education of public, advocacy, and research (teaching hospitals, pediatric departments, and University Affiliated Programs)
Private philanthropy	Special projects, all types

COORDINATION OF SERVICES

Interagency coordinating councils	These coordinating groups are required in all states that accept planning money under Part H of the Amendments to the Education for Handicapped Children's Act (P.L. 99-457). Under direction of the specified lead agency (usually Education or Health) all the elements of state government participating in the early education effort for children at risk of or with disability must meet regularly to share in the design of intended services
State advisory committees	The states participating in the awards from the Disability Prevention Program of the Centers for Disease Control are required to establish advisory committees with multiagency and consumer

TABLE 4-7 *Continued*

Program	Activity
	membership that monitor the progress of local efforts.
Citizen organizations	Many states that have created state prevention plans derive their original proposals under the stimulation and leadership of a special task force, study group, or governor's panel, with prominent representation by members of the Developmental Disabilities Council or Association for Retarded Citizens. Such committees usually remain in effect even after the state's Office for Prevention is operational and serve a valuable watchdog function in a voluntary setting

vices, and services for children with special health care needs. The programs of the Centers for Disease Control include injury control, lead poisoning prevention, childhood immunization, school health, and AIDS prevention. The new CDC Disabilities Prevention Program supports the planning, coordination, and evaluation of prevention services.

The Office of Human Development Services supports Head Start programs, state Developmental Disabilities Councils, and University Affiliated Programs for persons with developmental disabilities. The Health Care Financing Administration administers the federal contribution to Medicaid programs, which provide health care reimbursements for persons meeting state financial eligibility criteria.

Reimbursement for services in the Early Periodic Screening, Diagnosis, and Treatment Program is also managed by this agency.

Access to medical care and preventive services is an essential component of the prevention agenda. Persons who are socioeconomically disadvantaged need access to programs providing family planning information and comprehensive prenatal care. In addition, the private sector needs to be more active in programs to prevent developmental disabilities, as in the model to provide a "medical home" to children with disabilities that was developed by the Tennessee chapter of the American Academy of Pediatrics.

Professional Education

The rapid development of new technology makes continuing education of health professionals a challenge. University-based research groups supported by NIH, CDC, NIDRR, and MCH provide training settings for developmental disabilities researchers. Despite these programs, there is great need for additional epidemiologists with expertise in developmental disabilities. More leadership is needed in schools of public health to encourage program participants to enter this field. Development of coherent career tracts in universities and state health agencies is needed to keep capable researchers in the field.

Special professional educational programs are needed for practitioners and researchers in the area of developmental disabilities.

5

Prevention of Injury-Related Disability

In recent years, injury has begun to receive long overdue recognition as a major public health problem. Attention has focused primarily on the toll of lives lost and on the resultant economic costs.

INJURY IN AMERICA: MAGNITUDE OF THE PROBLEM

Each year more than 142,000 people in the United States are killed by injuries, the nation's fourth leading cause of death. Injury is the number one killer among people younger than age 45, who incur four-fifths of all injuries. In 1985, indirect costs of forgone productivity due to premature deaths caused by injury were estimated to total $47.9 billion (Rice et al., 1989).

The toll of injury-caused deaths would be much higher, however, if not for advances in the medical and surgical management of trauma and the regionalization of transport and treatment systems. These and other developments have substantially reduced the injury mortality rate during the last several decades. Between 1975 and 1988, the age-adjusted death rate due to unintentional injury decreased from 45.4 to 35.8 per 100,000 people (National Safety Council, 1989).

This impressive progress in averting death among injury victims does not translate into absolute success. Large and increasing numbers of survivors of once-fatal injuries sustain lifelong impairments and functional limitations that can greatly diminish their ability to carry out the major roles in which they had previously engaged. Consequently, gains in lives saved by advances in the care of injury victims have contributed to the prevalence of disabling conditions in the United States.

Each year an estimated 2.3 million Americans are hospitalized as the

147

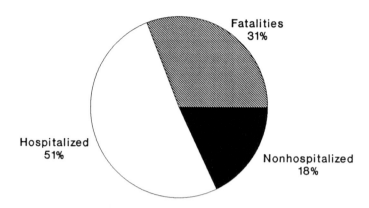

$158 Billion in Lifetime Costs

FIGURE 5-1   Cost of injury by class of injury in the United States, 1985. Source:
Rice et al., 1989.

result of injuries; an additional 54 million sustain injuries requiring outpatient medical care or resulting in one or more days of restricted activity
without medical attention (Rice et al., 1989). These figures translate into
16 injury-caused hospitalizations for every death due to injury in the United
States. Moreover, for every injury death an additional 381 people sustain
less severe injuries that do not require hospitalization.

A one-year accounting of the economic costs associated with the estimated 57 million people who sustain nonfatal injuries in the United States
provides some perspective on the enormity of the problem. Rice and colleagues
(1989) estimate that about $108 million, or two-thirds of the total cost of all
injuries incurred in 1985, could be attributed to nonfatal injuries (Figure 5-
1). Nearly 60 percent of these costs result from reduced or forgone productivity—
the market value of lost work and housekeeping days due to permanent or
temporary disability. Another way to assess this cost is to tabulate lost time
from work or other productive activity, a measure known as life years lost.
For every 100 injuries in a given year, the contributions of 9 life years are
lost in the same year. The bulk of this loss is attributable to the high
incidence of injury and injury-caused disabling conditions among people
between the ages of 15 and 44, which encompasses the most productive
period of the human life span. Injuries sustained by people in this age
group in 1985 resulted in 2.7 million life years lost, or $44 billion in lost
productivity.

In addition to high morbidity costs, nonfatal injuries result in significant direct costs spent for personal health care and rehabilitation. In 1985, $43.3 billion, or $764 per injured person, was spent for hospital and nursing home care, physicians' services, inpatient and outpatient rehabilitation services, and other health care expenditures related to the injury.

Although economic costs do not reflect the pain and suffering associated with injury or the burden placed on family and friends, they do provide a quantifiable measure of the public health significance of injuries and can be useful in guiding choices among competing programs of primary, secondary, and tertiary prevention. There is little question that nonfatal injuries represent a major economic burden to society.

Ranked by cause, cumulative losses are greatest for injuries incurred in falls and motor vehicle crashes, totaling $35.6 billion and $30.2 billion, respectively (Figure 5-2). Poisonings, burns, and injuries associated with the intentional and unintentional use of firearms are also costly to society, totaling $4.1 billion, $2.4 billion, and $2.2 billion, respectively. Nevertheless, these three categories account for a small percentage of the total economic costs of nonfatal injury relative to falls and motor vehicle injuries. Other common causes of injuries include stabbings and other assaults, injuries involving machinery, and sports-related injuries.

The ranking of costs according to causes of nonfatal injuries does not mirror the ranking of mortality costs associated with specific causes of injury (Figure 5-3). The two leading contributors to mortality costs are

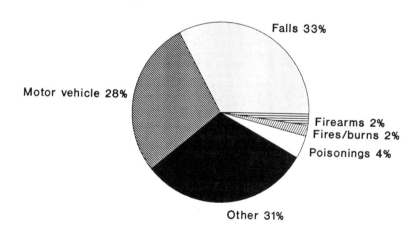

$108.2 Billion in Lifetime Costs

FIGURE 5-2   Lifetime costs of non-fatal injury, United States, 1985.

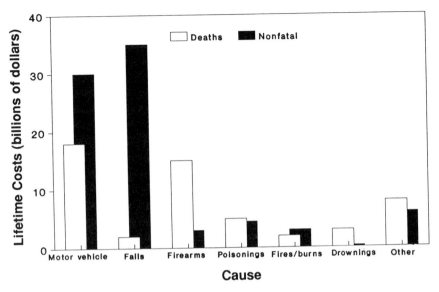

FIGURE 5-3   Lifetime costs of injury by cause—deaths vs. nonfatal injury, United States, 1985.

motor vehicle crashes ($18.4 billion) and incidents involving firearms ($12.2 billion). In contrast, falls, which rarely are fatal and account for less than 1 percent of the mortality costs of injury, are the major source of lifetime costs due to nonfatal injuries. Motor vehicle crashes are also a major source of costs due to nonfatal injuries, whereas firearm-related injuries account for about 2 percent of the total.

> *The role of firearms in contributing to the population of people with disabling conditions needs to be carefully evaluated. Improved data collection, discussed elsewhere in this report, is important to this evaluation and the development of effective interventions.*

CENTRAL NERVOUS SYSTEM INJURIES

The remainder of this chapter concentrates on spinal cord injury (SCI) and traumatic brain injury (TBI). Per-person economic costs associated with these traumatic injuries to the central nervous system are among the highest costs for injury-caused pathologies and impairments. Both types of injury often result in significant physical, neurophysical, and psychosocial deficits that cause long-term disabling conditions, which necessitate extensive treatment and rehabilitation of affected individuals. Although this chapter focuses on SCI and TBI, much of the discussion, such as that pertaining to the management of care, the development and evaluation of preventive interventions, the need for a stronger emphasis on behavioral and psychosocial determinants of disability, and the importance of tertiary prevention, is applicable to the broader fields of injury control and disability prevention. In addition, focusing on SCI and TBI is not meant to imply that disabling conditions resulting from injuries to other body systems merit less attention. Orthopedic injuries, for example, including serious injuries to the upper and lower extremities, result in significant impairment and disabling conditions. For many people with these injuries, recovery can be long and expensive, and even optimal treatment may not prevent permanent impairment involving chronic pain, loss of motion or contracture of joints, and deformity or loss of limb. Many of the strategies recommended in this chapter for reducing disability associated with TBI and SCI are relevant to the prevention of disability resulting from orthopedic injuries as well.

Traumatic Brain Injury: Incidence and Outcomes

Studies published within the past 15 years have reported incidence rates for traumatic brain injury in the United States ranging from a low of 180 per 100,000 people in San Diego County, California, to a high of 367 per 100,000 in the Chicago area (Annegers et al., 1980; Frankowski et al., 1985; Whitman et al., 1984). Differences in incidence are attributable to differences in case definition and case ascertainment methodologies, as well as differences in the age, sex, and, in particular, racial composition of study populations. The only national data available are from the National Head and Spinal Cord Injury Survey, which estimated a rate of 200 hospitalizations per year per 100,000 people (Kalsbeek et al., 1980). Applying this annual rate to the projected 1990 U.S. population yields an estimate of 500,000 expected new cases of TBI. Using an average of 10 percent mortality implies that each year approximately 450,000 people survive a TBI, the consequences of which range from slight to persistent vegetative state (Frankowski et al., 1985). Annual direct and indirect costs associated with traumatic head injury have been estimated at $12.5 billion (1982 dollars) (Grabow et al., 1984).

The acute severity of TBI has traditionally been measured using the Glasgow Coma Scale (GCS), a 13-point scale ranging from 3 to 15. GCS scores are based on three neurological responses: eye opening, verbal responses, and motor responses. In general, scores below 8 imply severe head injury; scores between 9 and 12 indicate moderately severe injury; and scores of 13 to 15 indicate mild or minor head injury. Although several studies have demonstrated a high correlation between GCS and chances of survival, the ability of the GCS to predict long-term quality of life is less clear (Uzzell et al., 1987) and requires further evaluation (Eisen berg, 1985).

The majority of individuals hospitalized for TBI are diagnosed as havin a mild, uncomplicated closed head injury. Very little is known about th consequences of these minor head injuries, although increasing evidenc suggests that they often result in persistent headaches and other physica symptoms, as well as significant psychosocial and behavioral problems including difficulty in performing at one's job (Casey et al., 1986; Dikme et al., 1986; Edna and Cappelen, 1987; Rimel et al., 1981; Wrightson an Gronwall, 1984). The most comprehensive study of mild head injury publishe to date indicates that of 424 individuals examined 3 months after injury, 7 percent complained of persistent headaches, 50 percent had difficulties wit memory, and 34 percent of those employed prior to the injury had not ye returned to work (Rimel et al., 1981). Given the high incidence of mino head injuries, their social and economic impacts are considerable.

Considerably more is known about the consequences of moderate an severe TBI. Each year approximately 70,000 to 90,000 individuals sustai moderate to severe TBIs that may result in lifelong potentially disablin conditions. The estimated 2,000 who sustain the most severe disablin conditions survive in a persistent vegetative state, a term referring to thei lack of response to external stimuli (Rice et al., 1989). Several studies hav documented the sequelae of severe TBI, leading to the characterization o TBI as the "silent epidemic" because sequelae are primarily neurobehaviora Although limitations in physical function can be significant following sever TBI, cognitive and psychosocial consequences are more common and contribut significantly to lifelong disabling conditions and poor quality of life (Bach y-Rita, 1989). Common cognitive sequelae include deficits in attention memory, general intellectual performance, and linguistic and perceptual functior A vast array of emotional disturbances and personality changes have als been documented, ranging from depression and withdrawal to disinhibitio and euphoria. Behavioral disturbances have become increasingly recognize as a major limiting factor in recovery and return to work following TB (Levin et al., 1982).

Estimates of the proportion of people who return to work following mod erate and severe closed head injury vary widely due to differences in injur definition, preinjury characteristics of the patient population, and lengths o follow-up. A recent study has shown that only 12 percent of patients wit severe head injuries had returned to work within 6 months; 29 percent ha returned within a year (MacKenzie et al., 1987). Other studies have demonstrate even lower rates for the most severely injured (Jacobs, 1988; Oddy et al. 1985; Weddell et al., 1980). Rates of return to work are somewhat highe for individuals sustaining moderately severe injuries, ranging from 30 percen to 50 percent at 3 to 6 months postinjury, and 50 percent to 60 percent at one year (Oddy and Humphrey, 1980; Rimel et al., 1982).

Profiles of individuals who are at highest risk of sustaining TBI are consistent in the research literature (reviewed by Annegers et al., 1980; Frankowski et al., 1985; and Whitman et al., 1984). Adults aged 15 to 24 years are at highest risk of sustaining a traumatic brain injury, but the elderly, aged 65 and over, and very young children are also at high risk. Compared with females, males are twice as likely to sustain TBI; thus, more than 70 percent of all TBIs occur among males. Demographic studies indicate that the incidence of TBI is highest for nonwhite, urban populations (ranging from 250 to 400 per 100,000). White populations living in rural and suburban areas, on the other hand, have the lowest rates (200 per 100,000).

Motor vehicle crashes constitute the leading cause of TBI, accounting for one-third to one-half of all new cases. The second leading cause of TBI is falls, accounting for an additional 20 percent to 30 percent of total incidence. Intentional injuries also represent a major cause, although the contribution of assaults to the overall incidence of head injuries varies among populations according to socioeconomic composition. Studies of inner city Chicago and Bronx County, New York, for instance, indicate that motor vehicle crashes and violence contribute equally to the incidence of head injury (Cooper et al., 1983; Whitman et al., 1984).

Given the force involved in motor vehicle crashes, resulting TBIs generally lead to a higher percentage of diffuse brain damage. Falls and blows to the head, on the other hand, are associated with a higher frequency of hematomas and focal paralysis.

Spinal Cord Injury: Incidence and Outcomes

The incidence of SCI is considerably lower than TBI; however, SCI substantially affects both the individual and society. Each year an estimated 10,000 to 20,000 people in the United States sustain an SCI (2.8 to 5 cases per 100,000 people). These incidence figures translate into a prevalence of approximately 200,000 people in any given year (Kraus, 1985). As with TBI, however, estimates of SCI incidence and prevalence vary considerably across studies because of differences in methods of case ascertainment and in characteristics of study populations. On average, lifetime costs for medical treatment and rehabilitation range from an estimated $210,379 to $751,854 (1989 dollars) per individual, depending on the extent of the injury. The average present value of forgone earnings due to premature death and disability ranges from $151,250 to $308,000 per person. Total lifetime costs of all new cases of SCI in 1989 will amount to an estimated $6 billion (1989 dollars) (DeVivo, 1989).

In contrast to TBI, the major impairments resulting from spinal cord

injury are muscle paralysis and loss of sensation. The distinction is made betwee
paralysis involving both the arms and the legs (quadriplegia) and that of th
legs only (paraplegia). Quadriplegia results from injury to one of the eigl
cervical segments or neck region of the spinal cord. Paraplegia resul
when the injury is confined to the thoracic, lumbar, or sacral regions of th
cord. In general, the higher the injury is to the cord, the more severe th
impairment will be. An estimated one-half of all SCIs result in quadripleg
(Stover and Fine, 1986). More than 95 percent of paraplegic individua
achieve independence in specific self-care activities and mobility in a wheelcha
(Young et al., 1982). Quadriplegic individuals often require frequent physic
assistance in performing personal care tasks such as feeding, dressing, an
bathing but may still be independent in the performance of communicativ
and cognitive activities such as operating a computer.

SCIs are also characterized according to the extent of neurologic injur:
Complete injuries, or plegia, result in complete loss of sensation or mote
control. In contrast, people with incomplete lesions, or paresis, may retai
some sensation and motor power, with the degree of impairment dependin
on the extent of the lesion. Overall, approximately one-half of all SCIs ai
complete lesions (Stover and Fine, 1986).

Studies of patients treated at Regional SCI Centers have reported 5-yea
employment rates ranging from about 14 percent for quadriplegics wit
complete lesions to 33 percent for paraplegics with incomplete lesions (Stove
and Fine, 1986). Again, estimates are influenced by the length of follow-u
and the preinjury characteristics of the patient population. A recent stud
(Whiteneck et al., 1989) reported that 63 percent of a select group of higl
level quadriplegic individuals on respirators had survived 9 years and wei
leading fulfilling lives.

Older adolescents and young adults are at highest risk of SCI. Compare
with females, males are at three to four times the risk of sustaining SC
Very little is known about the correlation between SCI injury and race ɑ
ethnicity. The few studies that have examined this relationship report cor
flicting results (Kraus, 1985).

Motor vehicle crashes of all types constitute the major cause of SCI i
the United States, accounting for between 30 percent and 60 percent of a
SCIs. Falls constitute the second leading cause, accounting for an additiona
20 percent to 30 percent of all cases. Acts of violence (primarily involvin
firearms) and sports or recreational activity also contribute significantly t
the incidence of SCI, each accounting for an estimated 5 percent to 2
percent of all SCIs. Diving is the major cause of sports-related SCI, bein
implicated in two-thirds of all sports-related SCI reported by the Mode
Spinal Cord Injury Systems Program. Football injuries also contribute greatl
to SCI in the United States (Stover and Fine, 1986).

The extent of injury is related to cause. Nearly one-third of all falls an motor vehicle-related spinal cord injuries result in incomplete quadriplegia; an additional 15 percent to 20 percent result in complete quadriplegia. SCIs due to acts of violence, on the other hand, more often result in neurologically complete paraplegia. Sports-related SCIs appear to be the most incapacitating; more than 90 percent result in quadriplegia, one-half of which are complete (Stover and Fine, 1986).

Temporal Changes in Patterns of Injury and Outcome

Medical and surgical advances in the acute management of trauma, combined with regionalization of transport and treatment systems, have contributed to a decrease in the injury fatality rate and accompanying changes in patterns of injury severity. For example, during the past 50 years, patterns of survival following SCI have changed dramatically. In the 1950s only those with low-level paraplegia were generally expected to survive. Today, even people who sustain high-level quadriplegia are surviving, and if properly cared for in a specialized, comprehensive program, can lead fulfilling lives (Whiteneck et al., 1989). Further, within the past 10 years, there have been discernible shifts in the proportion of patients with neurologically incomplete injuries. The National SCI Database has documented that while the proportion of all SCI patients who are quadriplegics remained fixed at about 50 percent between 1973 and 1983, the proportion with neurologically incomplete lesions increased from 38 percent to 54 percent. This increase is attributable, in large part, to improved emergency medical services, including better management of the patient at the scene of the injury and during transport to the hospital.

Only two studies have examined temporal trends in the incidence and outcome of head injury. One, an examination of the incidence of head injury in Olmsted County, Minnesota, between 1935 and 1975, found an overall increase in incidence rates but a constant mortality rate (Annegers et al., 1980). The increase was largest for less severe injuries, leading the authors to speculate that the trend resulted from an increased propensity over the years to treat or hospitalize people with minor head injuries. More recently, a study of people hospitalized for head injuries in Maryland reported an 18 percent increase in hospitalizations between 1979 and 1986. The greatest increase (nearly 200 percent), however, was among the most severely injured (MacKenzie et al., 1990). This increase was accompanied by a small decline in the hospital case fatality rate and an increase in the proportion discharged to extended care or rehabilitation facilities. Among those sustaining severe TBI, there was a decrease of 8 percentage points in the proportion discharged to home (from 31 percent to 23 percent) and a 5 percentage-point decrease in fatalities (53 percent to 48 percent). These changes were accompanied by a 15 percentage-point jump (9 percent to 24 percent), or a nearly threefold increase, in the proportion of patients discharged to extended care facilities.

Caution must be exercised in interpretation, but these trends are evidenc♦ that improvement in emergency medical services and acute management o♦ head injuries during the past 10 years has substantially increased the proportio♦ of individuals who survive with severe head injury, placing increased demand♦ on families, the health care system, and society at large.

SURVEILLANCE: COUNTING THE SURVIVORS AND ASSESSING THEIR NEEDS

The preceding review points to many inadequacies in our knowledge o♦ the incidence and outcomes of both TBI and SCI. Better data are needed t♦ identify important shifts in trends and patterns of injury and to build ♦ foundation for better planning and evaluation of injury control efforts. The♦ following discussion describes ongoing efforts to address these needs an♦ recommends areas for further research and development.

The Centers for Disease Control (CDC) has defined surveillance as the♦ "ongoing systematic collection, analysis, and interpretation of health dat♦ needed to plan, implement, and evaluate public health programs." The♦ timely collection and reporting of these data are important features of a♦ effective surveillance system (Centers for Disease Control, 1988a). Al♦ though originally developed to monitor and control epidemics of infectiou♦ diseases such as smallpox and cholera, surveillance systems are now applie♦ more broadly to study patterns of incidence and outcomes of noninfectiou diseases. As for infectious diseases, these efforts are intended to aid th♦ design of effective strategies for primary and secondary prevention of selecte♦ conditions in high-risk groups. Graitcer (1987) has outlined the specifi♦ attributes of injury surveillance systems and discusses the advantages an♦ limitations of alternative approaches.

Population-based information on injuries and events related to injuries i♦ available from a variety of sources. Examples of national injury data base♦ designed for the surveillance of injuries of specific etiologies include th♦ National Accident Sampling System, the National Electronic Injury Surveil lance Systems, the Survey of Occupational Injuries and Illnesses, and th♦ National Crime Survey. Although criticized for incompleteness of coverage limited content, and high cost, these surveillance systems have provide♦ important and useful epidemiological information on TBI and SCI, includ ing etiologies (National Research Council, 1987). Because these system♦ only track injuries of specific etiology, however, they do not provide com plete enumeration of all head and spinal cord injuries.

Surveys by the National Center for Health Statistics are another sourc♦ of data on nonfatal injuries, although they are not designed specifically fo the purpose of injury surveillance. Two specifically relevant surveys ar♦ the National Health Interview Survey (NHIS) and the National Hospita♦

Discharge Survey (NHDS). These instruments have the potential to provide uniform data on all neurological injuries of a general severity class regardless of cause or etiology.

The NHIS is a probability sample of households in the civilian noninstitutionalized population of the United States. The core survey provides data on the incidence of injury and acute conditions, duration and types of limitation of activity, persons injured, hospitalizations, physician visits, and the prevalence of selected chronic conditions. Although the NHIS is one of the few sources of population-based data on the incidence and outcome of minor or mild head injuries that do not result in hospitalization, it contains very little data on circumstances or cause of injury.

Injuries reported in the NHIS are classified into four broad categories: (1) injuries involving moving motor vehicles, (2) injuries occurring at home, (3) injuries occurring at work, and (4) other. This classification is clearly inadequate for identifying the major external cause of disabling injuries including falls, firearms, and injuries involving machinery. Also, there is inadequate information collected for classifying injuries as to their intent. Finally no attempt is made in the interview to ascertain the circumstances of the injury, for example, involvement of alcohol, use of protective devices such as seat belts, car seats, airbags, and special clothing and eyewear. Without this important information, it is difficult to appropriately identify and target interventions for reducing the occurrence of injuries.

The NHIS is also a potentially useful source of information on the use of and unmet need for rehabilitation services. Although the current survey asks questions pertaining to the frequency of physician visits and hospitalizations, it does not collect information about the use of specific inpatient and outpatient rehabilitation services.

The core NHIS survey should be expanded to include questions pertaining to the circumstances and cause of injury to help improve our knowledge of injury etiology. In addition, a comprehensive supplement to the NHIS on incidence, medical care, rehabilitation, and disability related to injury is needed and should be considered as one of the survey's annual special topics.

The NHDS is an important source of national estimates of the incidence of neurological injuries severe enough to require hospitalization. It consists of hospital discharge abstracts uniformly collected for a probability sample of approximately 200,000 patients treated in nearly 600 short-stay, nonfederal hospitals. Data conform to the Uniform Hospital Discharge Data Set. The recent development of a computerized conversion table that maps ICD-9CM coded discharge diagnoses into widely used scores denoting the severity of injuries (i.e., the Abbreviated Injury Scale) has enhanced the usefulness of this data base for studying patterns of injury specific to severity. A majc limitation of these data, however, is the lack of uniform coding of the externa cause of injury. Although a classification of external causes exists within th structure of the International Classification of Diseases (i.e., ICD E-codes hospitals vary in their use of these codes. Underreporting of E-codes i hospital discharge abstracts has been recognized as a major obstacle in the us of this valuable source of data for monitoring the causes and trends of injurie (National Research Council, 1985; Sniezek et al., 1989; U.S. National Committe for Injury Prevention and Control, 1989; Rice et al., 1989).

Although both the NHIS and the NHDS are potentially valuable tool for monitoring the epidemiology of TBI and SCI at the national level, thei utility for surveillance is limited by their mode of collection. Data ar collected and tabulated on an annual basis and published as much as a yea later. Such a design is inconsistent with some surveillance needs. With th increasing availability of statewide hospital discharge abstract data base: there are new opportunities for developing timely and cost-efficient surveil lance systems to monitor the incidence of TBI and SCI. Currently, 28 state maintain data bases that contain, at a minimum, the items incorporated i the Uniform Hospital Discharge Data Set. An important advantage of thes statewide data bases is that they include all hospital discharges and provid data specific to the state and its communities. In addition, many state publish timely data. Similar to the NHDS, however, information on caus of the injury is not uniformly collected for all discharges. A requiremer for E-code data elements in statewide data collection systems would help t solve this problem, and mandatory E-coding legislation has been introduce in several states. Implementing the use of E-codes will require the develop ment of guidelines for E-coding and the instruction of health care provider on the importance of recording data on the cause of injury (Sniezek et al 1989). Modifying current statewide hospital discharge abstract data to in clude E-codes would help provide timely information on the incidence o TBI and SCI.

Nationally collected E-code data for describing the external cause of injury are needed to enhance injury surveillance activities and improve the accuracy of data on the causes and trends of injury. This will entail the creation of a separate data field for E-codes in all hospital discharge abstract data systems. With respect to SCI and TBI, mandatory reporting is needed to improve incidence measures, to appropriately allocate resources, and to plan, implement, and evaluate the most effective interventions.

Another strategy for monitoring the incidence of TBI and SCI is to enac laws that require reporting injuries to the state health agency. Althoug mandatory reporting has been used successfully for monitoring the incidence of infectious diseases, it has only recently been recognized as an effective tool for surveillance of injuries. Seventeen states, including 12 where reporting is mandated by law, now have SCI registries. In 1987 the Council of State and Territorial Epidemiologists recommended mandatory reporting of acute, traumatic SCI to state health departments and to the CDC. The CDC, together with the Council of State and Territorial Epidemiologists, the American Spinal Injury Association, and other groups, is currently working to implement this resolution.

Similar efforts to identify head injury as a reportable condition are also being pursued. At least nine states have registries of persons with head injuries. However, surveillance of TBI is more difficult than surveillance of SCI, and may not be practical. The incidence of head injury is also much greater than that of spinal cord injury, making the development and maintenance of a surveillance system more resource intensive. In addition, TBI is more difficult to define, and standard case definitions are lacking. More work is needed to assess the costs and benefits of mandatory reporting of TBI. Evaluation of existing programs would be most helpful in this regard.

Resources should be allocated to implement and evaluate mandatory reporting of SCI to state health agencies. Mandatory reporting of SCI should be designed as part of a broader national surveillance program that would facilitate the development, implementation, and evaluation of effective interventions and countermeasures. Studies should be conducted to determine the feasibility and utility of mandatory reporting of TBI. Standard case definitions of TBI are needed and should be developed to facilitate this activity.

PRIMARY PREVENTION: THE STRATEGY OF CHOICE

An agenda for the prevention of disability associated with traumatic brain and spinal cord injury must place a priority on preventing the injury from occurring in the first place. Numerous interventions have been identified in the literature and have been shown to be effective in reducing the incidence and severity of traumatic injuries. Many of these interventions have not been implemented, however, because of a variety of social, economic, and political barriers. Still other interventions are promising but require further testing for efficacy.

As discussed, the causes of TBI and SCI are similar. Motor vehicle crashes are the leading cause of all nonfatal TBI and SCI, followed by falls, assaults, and sports or recreational injuries. The abuse of alcohol and drugs plays a major role in the incidence of all traumatic injuries, and TBI and SCI are no exceptions. For example, an estimated 50 percent of all motor vehicle deaths and homicides and one-quarter of all fatal falls have bee attributed to the abuse of alcohol (U.S. National Committee for Injury Pr vention and Control, 1989).

The literature is replete with examples of interventions that are known reduce the incidence and severity of injury. The U.S. National Committe for Injury Prevention and Control (1989) recently reviewed the state of tl art in injury control and concluded that, "while questions remain, we alreac know enough to act. Indeed, if the interventions recommended [in th report] were put in general practice, the result would be a dramatic savir in lives, health, and resources."

A recent review of the literature on the evaluation of injury preventic programs estimated that, for those interventions for which adequate data a available, the potential cost savings, after the cost of the injury contr programs, is in the billions of dollars (Rice et al., 1989). For example, promotional campaign developed in Australia to increase use of bicyc helmets has led to a documented 20 percent reduction in head injuries amor bicyclists. This translates in Australia into 178 fewer TBI fatalities eac year, 2,465 fewer head injuries requiring hospitalization, and 16,602 few nonhospitalized head injuries. The resultant cost savings is approximate $255 million (1985 U.S. dollars). In the United States, a similar 20 perce reduction in head injuries among bicyclists would result in a potenti savings of $183 million. Another dramatic example is the potential co savings from implementing motorcyclist helmet laws in states that do n now have this requirement. After deducting the cost of helmets and assumir that costs associated with law enforcement would be minimal (becau compliance with helmet laws is high), the savings due to fewer head injuri resulting from motorcycle crashes are estimated at $97 million. Analys such as these illustrate the potential cost savings of interventions ar provide the basis for more rational choices among alternative prograr and policies.

It is not possible in this report to evaluate the current state of knowled; regarding the effectiveness of alternative strategies for prevention. Tl reader is referred to the report of the U.S. National Committee for Injur Prevention and Control (1989) for a comprehensive review. To illustra the types of strategies available, however, Table 5-1 lists several interventio to reduce the incidence and severity of motor vehicle-related injuries. I terventions are classified as (1) those of proven effectiveness, (2) those th look promising but require more testing to establish their effectiveness or assess their feasibility or cost, and (3) those that require further resear and development.

A number of clear-cut, unassailable conclusions stand out from a revie of the literature. First, several studies have underscored the lack of a equate funding for injury prevention research and practice. As noted

TABLE 5-1   Interventions That Are Proven Effective, That Are Promising, or That Require More Research in Preventing or Reducing the Severity of Motor Vehicle-related Injuries Associated with Selected Causes and Conditions

	Effectiveness of Intervention		
Cause or Condition	Proven Effective— Implement and Monitor	Promising—Implement but Monitor Closely and Evaluate Outcomes	Require Further Research
Impaired driving	Administrative license suspension Enforcement of minimum legal drinking age laws Dram shop laws (civil liability of servers of alcoholic beverages) Implementation of compulsory BAC tests in traffic injury cases	Use of BAC of .05 g/ml or above as per se evidence of impaired driving Raising state and federal alcohol excise taxes to reduce alcohol availability Server training programs directed at waiters, waitresses, and bartenders Educational programs to prevent impaired driving among youths and young adults Use of road edgelines and wrong-way signs	Institute a lower BAC for teenage drivers Use of sobriety checkpoints Alcohol safety education schools for convicted drunk drivers Designated driver Ignition interlock systems Use of certain roadway countermeasures, including raised lane delineators, rumble strips, and herringbone patterns
Occupant protection	Enactment and enforcement of safety belt use laws Uniform, comprehensive laws requiring safety seat use for all children up to age 5 should be adopted in all 50 states Continued implementation and monitoring of child safety seat loaner programs targeted particularly at low-income parents	Requiring safety belt use by employees who drive in federal, state, municipal, or private fleet motor vehicles Local ordinances requiring taxicabs to have accessible and usable safety belts Requiring rental car companies to provide loaner child safety seats Educational and behavioral change interventions for increasing safety belt and child safety seat use	Improvement of safety belt systems to provide optimal protection and comfort for children under the age of 14 and the elderly Development and use of safety seats for low-birthweight infants

TABLE 5-1 *Continued*

	Effectiveness of Intervention		
Cause or Condition	Proven Effective— Implement and Monitor	Promising—Implement but Monitor Closely and Evaluate Outcomes	Require further Research
Vehicle design	Installation of integral rather than adjustable headrests in all motor vehicles	Integrating traffic safety information into health risk appraisals Lowering of bumper heights	
Motorcyclists and bicyclists	Enactment of helmet laws in all states	Use of conspicuity-enhancement measures and devices Motorcycle rider education Moped legislation Construction and maintenance of bicycle paths and lanes	Bicycle safety programs
Pedestrians	One-way street networks and conversion of two-way to one-way streets Adequate roadway lighting Use of roadway barriers Use of conspicuity-enhancement devices and materials by all nighttime pedes-trians and bicy-clists	Moving a transit bus or school bus stop location from near side to far side of an intersection Pedestrian safety education for children	Adverse effect of crosswalk markings Curb parking regulations Use of traffic signals and pedestrian indicator ligh Relative effecti* ness of vario* types of legis* tion to reduce pedestrian injuries Interventions targeted towa* the elderly pedestrian Adverse effects right-on-red la*

Note: BAC = blood alcohol concentration.

SOURCE: U.S. National Committee for Injury Prevention and Control, 1989.

Injury in America (National Research Council, 1985) and more recently in *Cost of Injury in the United States* (Rice et al., 1989), total expenditures for injury research amount to only 11 percent of the National Cancer Institute's obligations and 17 percent of the National Heart, Lung, and Blood Institute's obligations. Yet productivity losses associated with injury death alone (36 life years lost per death) exceed those associated with cancer (16 years lost), stroke (11 years), or heart disease (12 years). Deaths are only a small fraction of the injury problem, however. For every death an estimated 400 individuals survive an injury. Although considerable progress has been made in identifying injury as a public health priority, adequate resources for the prevention of injuries through application of existing knowledge and the development of new strategies are still lacking.

A second clear-cut conclusion is that, although numerous interventions have been shown to effectively reduce the incidence and severity of injuries, very few strategies have been broadly implemented. One of the major barriers to implementation has been the lack of evidence demonstrating cost savings (Rice et al., 1989).

Despite some estimates of large potential costs savings, implementation of interventions perceived as restricting individual liberties often meets strong resistance. A long-standing controversy in injury control concerns the right of governments to restrict individual liberty in the name of public health. Opponents of bicycle and motorcycle helmet laws have not challenged this basic principle, but they argue that the choice not to wear a helmet endangers only the individual and does not jeopardize the public. Yet the costs accrued as a consequence of injuries to those who do not wear helmets are substantial, and a significant fraction of these costs is borne by public agencies and society at large (U.S. National Committee for Injury Prevention and Control, 1989). It has been estimated that in 1985 nearly one-third of the costs associated with direct health care expenditures and 27 percent of transfer payments due to injury were paid by public sources (Rice et al., 1989). A better understanding of the real and perceived barriers to implementation will help ensure that the public benefits from the results of research and evaluation.

> *Research is needed to evaluate the benefits and costs of injury prevention programs and policies. This would include an assessment of the social, economic, and political barriers to implementation of prevention strategies. Implementation of those strategies that are shown to be cost-beneficial should be given high priority.*

As summarized in *Injury in America* (National Research Council, 1985), there are three types of strategies for preventing injuries: (1) persuading persons at risk to change their behavior, (2) requiring people to refrain from risky behaviors by law or administrative rule, and (3) providing automatic protection through product and environmental design. It is generally ac-

cepted that countermeasures involving the third approach are the most effective because individual behavior is minimally affected. Indeed, groups at
highest risk of injury are often the least likely to alter their behavior in
response to education or legislative mandate.

*The potential success of programs and policies aimed at changing
risky behavior should not be underestimated. Research is needed on
behavioral risk factors related to injury in order to develop and improve
effective interventions.*

Another conclusion that can be drawn from the literature is that com-
paratively little is known about the risk factors associated with falls; possible
countermeasures are rarely researched (National Research Council, 1985)
Falls rank highest among all nonfatal injuries in both incidence and cost
and constitute a leading cause of disabling conditions in the United States
nevertheless, there is limited information about the risk factors associated
with falls (National Research Council, 1985).

*More research is needed to identify and improve our understand-
ing of risk factors associated with falls and to develop effective
countermeasures that would reduce the number and severity of falls.
Necessary elements of such an approach include research, regulatory
change, and public education.*

Finally, the abuse of alcohol and drugs is known to be a major contribu
tor to injuries of all etiology. As will be discussed in later sections, alcohol
and drug use can also play an important role in recovery from major trauma
in the acute and rehabilitation phases.

*Research is needed to develop and implement a comprehensive,
coordinated approach to reducing the number of injuries resulting
from alcohol and drug abuse. A coordinated approach should involve
new legislation, regulatory change, and public education.*

A SYSTEMS APPROACH TO ACUTE
CARE AND REHABILITATION

Although primary prevention efforts should be given highest priority, the
is also a need to ensure that people who survive potentially disabling inju
receive adequate acute care and rehabilitation. Meeting this need is particular
important because of the growing number of survivors who sustain seve
injuries that result in significant physical and cognitive impairment, and f
whom the prevention of secondary conditions is important.

The Systems Approach

Universal access to coordinated systems of care that integrate treatment from the site of the injury through long-term community follow-up is recognized as essential for mitigating the short-term effects of SCI and TBI and for controlling the effects of long-term disabling conditions. The four basic elements of such a coordinated approach are summarized below:

• *Emergency Medical Services (and Acute Medical/Surgical Care)*: Prompt recognition and treatment of the injured person at the scene with rapid transport to a designated trauma center specifically designed to treat individuals with neurological injuries.

• *Acute (Medical) Rehabilitation*: Begins in the acute phase and continues with an integrated, comprehensive inpatient rehabilitation care facility specifically designed to care for SCI and TBI survivors and their families. These services focus on physical and cognitive restoration of the individual.

• *Psychosocial and Vocational Rehabilitation Services*: Services aimed at preparing the individual for independent living and community reintegration. Although initiated during the inpatient phase of acute (medical) rehabilitation, the majority of these services are delivered within the structure of a transitional living center, day program, or outpatient services.

• *Lifelong Comprehensive Follow-up*: Includes medical, social, psychological, and vocational follow-up on a regularly scheduled basis.

The scope and volume of services required at each stage of the system of care will, of course, depend on the nature and severity of the injury. However, some general statements can be made. For example, emergency services and acute care for an individual with SCI should be designed to prevent a second injury to the spinal cord, necessitating appropriate stabilization of the spine before arriving at the hospital. In the hospital, definitive stabilization of the spine and measures to prevent such complications as deep vein thrombosis, pulmonary emboli, pneumonia, contractures, and decubiti must be performed by experienced personnel. Medical rehabilitation services should begin immediately in the acute phase to minimize physical deterioration and prevent further impairment and functional limitation due to loss of strength and range of motion, bladder and bowel incontinence, and inadequate or inappropriate training and provision of equipment. Accurate assessment and preparation for return to work and independent living during acute care can help alleviate some of the feelings of hopelessness and depression that an injured person often experiences. Psychosocial and vocational rehabilitation should continue the effort to prevent medical complications and increase functioning. Upon returning to the community, the individual can benefit from proactive community outreach programs in housing, transportation, recreation, employment, and other activities.

Although a coordinated approach to the treatment of TBI patients shares many of the same elements as that for SCI patients, there are differences in the type and sequence of services required. As summarized previously, residual deficits associated with TBI are mainly cognitive, behavioral, and psychological. People with TBI require a constellation of cognitive rehabilitation services not typically needed by an individual recovering from a severe SCI. Also, TBI survivors often have difficulty generalizing what they learn to new situations or problems. Therefore, skills learned in an inpatient acute care or rehabilitation facility may not be transferable to community living. Transitional living centers, day treatment programs, and outpatient services become important components of a coordinated approach to caring for TBI survivors. The complexity of the care continuum in rehabilitation following TBI is discussed by Uomoto and McLean (1989) and is summarized in Figure 5-4. It is important to note, however, that persons sustaining mild or minor head injury may require initial treatment on an outpatient basis only. Appropriate follow-up of these individuals is important for identifying and treating potential late sequelae, including recurrent headaches, memory problems, and psychosocial and behavioral problems.

Significant progress has been made in developing comprehensive systems of care for individuals with SCI. With funding from the National Institute on Disability and Rehabilitation Research, 13 model systems have been established during the past two decades. Through uniform data collection these systems of care have documented "(1) the system's continually increasing national capture rate; (2) reduced time between injury and admission to the system; (3) reduced length of stays; (4) cost-containment efforts; (5) reduced complication rates; (6) reduced mortality statistics; (7) changes in patterns and extensiveness of neurological involvement; and (8) change in domestic and vocational patterns following spinal cord injury" (Stover and Fine, 1986). Although these data provide evidence in support of the effectiveness of SCI systems of care, it is important that comprehensive studies be conducted in which patient outcomes are compared with the outcomes of those who do not receive care within the system. Analyses to date lack appropriate controls and are not population based, due in part to a lack of mandatory reporting of SCI and its consequences.

Whereas systems of care for SCI patients have existed for almost two decades, TBI systems are still evolving. The number of dedicated rehabilitation programs for TBI has grown from 40 in 1980 to about 700 in 1988 (Dixon 1989), but federally funded systems of care for TBI patients have only recently been established and have yet to adopt a uniform data set (J. Thomas, Medical Sciences Programs, National Institute on Disability and Rehabilitation Research, personal communication, 1989).

The following sections review in more detail the four elements of coordinated systems of care for SCI and TBI that were summarized above. Attention

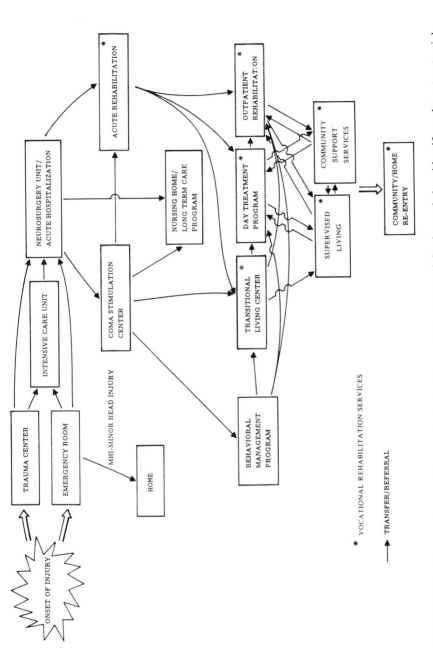

FIGURE 5-4 Care continuum in traumatic brain injury. Follow-up activity is needed to identify and treat potential sequelae in persons who initially require only outpatient treatment (see the box marked "Home"). Source: Uomoto and McLean, 1989. Reprinted with permission.

is focused on the potential for interrupting the chain of events leading from injury to impairment to functional limitation and disability. Table 5-2 summarizes what is known to be effective in minimizing impairment, maximizing functional capacity, and preventing disability, as well as what needs to be known to develop better and more efficient systems of care.

Emergency Medical Services

The nature of the trauma determines the initial severity of the injury to the central nervous system and to a substantial degree also determines the extent of the resulting impairment and functional limitation. Sufficient trauma to the brain may result in cardiopulmonary death, and direct injury to the upper cervical spinal cord may result in death due to paralysis of the muscles of respiration. Should the patient survive the primary injury, however, several other types of injury can occur and increase the extent and severity of impairment and functional limitation. These other types of injury (described below) are *secondary injury* to the central nervous system, additional *second injury* to the spinal cord, *associated injury* to other organs at the time of the initial event, and medical *complications* of other body systems. A primary role of emergency medical systems, acute care, and medical rehabilitation is to mitigate these effects and ensure maximum function. However, as the National Research Council (1985) and the U.S. Interagency Head Injury Task Force (1989) have noted, more information is needed on effective interventions.

Secondary Injury Primary injury to the brain results in focal hemorrhage or diffuse injury to axons and in hypoxia. The spinal cord, similarly, may sustain initial contusion, hemorrhage, and hypoxia associated with a disruption of the spine and surrounding structures (Becker and Povlishock, 1985). The cascade of events that follow the initial injury often results in further damage *(secondary injury)* to the nervous system. For example, diffuse brain swelling and space-occupying lesions resulting from TBI can contribute to increased intracranial pressure that can further contribute to ischemia and hypoxia—factors that contribute to impaired function and death. The mechanisms and pathophysiology underlying these changes remain unclear and in need of further research (National Research Council, 1985).

Second Injury The initial trauma of SCI can cause responses such as swelling, hemorrhage, and hypoxia. In TBI patients, drug treatment to remove focal hematomas and control swelling and pressure is helpful, but in SCI patients only modest improvements are achieved. Failure to adequately stabilize the spine during extrication, transport to the hospital, and in the hospital may result in a *second injury* to the spinal cord, converting an in-

TABLE 5-2 Current Knowledge and Knowledge Still Needed to Minimize Impairment, Maximize Functional Capacity, and Reduce Disability Through Improved Systems of Care for Persons with Spinal Cord Injury (SCI) and Traumatic Brain Injury (TBI)

Condition or System of Care	What Is Known	What Needs to be Known
SECONDARY INJURY TO CENTRAL NERVOUS SYSTEM	Control of intracranial pressure and early removal of blood clots is accepted treatment in TBI. International classification of severe TBI is accepted.	Basic research is needed into swelling of the brain and spinal cord postinjury. The methods and role of nutritional and neuroendocrine factors in TBI also need study.
	Increased understanding of pathophysiology has been gained in animal studies, as well as increased understanding of the mechanisms and dynamics of spine and spinal cord injury in animal models.	Evaluation is needed of current methods to stabilize the spine and their effects on neurological recovery in SCI.
		Evaluation is needed of the effectiveness of triage of patients with TBI and SCI to trauma centers in regard to reduction of secondary injury to SCI and appropriate management of associated injuries.
	Increased understanding has been gained of "post-concussion syndrome."	Development and refinement of methods should occur to determine the effectiveness of interventions in mild head injury.
COMPLICATIONS Neuro-musculo-skeletal	Exercises are effective in maintaining strength and range of motion. Drugs, surgery, and physical measures are of some benefit in control of spasticity and pain.	Newer methods of drug and electrical implantation devices need to be evaluated in spasticity. Electrical stimulation in prevention of atrophy and increase of strength requires further investigation. Effects of splints and phenol blocks need to be evaluated in treatment of spasticity in TBI. Clinical trials in treatment of heterotopic ossification are needed in SCI and TBI.

TABLE 5-2 *Continued*

Condition or System of Care	What Is Known	What Needs to be Known
	Effective methods for control of contractures, spasticity, and disuse weakness are known in the hospital phase.	Factors that contribute to progressive spasticity, contracture, and weakness with associated impairment posthospitalization need to be studied. Increased long-term incidence of arthritis in the shoulders and progressive weakness in the older SCI patient needs study.
Cardiovascular/ pulmonary	Prevention of deep vein thrombosis in SCI has recently been reported with use of electrical stimulation and heparin. Mechanisms of development of atelectasis/ pneumonia are better understood in SCI. High-level quadriplegic patients can be effectively managed on portable ventilators at home.	Larger clinical trials are needed to demonstrate the effectiveness of deep vein thrombosis and pulmonary embolus prevention. Studies on prevention of atelectasis/ pneumonia and risk factors of future pulmonary complications are indicated.
	Deep vein thrombosis, pulmonary embolus, and orthostatic hypotension are seldom a problem postdischarge.	Cardiovascular deconditioning needs to be studied in SCI and TBI individuals who are sedentary postdischarge.
Gastrointestinal/ genitourinary	Bowel training is effective in producing continence. Renal management can result in significant decrease in morbidity and mortality in SCI.	Clinical trials on the benefit of intermittent catheterization are needed. The value of drugs and electrical stimulation in the management of the neurogenic bladder should be determined. Long-term use of drugs and penile implants should be evaluated for treatment of impotence in SCI.
	Renal scans are an effective method to follow renal function and screen for complications in SCI.	Complications of the urinary tract in SCI need to be monitored postdischarge. Studies are needed as to the best methods of urinary tract prophylaxis for infection in SCI postdischarge.

TABLE 5-2 *Continued*

Condition or System of Care	What Is Known	What Needs to be Known
Integument (skin)	Pressure sores are preventable with proper attention to weight relief. Effective types of cushions and beds are available for longer-term prevention. Pressure sores can be effectively prevented in the hospital and postdischarge with adequate nursing care, patient education, and use of appropriate equipment.	Education of emergency medical services and trauma personnel is needed to apply known effective measures. New devices and electrical stimulation for prevention of pressure sores need further investigation. Factors that contribute to pressure sores postdischarge need further study to identify effective interventions.
IMPAIRMENT AND FUNCTIONAL LIMITATION	Recovery of motor power distal to the zone of injury is known in large groups, and recent information on recovery at the zone of injury is available in SCI. Recovery of motor power in TBI is not well appreciated. Some information exists on cognitive remediation in stroke patients but little in TBI. Clusters of cognitive disorders: attention, concept formation, executive functions, self-regulation of affect, and memory have been identified. Training of patients with SCI is effective, and large studies show significant gains in function from admission to discharge. Training of	More precise information on the extent and duration of motor recovery is needed to determine effectiveness of various interventions such as surgery, functional electrical stimulation, and other interventions on recovery and function. Motor recovery in TBI should be studied. Strength and fatigue studies should be correlated with upper and lower extremity function. Standardization of tests, categorization of patients, and potential interventions such as cognitive retraining devices need to be developed and evaluated. Various self-help devices and environmental control systems need to be evaluated. Precise relationship of strength to function in quadriplegic patients needs study. Effect of

TABLE 5-2 *Continued*

Condition or System of Care	What Is Known	What Needs to be Known
	patients with hemiplegia has been shown to be effective, but studies in TBI are limited.	self-care retraining with various categories of cognitive deficits in TBI needs evaluation.
	Mobility can be achieved in virtually all SCI individuals with training, orthotics, and manual or powered wheelchairs.	New developments in orthoses and functional electrical stimulation to assist ambulation in SCI need further refinement and evaluation. Centers for the development of advanced technology need to be identified to facilitate investigative interaction between rehabilitation professionals and engineers.
Neurobehavioral	Cognitive and behavioral factors limit function in self-care and community living.	Classification of cognitive/behavioral impairments and their natural course of recovery in TBI require study.
	Coma stimulation programs, day care, and transitional living programs have proliferated in recent years in response to the needs of a large TBI population.	Standard setting for and evaluation of the effectiveness of these alternative placement environments on cognitive/behavioral remediation are essential.
	Recent studies identify recovery from the persistent vegetative state (PVS) based on duration.	Costs and alternative care requirements need longitudinal assessment in PVS.
DISABILITY AND QUALITY OF LIFE		
Vocational	Return to work increases to 30% in paraplegic individuals 5 years postdischarge.	The disparity in capacity and actual return to work requires measurement and factor analysis in SCI and TBI.
	Barriers to employment have been identified, such as loss of health benefits and inadequate evaluation of retraining limits.	Effects of removal or reduced barriers to employment need evaluation.

TABLE 5-2 *Continued*

Condition or System of Care	What Is Known	What Needs to be Known
	Legislative authority for employment of people with disabilities was recently enacted.	The effect of legislative action should be evaluated in return to employment by people with SCI and TBI.
Psychological	Severe depression is uncommon in SCI in the hospital and early discharge period.	The incidence of depression, suicide, and other self-destructive behaviors over time is not known in SCI and TBI.
	Disruptive behavior that is disabling is common in TBI in the early discharge period.	The natural course of recovery from behavioral dysfunction in TBI requires study.
	Frustration and hopelessness are felt to contribute to medical complication in SCI and disability.	Interventions based on careful monitoring of psychological adjustment postinjury require study.
	Some behaviors that are disruptive to function are controlled with psychotropic agents.	The effects of psychotropic agents and other interventions require evaluation in TBI.
Social	Most individuals with SCI are quite active. High quadriplegic individuals on respirators may achieve a significant quality of life.	Normative data are needed for quality of life in SCI and TBI based on severity of impairment and disability.
	Severe SCI and TBI individuals are a significant burden of care for the family.	The longitudinal needs of attendant care and respite care based on severity of disability require study.
	Of SCI individuals in systems of care, 94% return directly to the community from rehabilitation hospitals. A great proportion of TBI individuals require alternative placement from the rehabilitation hospital.	Quality of life and cost differences for attentive placement in SCI need to be determined.
	Peer counseling through independent living centers has (perceived) value to individual adjustments.	Standards development and effectiveness measurement need to be carried out in TBI alternative care settings.

TABLE 5-2 *Continued*

Condition or System of Care	What Is Known	What Needs to be Known
	Cost data of longitudinal care will soon be available.	Factors such as assertiveness training, education, and advocacy which result in effective interventions should be studied Limitation of various categories of insurance for essential services and equipment should b« determined.

complete lesion into a complete lesion, which not only increases impair ment but also diminishes the prognosis for recovery (National Researc Council, 1985).

Associated Injury Persons with central nervous system trauma often hav« multiple injuries to other organs, and these *associated injuries* can contrib ute to further complications and impairment. For example, recent studie indicate that as many as 82 percent of patients with TBI sustain associate injuries (Bontke, 1989). These associated injuries include fractures of lon bones, skull, and spine; chest and abdominal injuries; and peripheral nerv damage (Stover and Fine, 1986). The high incidence of associated injurie is related to the major role that motor vehicle crashes play in causing cen tral nervous system trauma.

Finally, about 10 percent of TBI patients have associated SCI, and 1 percent of SCI patients have associated severe TBI. Compared with thos who damage only one organ of the central nervous system, both group sustain greater impairment and subsequent disability. A recent report indicate that up to half of SCI patients may have a mild head injury, but the inci dence of long-term impairment in these cases is not known (Davidoff et al 1988). A reduction in overall impairment and mortality may be achievabl by improving the skill with which TBI and SCI patients are managed (Nationa Research Council, 1985).

Complications (Secondary Conditions) The effect of medical compli cations on individual function is significant. Patients with SCI and TB often have similar complications that contribute to impairment and func tional limitation, including complications to the cardiopulmonary-vasculai neuromusculoskeletal, and genitourinary-gastrointestinal systems; howevei considerably more is known about the incidence and potential for interven tion in patients with SCI than in those with TBI (Young et al., 1982; Stover and Fine, 1986). In large part, this lack of information on TBI is attributable to a more mature system of neurological classification and data collection on SCI (Stover and Fine, 1986). For TBI, classification and data collection are relatively new and present more complicated problems (Bachy-Rita, 1989). Consequently, efforts to quantify the effectiveness of various intervention strategies in TBI lag behind similar efforts in SCI.

On closer inspection, certain types of complications that appear to be similar are substantially different in the SCI and TBI patient. For example, heterotopic ossification, a cause of contractures, occurs predominantly in the upper extremities in TBI, whereas it occurs predominantly in the lower extremities in SCI (Venier and Ditunno, 1971). Spasticity during the acute phase of TBI may frequently require casting to prevent contracture (Weintraub and Opat, 1989), but this is seldom required in SCI. Other complications are seen exclusively in TBI, such as cognitive dysfunction, linguistic and cranial nerve deficits, personality change, hydrocephalus, and seizures. Disseminated vascular clotting and neuroendocrine disorders are also prominent in TBI (Bontke, 1989; National Research Council, 1985).

Deep vein thrombosis is a very common medical complication and occurs in 80 percent to 100 percent of completely paralyzed SCI patients, leading to pulmonary embolism, one of the most frequent causes of early death. Recent studies provide evidence of effective methods of prevention, and these methods should be used more widely (Merli et al., 1988; Green et al., 1988). Occurring in 60 percent to 80 percent of high-level quadriplegic patients, pulmonary complications such as atelectasis and pneumonia are another major cause of mortality and morbidity. Improved understanding of the underlying mechanisms could point the way to more effective interventions (Fishburn et al., 1990).

Infection of the urinary tract is another common complication in SCI and TBI patients who use indwelling Foley catheters. However, advances in the use of intermittent catheterization and improved measures of follow-up in persons with SCI have been reported to reduce renal disease as a major cause of death in the long-term patient (Stover and Fine, 1986). Recurrent urinary tract infection and complications, however, continue to be a source of functional limitation and, at times, are associated with autonomic hypertension and increased spasticity. Impaired bowel function is common in both groups of patients because of immobility.

Contractures associated with muscle weakness and imbalance, spasticity, and heterotopic ossification constitute a type of medical complication that can lead to significant impairment and functional limitation. Limited shoulder motion resulting from contractures, for example, may make it impossible for an individual to put on a shirt or reach overhead; walking is severely compromised if strength recovers but the knees and hips are permanently fused in flexion, not allowing proper standing and ambulation. A recent study (Yarkony and Sahgal, 1987) reported an 85 percent incidence of contractures in craniocerebral trauma cases transferred to a rehabilitation unit; frequency was related to duration of coma. In SCI and TBI patients, contractures are most effectively prevented when bed positioning and therapies to maintain motion are instituted early and are continued throughout all phases of recovery.

Pressure sores are perhaps the most commonly cited medical complication associated with SCI. Nutritional deficiency, which may be prevalent early in the conditions of TBI and SCI patients, contributes to tissue breakdown and has been found to correlate with outcome (Ragnarsson, in press). Recurrent pressure sores do occur in a small proportion of patients after discharge, and improved strategies for prevention during this phase are needed. However, proper education and training in combination with assistive equipment can be effective in preventing this condition. SCI patients suffer severe pressure sores almost twice as often before arriving at a model system care facility as after entry into the facility (Young et al., 1982).

Basic and clinical research is needed in conjunction with improved surveillance data to develop and improve effective interventions for the prevention, management, and reduction of injury-related damage to the central nervous system. In particular, emphasis should be given to the reduction of medical complications that contribute to short- and long-term disability in persons with SCI and TBI.

Acute (Medical) Rehabilitation

Beginning a course of rehabilitation necessitates the assessment of a person's physical and mental status. In terms of the committee's disability model, it is important to establish the stage in the progression, the risk factors, and the relevant preventive interventions. Depending on the type of impairment, for example, different interventions can be used during rehabilitation to help prevent the development of functional limitations. In persons with SCI, reduced motor power is the major cause of functional limitation. Among persons with TBI, acute weakness of one side occurs in 18 percent of cases (Eisenberg, 1985) and usually improves without contributing to significant limitation. Most functional limitations associated with severe head injury are attributable to neurobehavioral impairments (Levin, 1985; Bleiberg et al., 1989; Diller and Ben-Yishay, 1989).

Virtually all studies of rehabilitation in SCI patients are concerned with the capacity for self-care and mobility and how they relate to the severity of the neurological deficit (Ditunno et al., 1987; Welch et al., 1986; Yarkony et al., 1988). Strengthening exercises have been shown to increase motor power in partially paralyzed muscles and are therefore important in preventing certain SCI impairments from progressing to functional limitations. In addition, recent studies (Ditunno et al., 1987, 1989a, 1989b) have shown sufficient recovery of motor power in the arms of quadriplegic patients to enable significant improvement in function during rehabilitation and at the time of one-year follow-up.

Recently reported research (Bracken et al., 1990) has demonstrated that treatment with methylprednisolone within 8 hours of spinal cord injury significantly improved the recovery of motor and sensory function. Because most people with acute SCI are admitted to a hospital within the critical 8-hour period, this intervention has great potential for reducing disabling conditions. The study, however, did not measure functional improvement.

Improved cardiovascular conditioning of paraplegic individuals is an important part of rehabilitation and can be achieved through aerobic exercises, especially in young people. Such conditioning enables many to participate in wheelchair sports and to walk in braces with crutches.

Functional electrical stimulation (FES) has been promoted as having several potential applications. These include increasing strength and endurance and preventing osteoporosis in paraplegic and quadriplegic individuals, although these claims have not been evaluated rigorously (Ragnarsson et al., 1988). Another application of FES is in implantable electrodes to enable upper extremity grasping and thus self-feeding by persons with high-level quadriplegia (Peckham et al., 1986). Applications of FES in ambulation (Marsolais and Kobetic, 1988) and prevention of pressure sores (Davidoff et al., 1988) show early promise but require further development and evaluation.

Individuals with complete paralysis of leg muscles can learn to get in and out of bed, bathe, dress, use the toilet, and dress without assistance by learning certain skillful maneuvers and using adaptive equipment. A high level of independence can be achieved with the aid of adaptive equipment and training in feeding, dressing, bathing, using a wheelchair, and driving a car. Even people with paralysis in all limbs can reduce dependency through the use of technology that permits such individuals to unlock doors, turn on lights, and operate a phone or a computer. The opportunity for enhancing functional capacity and independence in people with paralysis is great, meriting an expanded research and development effort on new assistive technologies.

Educational programs that help individuals perform self-care activities are an integral part of the rehabilitation process, which begins in the acute phase of injury and continues throughout the life course. Modification of procedures, tasks, and schedules according to the needs of the individual facilitates functioning on the job and in other social contexts. Eventually, these modifications should become the exclusive responsibility of the person with the potentially disabling condition. Another example is learning to control bladder and bowel dysfunction, which occurs in most individuals with injury to the spinal cord. Control of these functions is an important aspect of rehabilitation. With skillful training, more than 90 percent of SCI patients are capable of bladder and bowel continence. Training also includes education on how to avoid bladder infection and prevent other potentially disabling conditions.

People with TBI often have more extensive impairment of the nervous system than do people with SCI because TBI can result in focal or diffuse lesions in any part of the brain. Paralysis, spasticity and rigidity, ataxia, and other disorders affecting coordination in the hands or legs can lead to functional limitation. Posttraumatic involvement of the sensory, labyrinth, or cerebellar-mediated systems results in ataxia in 20 percent to 30 percent of people sustaining diffuse brain injury (Weintraub and Opat, 1989). In these cases, functional limitation is common because of difficulties in hand performance of fine motor skills and in gross motor skills such as walking.

Although the true incidence of cranial nerve involvement is unknown, loss of the sense of smell occurs in 7 percent to 25 percent of all head injury patients (Berrol, 1989). Because any of the cranial nerves may be involved, impairments caused by head injury include defective smell, vision, taste, and hearing and thus often limit the amount of information available from the environment; however, the effects of these impairments on function are unclear.

As many as 40 percent of all people with TBI experience problems in communication due to partial aphasia. Other linguistic limitations such as naming, sentence repetition, and word fluency occur in an additional 30 percent or more of cases (Levin and Goldstein, 1989). Because little is known about the natural course of these limitations, interventions that might improve function are lacking.

Assessment of the neurobehavioral impairments that contribute to the greatest functional limitations in TBI is a considerable research need. Cognitive impairments, which may be grouped into problems with attention, concept formation, executive function, self-regulation of affect, and memory, have been identified and occur in the majority of patients with head injury (Diller and Ben-Yishay, 1989). However, information on how these impairments affect function, particularly self-care, is very limited.

Finally, when motor impairment occurs along with neurobehavioral dysfunction, traditional instruments for evaluating function and the results of intervention may be of limited value. For example, the reason why some individuals do not dress themselves may not be because of paralysis but because they sit on the bed without initiating any movement (Diller and Ben-Yishay, 1989).

Although training individuals with cognitive deficits to become more functional has yielded some encouraging results, better tests to measure executive function, process function, and acceptance and awareness need to be developed (Diller and Ben-Yishay, 1989).

In summary, acute (medical) rehabilitation is an important component of the systems approach to acute care and rehabilitation. However, because impairments in strength, tone, coordination, and information transmission may be superimposed on cognitive and behavioral impairments, better indexes that integrate impairment, functional limitation, and disability need to be developed to determine the effectiveness of rehabilitation interventions. These assessments must be applied to the proliferating alternative treatment environments in TBI care, such as day treatment and cognitive rehabilitation.

Basic and clinical rehabilitation research is needed in the prevention, management, and reduction of the motor impairment associated with SCI and the neurobehavioral impairment associated with TBI. In particular, more thorough study is needed of motor recovery in SCI patients and the effectiveness of various interventions such as surgery, drugs, and rehabilitation in reducing impairment and improving function.

Future research should focus on potential applications of functional electrical stimulation, development and testing of new assistive technologies, and the causal relationships between TBI and the senses of smell, vision, taste, and hearing, as well as the causal relationship between TBI and aphasia.

Better tests to measure higher cortical function (e.g., executive function, process function, and acceptance and awareness) are needed to facilitate evaluation of rehabilitation effectiveness. These indexes should integrate measures of impairment, functional limitation, and disability.

An obvious need is for consistent classification and categorization of TBI severity. Such classification can serve as a basis for prognosis and permit reliable assessments of the effectiveness of therapeutic interventions in reducing impairments.

Psychosocial and Vocational Rehabilitation and Lifelong Comprehensive Follow-up

Psychosocial and vocational interventions during acute and rehabilitation phases are directed at helping the individual and family members cope with the sudden and potentially devastating effects of the affected person's altered self-image and self-esteem. Prior to the patient being discharged into the community, the goal of such interventions is to offer vocational opportunities, with early assessment, and prepare the individual and family members for the adjustment to the affected person's altered but possibly independent lifestyle.

As functional recovery improves during the first year or more after the injury, the focus of rehabilitation shifts from medical intervention and physical restoration to psychosocial and vocational adaptation. The ultimate goal of psychosocial and vocational rehabilitation is community reintegration. For children and adolescents, this may mean returning to school. For adults, returning to work is an important component of reintegration. It is important to emphasize that services aimed at community reintegration must consider not only attributes and limitations of the injured individual, but also the social, educational, and vocational systems in which the individual will function.

It has long been recognized that individuals vary greatly in their ability to adapt to a functional limitation. As discussed in Chapter 3, variability in outcome depends on a host of personal and environmental factors, some of which are mutable. Although a comprehensive review of the necessary components of an integrated, coordinated approach to community reintegration is beyond the scope of this report, a brief summary of some of the more important elements follows. The reader is referred to Chapters 18-20 of *Traumatic Brain Injury* (Bach-y-Rita, 1989) for a more complete discussion of the issues.

Transitional living centers offer community-based residential programs that provide an opportunity for individuals to relearn and practice, in a protected but real-life environment, the skills necessary for living independently and productively. Although most individuals who sustain SCI return home following inpatient rehabilitation, the individual with severe TBI often requires the services of a transitional living center after discharge from an acute rehabilitation center.

When the structure of a residential program (e.g., a transitional living center) is no longer needed, individuals may still require additional training and support from day programs designed to prepare them further for reintegration into society. For individuals who continue to require assistance with activities of daily living, in-home services may be required.

Vocational services are crucial for ensuring that return-to-work goals are achieved. These services may include counseling and work readiness evaluations, job training, job placement, work-site modification, and postemployment services intended to ensure satisfactory adjustment to employment.

Independent living centers offer valuable resources throughout the process of recovery from TBI and SCI. These centers are primarily staffed by individuals with disabling conditions and provide a supportive network for individuals who want to achieve an independent lifestyle. The importance of independent living centers to the welfare of people with disabling conditions cannot be overemphasized. (Independent living centers are described in more detail in Chapter 7.)

Providers and consumers alike express concerns that existing psychosocial and vocational services do not adequately meet the needs of clients (National Council on the Handicapped, 1986). This is particularly true for services required by individuals with TBI. Special education, for example, often focuses on the needs of children with developmental disabilities. The child coping with the effects of a head injury is thought to have needs different from those of the child with a developmental disability. Yet school systems often do not recognize these special needs and do not have the necessary resources to address them. Similarly, vocational rehabilitation specialists often are not trained to specifically respond to the needs of the head-injured adult who may have no physical limitations but, because of inappropriate behavior or memory problems, has difficulty keeping a job.

Existing and alternative strategies for psychosocial and vocational rehabilitation of individuals with SCI and TBI need to be developed and assessed for their effectiveness. This will require longitudinal studies to measure both outcome and program costs. Research on outcomes of psychosocial and vocational rehabilitation should include measures of quality of life and not limit the definition of successful outcome solely to return to work, school, or household maintenance. Community-based programs, independent living centers, projects with industry, and alternative programs should be considered in research and evaluation projects.

Despite some questions about the efficacy of the increasing number of alternative strategies for rehabilitating people with SCI or TBI, it is clear that a wide range of community services are needed. It is also clear that many people who need these services do not receive them, and that quality psychosocial and vocational rehabilitation services aimed at reintegrating persons with disabling conditions into the community and back to work should be available to those who need them. The number of day programs is increasing but is still insufficient to meet the more rapidly increasing demand for such services (Jacobs, 1988). A major conclusion of the Los Angeles Head Injury Survey was that the rehabilitation needs of many persons with traumatic brain injury go unmet because of the geographic and financial inaccessibility of services. The shortage of services is even more acute in rural areas of the country.

Rehabilitation, especially neurobehavioral rehabilitation and psychosocial services, is rarely covered by private health insurance. The extent of coverage under Medicaid varies greatly from state to state, but, generally, Medicaid funding is restricted to inpatient medical rehabilitation and physical therapy. Financial support for transitional living centers and vocational

rehabilitation is more limited. Strict and often confusing eligibility require
ments for vocational rehabilitation programs further limit accessibility t
these services, especially for those with TBI.

> *Means for removing financial barriers that limit accessibility to
> rehabilitation services need to be studied. Such studies should evaluate
> the extent to which current public and private compensation pro-
> grams create nonproductive disincentives for rehabilitation and re-
> sumption of a productive role in society. In addition, the lack of
> public and private insurance coverage for neurobehavioral rehabilitation
> and psychosocial and vocational services should be examined.
> Multidisciplinary research is needed to develop a better understand-
> ing of the multiple factors, both medical and nonmedical, that contribute
> to disability and the overall quality of life following TBI and SCI.*

Given the problems associated with the availability and accessibility o
services, the family often assumes the major responsibility for providing
care and support to individuals with SCI or TBI (Jacobs, 1988). Thi
responsibility, often lifelong, may have a major impact on members of the
family, as well as on the family unit as a whole (Bach-y-Rita, 1989). Separation and divorce and financial difficulties are among the problems commonly
reported by families of persons who have sustained major trauma. These
problems are especially acute for families of persons with TBI (Brooks
1984). Additional problems arise when the primary caregiver dies.

Society must face the challenge of providing appropriate and adequate
support to individuals with major physical and neurobehavioral disabling
conditions. Addressing this need will require educating employers of the
rights and capabilities of people with disabling conditions associated with
TBI and SCI.

> *Expanded education programs are needed to inform the public
> about the legal rights of people with disabling conditions, including
> their rights to work and their guarantees of full participation in
> society, as is consistent with provisions of the Americans with Disabilities
> Act. Education programs are also needed to instruct employers in
> the special capabilities and needs of persons with TBI and SCI.*

In summary, there is a growing consensus that universal access to coordinated systems of care that integrate treatment from the site of injury
through long-term community follow-up is essential for mitigating the short-
term effects of SCI and TBI and for reducing long-term disability. However, the establishment of national and regional networks of SCI and TBI
systems of care that link state and local systems will need to be tested. For

TBI, testing of the entire system, its components, and overall effectiveness is needed; for SCI, more rigorous control is required. Closer working relationships between industry and vocational rehabilitation programs should also be fostered.

Coordinated systems of care that integrate treatment from the site of injury through long-term community follow-up are needed for mitigating the short-term effects of SCI and TBI and for reducing long-term disability.

Several studies have underscored the lack of adequate funding for injury prevention research and practice (National Research Council, 1985; Rice et al., 1989). Although considerable progress has been made in accurately describing and establishing injury as a major public health concern, greater resources must be directed to the prevention of injuries by applying existing knowledge and by developing new intervention strategies.

Available resources for injury prevention research and practice should reflect the importance of injury as one of the leading causes of disability. Consonant with the recommendations included in **Injury in America** *(National Research Council, 1985),* **Cost of Injury in the United States** *(Rice et al., 1989), and* **Injury Prevention** *(U.S. National Committee for Injury Prevention and Control, 1989), a Center for Injury Control is needed and should be established within the Centers for Disease Control to serve as a focal point for national injury prevention programs and activities. This would be an important component of a national disability prevention program.*

6

Prevention of Disability Associated with Chronic Diseases and Aging

Disease prevention and health promotion have been a strong focus of interest among policymakers, researchers, and practitioners in recent years. Demographers and epidemiologists have documented convincingly one significant outcome of disease prevention and health promotion: the revolutionary change in average life expectancy during the past two centuries. The first revolution in public health occurred when the basic principles of sanitation were understood and implemented and when basic nutritional needs could be met reliably in modernizing societies. In the eighteenth and nineteenth centuries, coping with acute bacterial and virus-related diseases ultimately led medical practitioners to better understand the importance of sanitation, adequate nutrition, and, eventually, medical immunization.

This first revolution has had at least two consequences: the age structure of modern society shifted as a result of increased average life expectancy, and acute disease was joined by chronic disease as a focus of public health attention. Chronic disease and its related disabling conditions, however, have not been responsive to the traditional public health interventions that were so successful in the first revolution. The continuing challenge of coping with chronic disease sets the stage for the second revolution in public health, which focuses on behavior and lifestyle modification as key components in health promotion and disease prevention.

The Canadian Lalonde report (1974) and the U.S. surgeon general's reports (U.S. Department of Health, Education, and Welfare, 1979; U.S. Department of Health and Human Services, 1980a) were notable public statements of a belief in the modifiability of risk factors with a specific focus on the potential benefits of behavioral and lifestyle modifications. The surgeon general's reports used the life course approach to set specific health objectives to be achieved by the year 1990 among children, adolescents, adults, and older persons. These reports noted the relevance of genetics, medical care, and toxic factors in the environment; however, behavior and lifestyle change were clearly the major foci. The reports were notable for their inclusion of older adults in the health objectives, affirming that although age and disease are associated, the association is conditional and modifiable.

Recent federal initiatives have focused on the older population as a target group for preventive care and health promotion activities. For example, the surgeon general sponsored a Workshop on Health Promotion and Aging (U.S. Department of Health and Human Services, 1988b), which documents the benefits of several interventions to lower existing risks among the elderly (see the discussion later in this chapter). The recent Healthy People 2000: National Health Promotion and Disease Prevention Objectives (U.S. Department of Health and Human Services, 1990) employs the life course approach in setting objectives, including goals to increase average life expectancy to 78 years, to reduce disability caused by chronic conditions to a prevalence of no more than 6 percent of all people, and to increase years of healthy life to at least 65 years. In the area of research, the National Institute on Aging is supporting studies to understand the aging process; to improve the diagnosis, treatment, and prevention of diseases that affect older people; and to improve their quality of life (National Institute on Aging, 1989).

There are several reasons for adopting a health promotion and disease prevention approach for older adults. Life expectancy is increasing, and it is desirable to enhance health status during these additional years of life. In addition, there is increasing evidence that some harmful habits and behaviors are amenable to modification or reversal when interventions occur in later years. This capacity for modifying physiological or pathological conditions has been referred to as the plasticity of the aging process (National Research Council, 1988). Finally, the high incidence of chronic disease and disabling conditions among the elderly and the burden disease places on individuals and society dictate the need for effective methods to ameliorate the deleterious effects of illness and disabling conditions that require costly medical care services.

The public perceives aging as a process of steady deterioration, which results in subtle discrimination that is sometimes referred to as ageism. The perception that age, chronic disease, and disability are equivalent conditions prevents our society from realizing the potential benefits of a disability-free life even among older persons. This perception has also influenced the social policies and social support networks developed in our society.

The public needs to be educated about the potential for modifying the aging processes through individual lifestyle change and through social policies ensuring adequate income, educational opportunities, and social support during a person's life course.

MAGNITUDE OF THE PROBLEM

The magnitude of disability associated with chronic conditions and aging can be measured from a variety of perspectives. Three of these perspectives—prevalence of chronic conditions and their risk of disability, prevalence of multiple chronic conditions, and limitation in basic life activities—will be discussed here. Because some chronic diseases occur before age 65, and because a life course perspective is important for considering chronic disease, aging, and disability, the data presented are not limited to the elderly.

Prevalence of Chronic Conditions

Although the prevalence of chronic illness increases with age and is a major cause of disabling conditions, many elderly persons are healthy and function independently. In 1988, 33.1 million people in the United States, or 13.7 percent of the noninstitutionalized population, reported some limitation of their activities as a result of chronic disease or impairment; 4.3 percent were limited, but not in their major activity; 5.4 percent were limited in the amount or kind of their major activity, and 4 percent—"the most severely disabled"—were unable to carry on their major activity (Table 6-1) (National Center for Health Statistics, 1989a). The prevalence of all three levels of activity limitation increases with age except for those with "severe disabilities," for whom the rates rise from less than one-half of 1 percent for those under 18 years to 16.2 percent for the 65- to 69-year-olds. For those 70 years and older, however, the prevalence rate falls to 7.6 percent. This reduction may be the result of the oldest old population entering institutions when they become severely disabled.

The prevalence of most chronic health conditions varies by age group. Table 6-2 presents estimates from the 1988 National Health Interview Survey (NHIS) of the number of chronic conditions and the rate per 1,000 persons for all noninstitutionalized persons and for the population aged 65 and older. The conditions are ranked according to their prevalence in the total population. The five most prevalent chronic conditions for all ages are chronic sinusitis, arthritis, high blood pressure, deformity or orthopedic impairment, and hay fever. For the elderly population, arthritis ranked highest with almost half (49 percent) reporting this condition, followed in rank order by high blood pressure (37 percent), hearing impairment (32 percent), heart disease (30 percent), and chronic sinusitis (12 percent) (Figure 6-1). The relative ranking of conditions depends on how the conditions are grouped. For example, if deformities of the back were shown separately, they would rank eighth for all ages and eleventh for the elderly. When combined with deformities or orthopedic impairments of the upper extremities, as shown in Table 6-2, they rank fourth for all ages and seventh for the

TABLE 6-1 Number and Distribution of Persons by Degree of Activity Limitation Due to Chronic Conditions and Age, 1988

Age	All Persons	With No Activity Limitation	With Activity Limitation	Limited But Not in Major Activity	Limited in Amount or Kind of Major Activity	Unable to Carry on Major Activity
Number (in thousands)						
Under 18 years	63,569	60,175	3,394	898	2,235	261
18-44	103,066	94,230	8,835	2,772	3,562	2,502
45-64	45,573	35,347	10,225	2,518	3,806	3,901
65 yrs and over	28,683	18,080	10,602	4,118	3,466	3,018
65-69	9,801	6,305	3,496	744	1,167	1,585
70 yrs and over	18,882	11,775	7,107	3,374	2,299	1,433
Total	240,890	207,833	33,057	10,305	13,069	9,682
Percent distribution						
Under 18 years	100.0	94.7	5.3	1.4	3.5	0.4
18-44	100.0	91.4	8.6	2.7	3.5	2.4
45-64	100.0	77.6	22.4	5.5	8.4	8.6
64 yrs and over	100.0	63.0	37.0	14.4	12.1	10.5
65-69	100.0	64.3	35.7	7.6	11.0	16.2
70 yrs and over	100.0	62.4	37.6	17.9	12.2	7.6
Total	100.0	86.3	13.7	4.3	5.4	4.0
Percent distribution by age						
Under 18 years	26.4	29.0	10.3	8.7	17.1	2.7
18-44	42.8	45.3	26.7	26.9	27.3	25.8
45-64	18.9	17.0	30.9	24.4	29.1	40.3
65 yrs and over	11.9	8.7	32.1	40.0	26.5	31.2
65-69	4.1	3.0	10.6	7.2	8.9	16.4
70 yrs and over	7.8	5.7	21.5	32.7	17.6	14.8
Total	100.0	100.0	100.0	100.0	100.0	100.0

SOURCE: National Center for Health Statistics, 1989a.

TABLE 6-2 Chronic conditions with highest prevalence in noninstitutionalized population, all ages and 65 years and older, 1988

Condition	All Ages			65 Years and Older		
	Rank	Number of Conditions (thousands)	Rate per 1,000 Persons	Rank	Number of Conditions (thousands)	Rate per 1,000 Persons
Chronic sinusitis	1	33,658	140	5	4,961	173
Arthritis	2	31,292	130	1	13,930	486
High blood pressure	3	29,257	122	2	10,698	373
Deformity or orthopedic impairment	4	26,878	112	7	4,621	161
Hay fever or allergic rhinitis without asthma	5	22,413	93	12	2,047	71
Hearing impairment	6	21,864	91	3	9,040	315
Heart disease	7	20,258	84	4	8,484	296
Chronic bronchitis	8	11,894	49	13	1,859	65
Hemorrhoids	9	11,031	46	14	1,849	65
Asthma	10	9,934	41	21	1,188	41
Migraine headache	11	9,222	38	41	529	18
Dermatitis	12	9,025	38	32	781	27
Visual impairment	13	8,365	35	9	2,602	91
Varicose veins of lower extremities	14	7,632	32	11	2,301	80
Tinnitus	15	6,361	26	10	2,407	84
Diabetes	16	6,221	26	8	2,649	92
Cataracts	17	6,105	25	6	4,810	168

SOURCE: National Center for Health Statistics, 1989b.

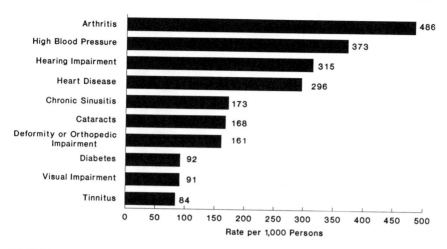

FIGURE 6-1 Prevalence to top 10 chronic conditions, age 65 and over, 1988. Source: National Center for Health Statistics, 1989a.

elderly (National Center for Health Statistics, 1989a). As noted in Chapter 2, however, one limitation of the NHIS data is that they are self-reported with no objective measurements.

Because of the large and significant contribution that chronic disease and aging make to disability, an in-depth study of this relationship is warranted. It should focus on disability prevention, health promotion, quality of life, and implications for public health.

Chronic Conditions Causing Disability

The higher-ranking prevalent chronic health conditions are not necessarily those that cause the most disability (defined here in terms of activity limitations). For example, a recent analysis by LaPlante (1989b), based on four years (1983-1986) of the NHIS, showed an inverse relationship between the prevalence of chronic health conditions and the risk of disability. As shown in Figure 6-2, conditions with high prevalence have low risks of disability, whereas conditions low in prevalence have high risks of disability. For example, sinusitis ranks highest in prevalence for all ages, but less than one-half of 1 percent of the persons with this condition report being limited in activity. By contrast, the three least prevalent conditions—absence of arms and/or hands, multiple sclerosis, and lung or bronchial cancer—have significantly higher risks of disability. Three-fourths of those with lung or bronchial cancer report being limited in activity.

Current data on chronic and disabling conditions are restricted to na-

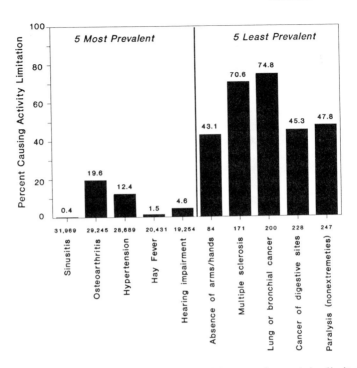

FIGURE 6-2 Percent of specific chronic conditions causing activity limitation for the five most prevalent and five least prevalent conditions, 1983-86. Source: LaPlante, 1989b. Reprinted with permission.

tional samples derived from cross-sectional surveys and provide only basic measures of activity limitation. Because most health and social service programs are coordinated at the state level, the lack of state-specific data hampers planning of services. Existing data systems are insensitive to changes in the prevalence of impairment and disability over time, and they do not measure the degree of limitation and disability that results from specific chronic diseases and mental illnesses, also undermining planning of prevention strategies.

Data collection reflects this nation's emphasis on acute care. It is episodic, and fixed on single points in time. In contrast, chronic diseases, by definition, are long-term conditions, and their impacts change over time.

Surveillance methods do not permit us to track the series of changes in health status, functional capacity, and quality of life that people with chronic disease are likely to experience. National and state systems of surveillance of disabling conditions should be refined so that functional limitation and disability resulting from chronic diseases and mental disorders can be measured and changes in the prevalence of these conditions can be monitored over time.

Multiple Chronic Conditions

Multiple chronic conditions have a significant impact on disability status. Many people, especially the elderly, have multiple chronic and potentially disabling conditions. Data from the NHIS for the three-year period from 1979 to 1981 indicate that multiple chronic conditions causing limitation of activity increase with age. For example, among those who report chronic conditions that cause limited activity, only 15 percent of the group under age 17 reported more than one condition; this proportion increased to 40 percent for those aged 75 and older (Rice, 1989).

In recent years, more people are reporting that they have chronic conditions that limit their activities. Analysis and comparison of the NHIS data from two three-year periods, 1969-1971 and 1979-1981, showed that the prevalence rate of limitations in activity increased significantly (Rice and LaPlante, 1988a). The rate increased more than one-fifth, from 119 to 145 per 1,000 persons, for the entire noninstitutionalized population, with greater increases for women than for men. The largest increases occurred for children and youth and for middle-aged persons, 45 to 64 years of age, especially for the "most disabled"—those unable to carry on their major activity. The prevalence rate of limitation declined slightly in later years (ages 75 and over), indicating that the health of the very old living in the community may have improved slightly. Comparison of health indicators over time for the very old, however, must account for changes in institutionalization, and this factor was not addressed in that report.

People with disabling conditions reported more chronic conditions and more days of restricted activity over the ten-year period 1969-1971 to 1979-1981. The number of chronic conditions per person causing limitation of activity increased 12.5 percent, from 1.32 to 1.48 per person with increases reported for all ages (Rice and LaPlante, 1988a). The greatest increase was for noninstitutionalized persons aged 85 and older, suggesting worsening health as the probable explanation. In general, the more severely limited population reported the greatest increases in multiple chronic conditions, which suggests that persons may be living longer with severely limiting chronic conditions.

Other researchers have found similar trends. Verbrugge (1984) analyzed past trends in specific chronic conditions, in disability (as defined by activity limitation), and in mortality for middle-aged and older persons reported in the NHIS over a 23-year period, 1958 to 1981. For middle-aged people, 10 of the 11 chronic diseases with high mortality rates had become more prevalent; over the same period, however, mortality rates declined for 8 of those diseases. Increased morbidity and declining mortality trends in chronic conditions for the elderly were similar. Verbrugge also noted an increase since the late 1960s in limitation of activity. She suggests that these increases may be caused by a variety of factors: there may be changes in "true" incidence and survival rates, individuals may be more accepting of and accommodating to their conditions, and they may be more likely to adopt the sick role than in the past.

Using data for nine commonly reported chronic conditions from the 1984 Supplement on Aging of the NHIS, Guralnik and colleagues (1989b) showed that the prevalence of comorbidity (multiple conditions) is substantial among the population aged 60 and older. High rates of comorbidity were reported for women, with prevalence rates rising from 45 percent in the age group 60 to 69 years to 70 percent in those 80 years and older. For those 60 years of age and older who had no chronic conditions, only 2.1 percent of men and 2.3 percent of women required assistance in performing one or more activities of daily living (ADLs). These rates increased to 8.6 percent for men and 6.9 percent for women who had 2 chronic conditions and to 22 percent for men and 15.7 percent for women who had 4 chronic conditions. In addition, there was a clear association between the number of conditions and the proportion of people with disability as assessed by inability to perform activities or self-care. The authors found that, for the most commonly reported pairs of comorbid conditions (i.e., high blood pressure and arthritis), the observed coprevalence was consistently higher than expected. Possible explanations for this finding include (1) detection bias (those with one condition may have more contacts with the medical care system and a greater likelihood of being diagnosed with a second condition); (2) response patterns (people who report one disease may be more likely to report having other diseases); and (3) biological basis (genetic and environmental factors may increase susceptibility to disease).

Limitation in Basic Life Activities

Measures of functioning in basic life activities, including ADLs and instrumental activities of daily living (IADLs), are important indicators of health status and disability. Analysis of data from the 1979 and 1980 Home Care Supplement to the NHIS shows 5.4 million persons who reported needing assistance in ADLs or IADLs; of this total, 43 percent were under age 65 (LaPlante, 1989b). Middle-aged adults who need assistance are somewhat more likely than either children or older adults to use equipment and to be less dependent on help from others. Children and people aged 85 and older are also more likely to need assistance in multiple activities and to need help from others more often.

Nonelderly and elderly persons with assistance needs living in the community have very similar levels of disability and use of health services. Of persons who need help in basic life activities, however, the elderly are more likely than the nonelderly to need someone with them at home all or most of the time. LaPlante (1989a) concludes that if rates of assistance needs are not reduced in successive age cohorts during the next several decades, the population with assistance needs will grow as these cohorts become older.

LIFE COURSE PERSPECTIVE ON DISABILITY AND ITS PREVENTION

The life course provides a useful framework for considering disabling conditions and their prevention. For persons 60 years of age and older, 8 out of 10 have one or more chronic diseases or impairments (Guralnik et al., 1989b). Roughly 40 percent of the elderly population have some activity limitation, and about 17 percent need assistance in basic life activities (LaPlante, 1989b).

The age gradient for assistance in basic life activity measures (ADLs and IADLs) is particularly evident from age 55 onward. By age 85, the risk of significant disablement approaches 50/50. The older population, therefore, constitutes a particularly important group for studying the potential limits of preventing or minimizing disability. Not only is the risk of disability in late life great, but the population aged 65 and older is also large and growing. An estimated 12.7 percent of the total U.S. population in 1990, 31.7 million persons, are 65 years of age or older; this population group is forecast to grow by the year 2020 to 51.4 million, or 17.3 percent of the total population, and to 67 million persons, 21.7 percent of the total, by 2040 (U.S. Bureau of the Census, 1984). Thus the incidence and prevalence of disability will rise significantly in the foreseeable future.

A Dynamic View of Disability as a Process

During the past two decades, the potential for modifying some processes of aging and for reducing disabling conditions in older populations has been identified in both research and practice. Gerontological and geriatric research and practice have laid a solid foundation for therapeutic optimism regarding the prevention of excessive disability and the rehabilitation of older individuals. Indeed, the notion that prevention or reduction of disability is relevant only early in the life course can no longer be defended (Maddox, 1985; Rowe and Kahn, 1987; Riley and Riley, 1989). Research on disability as a dynamic process, not just a static condition, has contributed greatly to the emergence of an optimistic perspective on reducing disablement during adulthood. For example, in a longitudinal study of disabling conditions in a large sample of people 65 years of age and older with ADL and IADL impairments (the National Long-Term Care Survey), the stereotypical view of age-related monotonic decline in functional capacity was clearly contradicted (Manton 1988). In the first two years of this continuing study (1982-1984), 81.6 percent of the older adults who in 1982 did not have disabling conditions remained free of them two years later. Of the persons who had chronic disabling conditions in 1982, notable proportions were significantly improved two years later. For example, 22.2 percent of the persons who were most limited (5 to 6 ADL impairments) and 23.7 percent of those who were moderately limited (3 to 4 ADL impairments) showed an improvement in functional status two years later.

Research evidence is accumulating that a broad range of interventions have demonstrable beneficial effects in reducing the risk of disability associated with aging. Riley and Riley (1989) provide an excellent collection of relevant articles that review the research documenting the modifiability of some aging processes. Some cognitive loss, for example, typically described as an inevitable concomitant of aging, is known to be reversible under a variety of conditions. Conceptions of self can be improved, as can an individual's sense of empowerment to take interest in, and some responsibility for, self-care, even in very old institutionalized individuals with severe limitations. In addition, the capacity of older adults to benefit physically from systematic exercise has been repeatedly demonstrated (Fries, 1988). Older adults constitute, in sum, an interesting case of the modifiability of disablement from chronic diseases and impairment over the entire life course through risk factor reduction. A related question to be pursued in future research is the effect of not sustaining previously developed healthy lifestyles in later years. Without further evidence, old age cannot be assumed to provide immunity from the risks of unhealthy lifestyles.

Some of the beneficial interventions to prevent or reduce disability are self-initiated, such as adopting and maintaining healthy lifestyles. Research indicates that healthy lifestyles are as characteristic of older adults as they are of adults generally (Berkman and Breslow, 1983; Kaplan and Haan, 1989). Health professionals, however, can and do play an important complementary role in limiting or reversing the consequences of potentially disabling disease or impairment. Timely access to geriatric assessment with appropriate follow-up services has, in randomized controlled trials, proved to be beneficial in improving both functional capacity and more effective use of health resources among older patients (Chernoff and Lipschitz, 1988). The ultimate supporting evidence of improving functional status through systematic intervention is found in geriatric rehabilitation. Even difficult problems in later life, such as those related to incontinence and osteoporosis, have in many instances proven to be amenable to skilled rehabilitative intervention. Beneficial outcomes are known to be more likely in geriatric rehabilitation when attention is given to the psychosocial variables of personal and social resources (Riley and Riley, 1989).

The widely varying needs of persons with disabling conditions demand a multidisciplinary collaborative approach among many professionals and organizations. The interventions should be determined by the needs of each individual rather than by rigid definitions of disabilities.

Collaborative projects involving primary care providers, public health agencies, voluntary associations, and the community should be developed to coordinate disability prevention programs that implement interventions centered on individual needs with a goal of improving an individual's physical, mental, and social well-being over the life course.

Aging Differently

Research has demonstrated the error in thinking that older adults are all alike or that they become more alike as they age (Maddox and Lawton, 1989; Rowe and Kahn, 1987). For example, among those 65 years of age and older, the risk of acquiring a disabling illness differs significantly among the categories of the younger old (65-74), the old (75-84), and the oldest old (85 and older). Patterns of disability, morbidity, and mortality also differ significantly between males and females, and the risk of disabling conditions among older adults is known to be associated with poverty, inadequate education, and social isolation (see Chapter 2). The increased awareness of the diversity of health status in later life has had a salutary effect on health and welfare professionals who are increasingly less likely to use "being older" (i.e., over 65) as an explanation of disability or as a justification for failing to intervene in the interest of improving the quality of life among impaired older adults.

DEVISING APPROACHES TO PREVENTION

Disease prevention and health promotion must be pursued throughout life. It is now well recognized that chronic conditions often can be prevented. For example, it has been estimated that 70 percent of all cancer cases are preventable through changes in lifestyles (e.g., cessation of smoking). Nonetheless, it would be naively optimistic to assume that all chronic disease can be prevented, even though the risk of developing these conditions can be reduced. Mounting evidence clearly indicates, however, that adopting healthful behaviors even late in life can be beneficial, perhaps preventing the progression of impairments to functional limitations and disability. In addition, it is clear that existing knowledge points the way to effective approaches to averting or mitigating the potentially debilitating consequences of some chronic diseases. For example, much can be done to reduce the risk of disabling conditions for people with diabetes, but as the box entitled Preventing Diabetes-Related Disability explains, the disease persists as one of the leading causes of disabling conditions.

Thus, although much is known about the prevention of certain chronic diseases and associated disabling conditions, sometimes the preventive and rehabilitative interventions that are used are not underlain by sufficient understanding, and their effectiveness has not been thoroughly evaluated. Moreover, prevention efforts are hampered by limited understanding of the natural histories of many chronic diseases, of the aging process, and of the relationships among chronic disease, aging, and functional outcomes. Thus, it must be recognized that our knowledge has limits and that we often fail to translate existing knowledge into practice.

The limitations of care delivery systems must also be recognized. The needs of people with long-term conditions mesh poorly with a health care system that is oriented toward the treatment of acute conditions, where care is akin to crisis management. People with chronic conditions require continuity of care and their needs are diverse, encompassing more than medical treatment. If, for example, social support is lacking, a person's well-being may deteriorate despite the availability of adequate health care. Unfortunately, systems for the delivery of social services are fragmented and fail to achieve the continuity that people with chronic conditions often require.

The remainder of this section describes an approach for conceptualizing disability prevention during the life course among people with chronic disease, summarizes some opportunities for prevention, and discusses shortcomings in current systems for the delivery of health care and social services. Much of the discussion focuses on the prevention and management of chronic disease in the elderly.

Perspective on Preventing Disability Among People with Chronic Disease

Unlike acute conditions and injuries, chronic diseases often do not have an identifiable point of onset, and they frequently entail gradually progressive declines in functional capacity. In terms of the committee's model of the disabling process (see Chapter 3), people with chronic diseases are usually first identified when their condition is at the impairment stage (i.e., with a loss or abnormality of physiological, psychological, or anatomical structure or function).

People with chronic disease are at increased risk of functional limitation and disability, and, absent effective preventive measures, the quality of their lives is also likely to decline. In the minds of many—layman and professional alike—the aging processes during the later stages of adulthood are virtually synonymous with chronic disease, and prospects for improve-

PREVENTING DIABETES-RELATED DISABILITY

Diabetes is a leading cause of disability, particularly among the elderly. Approximately 7 million people in the United States have been diagnosed with diabetes, and an additional 5 million may unknowingly have the disease. The prevalence rate of diabetes increases with age; about 10 percent of persons 65 years or older have been diagnosed with diabetes. Disability from diabetes result from the major complications of the disease—cardiovascular disease, peripheral vascular disease, and neuropathy, blindness, and kidney failure. These conditions are largely preventable (Herman et al., 1987).

Most people with diabetes have non-insulin-dependent, or type II, diabetes. The disorder usually appears after age 40 and is frequently associated with obesity. Prevention and control of obesity may be effective in the primary prevention of diabetes; however, a successful strategy for primary prevention has not yet been demonstrated. Existing approaches to reducing disabling conditions and premature mortality caused by diabetes rely on secondary and tertiary prevention of complications.

Cardiovascular disease is a leading cause of mortality among people with diabetes, accounting for half of all diabetes-related deaths. Reducing the rest of cardiovascular disease among diabetic persons primarily entails eliminating or reducing the traditional risk factors associated with the disease, such as cigarette smoking and hypertension. About half of people with diabetes have uncontrolled hypertension, and 27 percent smoke cigarettes. Elimination of these risk factors could decrease deaths due to cardiovascular disease by more than one-fourth (Centers for Disease Control, 1989a).

About half, or 50,000, of all nontraumatic amputations in the United States are performed on people with diabetes. Half of all lower-extremity amputations can be prevented through proper foot care and by reducing risk factors for peripheral vascular disease and neuropathy. These risk factors include hyperglycemia, cigarette smoking, and uncontrolled hypertension (Herman et al., 1987).

Diabetes is the leading cause of new cases of adult blindness. Clinical trials have demonstrated that approximately 60 percent of diabetes-related blindness can be prevented with early detection and treatment (Herman et al., 1987).

Since 1983, the number of patients initiating treatment for end-stage renal disease (ESRD) attributable to diabetes has been increasing by about 10 percent per year. About 20,000 people with diabetic ESRD are sustained through maintenance dialysis. Control of hyperglycemia and hypertension are recommended for preventing and slowing the progression of diabetes-associated renal disease (Herman et al., 1987).

Blacks, Hispanics, and Native Americans are at increased risk for diabetes and many of its complications, making these groups prime targets for preventive efforts. To reduce disability from diabetes, all people with the disease must have access to sustained preventive care. Access to qualified health care providers and referral to appropriate facilities with adequate resources must be improved, particularly for minority populations.

ment are dismissed as highly doubtful. The elderly are viewed as being in a state of inevitable physical and mental decline, resulting in a deteriorating quality of life and, eventually, total dependence. Indeed, about 80 percent of people age 60 and older have at least one chronic disease (Guralnik et al., 1989b), and about 40 percent of those age 65 and older have an activity limitation, including the 17 percent who require assistance in performing some basic life activities (LaPlante, 1989b). Yet to view people in late adulthood as being in an irreparable state of decline is to ignore the tremendous diversity among individuals who are collectively identified as the elderly.

As the committee's model of the disabling process suggests, there are numerous opportunities for intervening and modifying the risk factors that predispose people with chronic diseases to disability. Obviously, the goals of preventing, or at least delaying, the onset of disability and of minimizing the severity of its consequences become more challenging as the age of the target population increases and as the risks of chronic disease, comorbidity, and functional limitation also increase. As mentioned earlier, from age 55 onward, the risk of requiring assistance in basic life activities rises sharply, and by age 85 the risk of disability approaches 50 percent. Still, disability is not a fait accompli even among the oldest of the elderly.

At issue is not whether preventive interventions are beneficial but rather what those interventions should be and how they should be evaluated. Traditionally, the evaluative standard has been improvement in health status. But this standard, borrowed from acute care, is too confining to guide development and assess the effectiveness of prevention measures for chronic disease and disability. A more appropriate standard is quality of life, of which health status is one component. Even when functional capacity cannot be restored, it is indeed possible to improve well-being and to facilitate personal autonomy by addressing factors in an individual's social situation.

The fields of gerontology and geriatrics recognize the importance of interventions to achieve the broader goal of improving quality of life. In these fields, the concept of successful aging has been advanced to expand the focus of practitioners beyond health status to include assessments of the quality of day-to-day life. Successful aging, or aging well, does not imply freedom from disabling conditions. One is aging well when one maintains a satisfying sense of continuity and can fulfill expectations of personal independence and social participation. Despite the physiological and psychological stresses that can accompany advancing age, many older adults have the vitality and resilience to function at a high level. Moreover, frailty and dependence need not preclude a reasonable quality of life. Conversely, a low quality of life can affect the likelihood of developing a disability. Just as among younger age groups, the risk of disability among the elderly is associated with poverty, inadequate education, poor housing, and social isolation.

Therefore, effective management of chronic disease requires an approach that comprehensively addresses not only the individual's health condition but also his or her total social situation. Indeed, beneficial outcomes have been shown to be more likely when personal and social variables are taken into account in geriatric rehabilitation programs (Riley and Riley, 1989).

The concept of quality of life requires considerable refinement before it can become a widely accepted methodological construct. Nevertheless, even if formulated only in general terms, quality of life as an evaluative standard provides a cohesive, transcending concept that can guide the composition, organization, and integration of prevention services for people with chronic disease and for the elderly.

Needs and Opportunities

Although the past 25 years have seen considerable progress in health promotion and the prevention of chronic disease, the need remains for further development and critical evaluation of primary, secondary, and tertiary prevention efforts. Health promotion and other primary prevention efforts that begin at the earliest stages of life are among the most effective and are applicable not only to those who are free of disease or impairment but also to those with disease and disabling conditions. Moreover, risk-reducing, health-promoting activities are important for the elderly with chronic disease because they are already predisposed to functional limitation and disability. In this regard, it should be noted that the Health Care Financing Administration is currently conducting several Medicare prevention demonstration projects. The second interim report on these projects is due to Congress in the spring of 1991, with the final report scheduled for 1993.

Secondary prevention measures, which seek to halt, reverse, or at least retard the progress of a condition, and tertiary prevention measures, which concentrate on restoring function and increasing personal autonomy in people who are already limited in functional capacity, are especially important for people with chronic disease. Combined with appropriate health promotion efforts, these measures constitute the building blocks of chronic disease management. Although the particular elements are dictated by the type and number of conditions present and their predicted course and by the features of an individual's social and environmental surroundings, the management of chronic disease focuses on quality of life, not just health status, and involves self-care, measures to prevent disease complications, counseling and other measures to foster psychosocial coping, and modification of the environment to accommodate functional limitations.

Researchers and service providers have little epidemiological data to guide their efforts to identify effective interventions on which to build chronic disease management plans. The information that is available describes the

prevalence of disabling conditions but does not yield insights into the fac
tors that underlie the results. Nor is it useful in identifying populatio
groups that have a higher-than-average risk of developing disability. Greatl
needed is longitudinal epidemiological research that tracks the progressio
to disability and identifies the contributing risk factors.

*Longitudinal studies are needed to help define the dynamic nature
of pathology, impairment, functional limitation, and disability, and
to describe the natural history of chronic diseases and aging in terms
of these conditions.*

Given the paucity of epidemiological analysis, it is not surprising tha
many secondary and tertiary interventions have evolved without rigorou
scientific evaluation of their effects on functioning and on quality of life
There is a pressing need for studies of the effectiveness and outcomes o
disability prevention measures. An associated need is to incorporate exist
ing knowledge and the results of evaluative studies into consensus guideline
and protocols for preventive health care services.

Despite the serious weaknesses in the foundation upon which disabilit
prevention strategies are built, recent research points to many importan
opportunities for prevention. Several studies contradict the stereotypica
view of age-related monotonic physical and mental decline. An analysis o
data from the National Long Term-Care Survey, one of the few longitudina
studies of disabling conditions, clearly documents the dynamic nature of th
disabling process and thus suggests opportunities for intervention. In additio
the potential for older adults to benefit from regular exercise, good nutrition
and smoking cessation has been reported in several studies (Berkman an
Breslow, 1983; U.S. Department of Health and Human Services, 1988b
Hermanson et al., 1988). A partial summary of conditions amenable t
prevention is presented in Table 6-3 (German and Fried, 1989).

Concurrent with this committee's study, another committee of the Insti
tute of Medicine reviewed research on the prevention of disability after ag
50. The IOM Committee on the Prevention of Disability in the Secon
Fifty has focused on specific chronic diseases and on specific behaviora
and social risk factors that predispose individuals to disability (Institute o
Medicine, 1990b). Topics investigated by the committee include hyperten
sion, medications, infection, osteoporosis, sensory loss, oral health, cancer
nutrition, cigarette smoking, depression, physical inactivity, social isola
tion, and falls. Based on that committee's report, Table 6-4 presents ;
summary of what is known about the prevention of disability in each o
these areas and of what must be learned to improve the effectiveness o
disability prevention efforts.

Even though Table 6-4 is only a partial listing, it suggests several poten

TABLE 6-3   Areas Potentially Amenable to Preventive Health Care in the Elderly

Primary	Secondary	Tertiary
Health habits	Screening for	Rehabilitation
Smoking	Hypertension	Physical deficits
Alcohol abuse	Diabetes	Cognitive deficits
Obesity	Periodontal disease	Functional deficits
Nutrition	Dental caries	
Physical activity	Sensory impairment	
Sleep	Medication side effects	Caretaker support
	Colorectal cancer	Introduction of
Coronary heart disease risk	Breast cancer	support necessary
factors	Cervical cancer	to prevent loss
	Prostatic cancer	of autonomy
Immunization	Nutritionally induced	
Influenza	anemia	
Pneumovax	Depression, stress	
Tetanus	Urinary incontinence	
	Podiatric problems	
Injury prevention	Fall risk	
Iatrogenesis prevention	Tuberculosis (high risk)	
Osteoporosis prevention	Syphilis (high risk)	
	Stroke prevention	
	Myocardial infarction	

SOURCE: German and Fried, 1989. Reproduced with permission from the *Annual Review of Public Health*, Vol. 10. Copyright, 1989, by Annual Reviews, Inc.

tial targets for disability prevention. For example, inappropriate prescribing of medications by physicians and improper use of drugs among the elderly pose serious risks to physical and mental health. Certain medications can cause drowsiness or impair coordination, increasing the likelihood of falls and injuries; they can also reduce appetite, resulting in nutritional deficiencies. Thus improved education and training of physicians that places greater emphasis on prescribing and drug-monitoring practices that are tailored to the elderly would be beneficial in preventing these conditions. Also needed are public education programs and drug labeling practices that foster greater awareness of proper use of medications, particularly when multiple drugs are involved (Montamat et al., 1989).

Injury prevention is especially important for the elderly. The incidence of falls increases greatly after age 65. Combined with the high prevalence of osteoporosis among the elderly, falls are responsible for a large portion

TABLE 6-4   Known vs. Needed Information on Preventing Chronic Disease and Disability Associated With Aging

Risk Factor	Known/Available	Unknown/Needed
Hypertension	Treatment of moderate to severe diastolic hypertension in older people is warranted, but treatment of mild diastolic hypertension may be of marginal benefit. Systolic/diastolic hypertension and isolated systolic hypertension are important risk factors in persons 50 years of age and older.	Cost-effectiveness of anti-hypertension treatment. Data on effectiveness of treatment of isolated systolic hypertension, especially in persons aged 80 and older (the "old" elderly). Toxicity of antihypertensive medication, particularly in the "old" elderly; effect of anti-hypertension therapy on quality of life.
Medications	The older the patient, the less a physician can predict optimal dose based on lab tests and clinical judgment. Many adverse drug effects can be eliminated through more judicious prescribing.	Drug testing in older persons; how the effects of medication are magnified by the physiology of normal aging. Effect of drugs on quality of life and functional capacity in the elderly. Risks and benefits of individual prescription drugs for the elderly.
Infection	23-valent pneumococcal vaccine is effective in preventing pneumococcal diseases. Influenza vaccine is 70% effective in preventing influenza.	Alternative influenza vaccines that provide protection that will last longer than current period of one year. Ways to reduce infection in long-term care facilities. Safer preventive therapy and better early case detection for tuberculosis.
Osteoporosis	Osteoporosis is responsible for a substantial portion of the 1.3 million hip fractures occurring annually, resulting in a 5-20% reduction in survival and increased dependence.	Identification of populations at high risk of fractures through a surveillance system to monitor osteoporosis prevention efforts. More refined data on specific types and causes of injuries to develop effective interventions.

TABLE 6-4 *Continued*

Risk Factor	Known/Available	Unknown/Needed
	Identification of at-risk women can be achieved accurately using non-invasive tests: single-photon absorptiometry, dual-photon absorptiometry, dual-energy X-ray absorptiometry, and quantitative computed tomography. Estrogen replacement therapies (ERT) significantly retard bone loss; but once lost, before ERT, bone mass is irretrievable.	Better therapies to prevent postmenopausal bone loss and new drugs for osteoporosis prophylaxis that do not have estrogen replacement therapy (ERT) side effects or complications (biphosphonate, etc.).
Sensory loss	Approximately one-third of the elderly population suffers hearing or vision loss of varied etiology. Case studies of people with sensory loss show that there is a strong association with psychiatric illness.	Association between sensory loss and physical limitation to determine risk factors for those with hearing and sight loss. Extent to which hearing and sight loss cause emotional and social problems and how they can be avoided. Evaluation of rehabilitation techniques that can be effective for the elderly in reducing handicap due to sensory loss.
Oral health	Oral diseases in old age are exacerbated by medications, physical and financial limitations that restrict dental care, and systemic disease. Edentulous people face psychological, social, and physical problems: soft tissue lesions, speech limitations, chewing limitations, and prosthedontic limitations.	Longitudinal data on the natural history and microbiology of oral diseases. Determination of effective secondary prevention and early detection of oral cancer. Prevalence, incidence, cohort differences, and risk factors of oral dysfunction in older adults (e.g., tooth loss, oral cancer, oral mucosal conditions, oral sequelae of systemic diseases, chronic orificial pain, trauma, salivary gland dysfunction, and aspects of caries and periodontal diseases).

TABLE 6-4 *Continued*

Risk Factor	Known/Available	Unknown/Needed
Cancer	Women aged 60-80 years benefit from cervical cancer screening as much or more than younger women. Hemoccult testing for colorectal cancer improves predictive value with increasing age. New immunology-based tests may provide an alternative to sigmoidoscopy, which is variously tolerated in the elderly. With advancing age, there is a marked decline in the benign-to-malignant ratio of biopsies in screened women and an improvement in the positive predictive value of mammography, 45% to 85% in women over 65 years.	Efficacy of screening for cancer in the elderly. Assessment of elderly tolerance for hemoccult testing and for flexible sigmoidoscopy to 35 and 60 centimeters, and the rates of complication of endoscopy. Evaluation of recent modifications for specificity in fecal occult blood testing. Epidemiologically grounded methodologic research to incorporate nonmortality measures of screening efficacy that reflect impairment, disability, and handicap.
Nutrition	Poor nutrition is a risk factor for many common chronic diseases—coronary artery heart disease, hypertension, stroke, and certain cancers. Nutritional requirement for energy decreases 6% from 51 to 75 years and another 6% thereafter.	Clarification of the associations between nutritional requirements and function. Optimal activity rate for those over 50 to preserve lean body mass and keep metabolic rates high, thereby maintaining high energy needs. Methods for maintaining independent functioning with respect to nutrition among individuals living at home participating in meals programs (e.g., Meals on Wheels and congregate dining). Methods for screening nutritional risk that are reliable, valid, and predictive of later maintenance of independent function.

TABLE 6-4 *Continued*

Risk Factor	Known/Available	Unknown/Needed
Cigarette smoking	21% of coronary heart disease, 82% of chronic obstructive lung disease, and 90% of cancer can be attributed to smoking. Smoking may also be a significant risk factor for stroke. Cessation of smoking decreases risk of all these chronic diseases, particularly coronary heart disease, even after age 50. Past age 50, smoking continues to diminish life expectancy and increase morbidity, and remains a good predictor of lung and other cancers.	Assessment of patients' motivation for smoking cessation. Effective means of smoking cessation and elimination of smoking initiation.
Depression	Elderly who are physically ill are 4-5 times as likely to be depressed as nonill elderly. Depression commonly manifests differently in the elderly than in the young. Older people respond extraordinarily well to treatment of depression.	Criteria for the diagnosis and treatment of depression. Data on prevalence, incidence, and symptom severity of depression in the elderly. Innovative psychosocial measures, particularly in the community, for the restoration and preservation of morale during stressful periods, such as bereavement. Assessment of the efficacy, safety, and indications for the use of electroconvulsive therapy in the elderly.
Physical inactivity	50% of the decline in physical activity in those over age 50 is due to disuse atrophy, not to physiological aging; physical activity is crucial to the ability to maintain independent function. The elderly present a heterogeneous population and therefore require physical activity programs adapted to the individual.	Longitudinal studies that trace the determinants of exercise maintenance at particular stages. The relevance to the individual of cognitive, behavioral, and physical abilities; that is, the kind of interactions that are necessary for initiation, the perception of barriers, and the relationship of other health risks to physical inactivity interventions.

SOURCE: Institute of Medicine, 1990b.

of the 1.3 million hip fractures that occur annually. Hip fractures, in turn, often result in premature death or increased dependence. A number of age-related factors have been implicated in injuries among the elderly: poor eyesight and hearing, arthritis, neurological diseases, and poor coordination and balance. In addition, medications and preoccupation with personal problems may result in distractions or drowsiness that leads to injury. Environmental factors such as poor lighting, uneven floor surfaces, and lack of safety equipment also increase the risk of injury. Most of these risk factors can be reduced by modifying the home environment, monitoring drug usage, and training people to compensate for physical limitations.

Oral health is a neglected area of care for the elderly, even though loss of teeth and oral disease are among the most common impairments in late adulthood. The impact of these impairments on personal health and on psychological and social well-being often goes unappreciated. Difficulty in eating and speech limitations are two examples of how dental impairments can exacerbate existing physical and mental conditions. The importance of preventive dental care for the elderly warrants much greater consideration from service planners.

Although about two-thirds of nursing home residents have a mental disorder (National Center for Health Statistics, 1989b), the role that mental impairment plays in the occurrence of disability among the elderly, as well as among younger segments of the population, is an important area for continued investigation (box follows). The research conducted thus far suggests a strong correlation between physically disabling conditions and mental illness, especially depression. Wells and colleagues (1989) found that, compared with patients with physical disorders only, depressed patients reported greater bodily pain, had a lower perception of their health status, and performed more poorly in physical and social activities. Poor functioning attributed solely to depressive symptoms was comparable to the level of functioning associated with cancer, cardiovascular disease, and six other major chronic conditions. Given that the likelihood of depression is high among elderly people who have a physical illness, these findings underscore the potential health benefits that are likely to result from the provision of appropriate mental health services. Research strongly indicates that depressed older adults are very responsive to interventions, especially those that focus on fostering socially supportive contacts and activities (U.S. Department of Health and Human Services, 1988b).

As mentioned above and discussed in a recent IOM report (1990b), social isolation is considered an important risk factor in the development of disease and disability. A consideration of social isolation usually occurs in the context of social support, and both concepts are often used interchangeably.

Clearly, many simple interventions can have a broad, positive impact on the health of the elderly. Yet despite advances made in clinical research

DISABILITY FROM CHRONIC MENTAL DISORDER

The causes of most of the serious mental disorders are not well understood. Substantial evidence suggests, however, that secondary conditions associated with these disorders can be prevented or at least reduced in severity through appropriate management and rehabilitation efforts. Appropriate medication and aggressive community treatment have been shown to limit the severity of limitations associated with major disorders, improve social functioning, and enhance the quality of patients' lives (Mechanic, 1989). Many of the conditions affecting motivation, behavior, and social participation seen among the mentally ill result from poor medication management, impoverished environments, social isolation, neglect, and homelessness.

There is broad neglect of patients with mental illness at all levels of our health care system (Mechanic and Aiken, 1987). Patients with depression often go unrecognized and receive no treatment, resulting in needless disability. People with depression, however, typically respond favorably to treatment. Failure to recognize depression and provide treatment may result in alcohol and drug abuse, suicide, work absenteeism, and family disruption.

Even in the case of schizophrenia, one of the most disabling mental illnesses, recent research suggests hopeful prognoses (Harding et al., 1987). Aggressive, sustained treatment can prevent deterioration, allowing many patients to lead constructive lives. Assertive community care has been demonstrated to promote function and make reasonable levels of social participation and satisfaction possible (Stein and Test, 1985). Fourteen studies, most with random assignment, show that organized alternatives to hospitalization result in superior outcomes across a range of patient populations (Kiesler and Sibulkin, 1987).

Patients with chronic schizophrenic symptoms are commonly neglected, which may exacerbate their symptoms and lead to a variety of secondary conditions, including sometimes violent acting-out behavior, social isolation, withdrawal from everyday activities, malnutrition, substance abuse, imprisonment, and homelessness. A recent IOM report found that the proportion of homeless populations with an acknowledged history of prior psychiatric hospitalization ranged from 11.2 percent to 26 percent (Institute of Medicine, 1988a). Many more of the homeless without such a history suffer from serious mental disorders as well. The lack of adequate housing constitutes one of the most significant barriers to implementing appropriate mental health care, contributing to a continuing cycle of neglect and disability.

Responsibility for the services necessary to prevent disability and secondary conditions among the mentally ill is distributed among a variety of categorical agencies at several levels of government and in the private sector. These programs suffer from fragmentation, lack of coordination, and large gaps in essential service components. It has been demonstrated repeatedly that the seriously mentally ill often require not only medical and psychiatric

Continued on next page

treatment but also assistance in obtaining welfare benefits, help in structuring daily activities, psychosocial education, vocational rehabilitation, and housing. Delivering such services requires a point of focused responsibility and accountability on a continuing basis, and the ability to direct funding to ensure that patients receive the care they need. An example of this type of service delivery is the Training in Community Living Model developed in Madison, Wisconsin, and adopted in other localities (Stein and Test, 1980a, 1980b, 1985). In most communities, however, responsibility and authority for mental health rehabilitation are diffused across many agencies, and many patients suffer from neglect and inappropriate care.

and efforts to disseminate these results through consensus guidelines for preventive services, the standard practice of clinical medicine is slow to change and incorporate these approaches. Because of the complexity of chronic diseases and their interactions, optimal treatments that will lead to the highest levels of quality of life and functional outcome are not well standardized and evaluated.

> *Both standardized protocols for the management of chronic diseases and mental disorders, and guidelines for preventive services need to be developed and widely disseminated with the goal of preventing disability.*

The increased life expectancy for persons with developmental disabilities, chronic diseases, or injury-related conditions, for example, mandates an emphasis on their inclusion in the national disabilities prevention program. For example, while most persons with Down syndrome used to die before age 40 only two decades ago, many now live into their sixties and seventies. These individuals have both social (residential, work, retirement) needs as well as health needs.

> *Additional study is needed of the relationship between chronic disease, disability, and aging in terms of health promotion, quality of life, and access to services. Such study should include issues related to age-related disability, as well as aging with a disability.*

Composition and Organization of Services

The preceding discussion described some of the promising avenues leading to the goal of disability prevention among the elderly and among younger people with chronic disease. By themselves, however, individual preventive strategies—whether in health care or in social services—are not likely to accomplish much. As in other areas of disability prevention, success will depend on the whole of the effort—on the composition of services, on the availability and organization of services, on the contributions of formal and informal caregivers, and on much, much more. Thus the execution and integration of services are as important as the composition of the particular range of services provided.

This is not meant to minimize the importance of individual service elements. For most people, the range of available preventive services is deficient. For example, accumulating research evidence clearly demonstrates the significant impact that mental health has on functional status and on quality of life. Yet mental health services are not available to many people, or the types of services that are available are inconsistent with their needs because of insurance restrictions or other factors. Similarly, many of the environmental modifications known to reduce the risk of falls and other injuries in the home do not qualify for reimbursement. More examples could be cited, but each has a common thread. Most of the needs of people with chronic disease fall outside the scope of a health care system oriented to the treatment of acute conditions.

Even with diagnostic-related groups, the Medicare system favors acute care treatment in hospitals. As Patricia P. Barry of the University of Miami School of Medicine has explained, "[P]rimary care practitioners struggle to receive adequate reimbursement for lengthy home visits, assessment, family counseling, and multidisciplinary teamwork, while their technologically oriented colleagues have no problem collecting for radiologic or laboratory studies, or invasive tests that may not only be uncomfortable but also pose risks to the patient" (Institute of Medicine, 1989b).

Today, much of the gap between needs and available services is being filled by informal caregivers. The committee recognizes the importance of personal responsibility in health care and of the contributions of family and friends in the provision of needed services; however, it also recognizes the dangers of abdicating total responsibility for care to individuals and informal caregivers, a situation that can result from current reimbursement systems that provide no other option.

The 1982 Long-Term Care Survey showed that approximately 2.2 million caregivers (age 14 or older) provided unpaid assistance to 1.6 million elderly people who required help with one or more basic life activities. The average age of the informal caregiver is 57; a quarter of these caregivers are between the ages of 65 and 74, and 10 percent are older than 75. Many of these caregivers make substantial commitments, which often preclude employment and reduce the time available for other responsibilities. Indeed, 80 percent of informal caregivers devote at least 4 hours a day, 7 days a week, to providing assistance (Stone et al., 1987).

Because of the post-World War II baby boom, the number of offspring available to provide care to parents will increase, but so will the number of elderly. The ratio of people older than age 80 to children will peak in the year 2000, decline somewhat over the next two decades, and then soar to an even higher peak in the year 2030 (Institute of Medicine, 1989b).

These predicted trends and the mismatch between today's health and social service system and the needs of the elderly and of younger adults with chronic disease and disabling conditions should compel policymakers and service planners and providers to rethink current approaches to care. Driven by concerns about escalating expenditures, such a reappraisal is taking place, but too little attention is being paid to access to care and, in particular, to quality of care. As a result, changes implemented in the name of controlling costs are generating new issues in their aftermath. Health care practitioners, noting that the average hospital stay in the United States is shorter than in any other nation, complain that patients are being discharged from hospitals not only quicker but also sicker, although research on this issue has produced equivocal results. Also motivated largely by cost concerns, many people are placing greater emphasis on home and community care as an alternative to institutionalization. Although this shift is often viewed positively, lack of standards for home care, questions about the competency of providers, restrictions on reimbursement for services, and other concerns suggest considerable variability in the effectiveness of this approach.

Robert L. Kane contends that many of these new issues and problems are the product of an "alternatives mentality" (Institute of Medicine, 1989b). Home and community care, for example, has been advanced as a means of keeping the elderly and chronically ill out of nursing homes, but other than the goal of avoiding institutionalization, objectives have not been established for community care. "We have not addressed more fundamental questions," Kane maintains, "such as, Is community care a legitimate and important vehicle for providing care on a long-term basis" (Institute of Medicine, 1989b). Moreover, if avoiding institutionalization is the sole aim, then attention is distracted from improving the quality of care in nursing homes, which will continue to be needed.

If social and health care issues related to disability and its antecedent conditions are not addressed coherently at the policy level, it should not be surprising that current approaches to prevention lack necessary comprehensiveness, continuity, and coordination. An essential first step toward achieving the requisite "3 C's" is to redefine the standard by which we judge our efforts.

Quality of life, not just physical functioning, should guide the design, organization, and integration of services. Although quality of life is a subjective concept, valid measures exist for assessing many of its components, including physical, cognitive, psychological, and social functioning. By broadening our attention to embrace all of these determinants of individual well-being, we are more likely to develop service delivery systems that prevent needless impairment and disability.

Overcoming the fragmentation, lack of coordination, and large gaps in essential service components that now characterize health care and social service programs will not be easy. However, effective delivery of services requires a focal point of continuing responsibility and accountability. It also requires freeing up funding from overly restrictive and overly rigid reimbursement schemes so that the particular service needs of individuals can be accommodated. For insurers and other third-party payers, this will necessitate determining how to work with providers of social support services and other services that are now excluded from the traditional medical model upon which most insurance coverage is based.

Thus it seems obvious that new funding arrangements are needed, as are new relationships among service providers. It is not clear what forms these new arrangements and relationships should take, although several models probably will be needed.

Primary care providers, public health agencies, private insurers, voluntary associations, and community organizations should undertake the development and evaluation of collaborative demonstration projects that are designed to provide comprehensive, coordinated disability prevention programs. Interventions should focus on individual needs, with the goal of improving quality of life and physical, mental, and social well-being.

Education

Stereotypes are slow to die. In the area of disability prevention, however, clinging to outdated service delivery models and to disproved notions about the chronically ill and the elderly makes the prospects for progress quite poor. New thinking is required, and this can be achieved only through public and professional education.

More must be done in schools and in the home to instill in the young the importance of healthful behaviors. Health promotion, however, is relevant to all stages of life, and the themes are often the same (e.g., regular exercise, proper diet, avoidance of substance abuse, and injury prevention). Reinforcing messages in the community, the school, the workplace, and the physician's office can help create a social context that promotes healthful lifestyles. The change in public attitudes toward cigarette smoking clearly demonstrates that such constant reinforcement can have a positive impact on individuals, resulting in benefits for all of society.

Public attitudes toward the aging process have fostered an unduly pessimistic view of the late stages of adulthood. Attention has focused on the health risks associated with aging. It would be far more constructive for society to concentrate on preventable extrinsic factors that underlie these increasing health risks. The public must be made aware of the potential for modifying the aging process and of the physical, psychological, environmental, and social determinants of the quality of life in late adulthood.

The thrust of educational programs for health care and social service professionals should be similar with regard to disabling conditions. However, medical education and training continue to emphasize the diagnosis and treatment of acute diseases. Consequently, treatment is usually fixed on the short term, whereas the needs of people with chronic disease and of the elderly are long term, and rates of cure and survival are the primary gauges of the success of therapeutic interventions. Moreover, underappreciation of other aspects of personal well-being and of the contribution of psychological, social, and economic variables to health status can result in inappropriate care. As a consequence, high-technology medicine tends to be favored even when low-tech services are likely to be more beneficial, and providers of health care and social services operate in isolation rather than as multidisciplinary teams.

The potential exists for modifying the quality of life associated with aging and chronic disease processes through individual lifestyle change and through social policies that ensure adequate income, educational opportunities, and social support across a person's life course. Broader measures that are more relevant for the individual, such as functional limitation and quality of life, are not integrated into professional education programs. In addition, health financing systems do not reward counseling, chronic disease management, and preventive measures in clinical practice.

Professional education should foster a quality-of-life perspective, one that does not treat all needs as medical in nature. Geriatric assessments provide a useful model that should be incorporated into the training of all health care professionals. Such assessments evaluate a patient's total situation, considering a broad range of functional abilities and analyzing the availability of social support.

On the basis of this type of comprehensive appraisal, a physician, nurse, or social worker can determine the elements of a comprehensive long-term program of care. For many elements, several options are possible, and most are likely to qualify as low technology. In addition, geriatric assessments have a follow-up component that fosters continuity.

Finally, while integration and continuity imply complexity, new information technologies offer opportunities to simplify case management and ensure coordination. Lap-top computers and bar code readers, for example, can be used to create patient data bases that provide a continuing record of the administration of medications, the type of services received, and other information relevant to the care and well-being of individuals. In addition, information technologies should make more accessible the guidelines for preventive services and clinical protocols that are emerging from ongoing research on the effectiveness and outcomes of interventions. If this information were compiled in easy-to-use data bases, adoption of these consensus guidelines and protocols by health care professionals would be accelerated.

7

Prevention of Secondary Conditions

Traditionally, rehabilitation has been viewed as the major type of health care intervention for people with disabling conditions, with recovery of function as the sole aim of treatment. A consequence of this perspective is that disabling conditions are categorized as static entitities (Marge, 1988). One commonly held view is that once recovery reaches a plateau and treatment ceases, the person with a disabling condition is likely to remain permanently at this level of health status and functioning.

This long-held view fails to recognize the true nature of disabling conditions: they are long-term, dynamic conditions that can fluctuate in severity during the life course. Moreover, people with disabling conditions often develop additional conditions that are causally related to the primary disabling condition and that may be more debilitating. Much of the literature refers to these conditions as secondary *disabilities*. In the interest of conceptual clarity, however, the committee has adopted the term secondary *conditions* because many of the conditions that occur are not disabilities per se but pathologies, impairments, and functional limitations. Thus a *secondary condition* is a condition that is causally related to a disabling condition (i.e., occurs as a result of the primary disabling condition) and that can be either a pathology, an impairment, a functional limitation, or an additional disability.

The existence of a potentially disabling (primary) condition is a strong risk factor for certain secondary conditions; by definition, the secondary condition would not occur in the absence of the primary condition. This causal relationship between primary and secondary conditions lends itself to preventive interventions that are designed to reduce the risk of developing secondary conditions and the concomitant potential for additional deterioration in health status and quality of life.

According to Marge (1988), among the most commonly reported secondary conditions are pressure sores, contractures, urinary tract infections, and depression (Table 7-1), each of which can cause additional impairment, functional limitation, and disability. Specific examples of the relationship between a primary disabling condition and resultant secondary conditions include decubitus ulcers and contractures that develop because of lack of movement in a person with paraplegia, and depression that develops as a result of spinal cord injury.

Health promotion and amelioration of the primary disabling condition—the traditional aim of rehabilitation—are the principal strategies for minimizing the risk of a secondary condition. Because the presence of a disabling condition and, consequently, vulnerability to secondary conditions are lifelong, approaches to prevention should focus on the long term and the whole person. Critical elements of interventions include regular monitoring of health status, continuity of care, availability of appropriate assistive technology, training in coping with limitations, and community support including measures that ensure access to transportation, housing, and opportunities for employment.

MODEL OF SECONDARY CONDITIONS

All primary disabling conditions entail increased vulnerability to secondary conditions that can arise in many ways. A model of the process that leads to a secondary condition is depicted in Figure 7-1. Added to the nexus of interactive risk factors in the previously described model of the disabling process (Figure 3-3) is the existence of a primary disabling condition. Collectively, the presence of risk factors predisposes a person to a progression that begins with a new, or secondary, pathology and that can end with additional disability. Thus opportunities to intervene exist at several stages.

The committee has defined the relationship between the primary disabling condition and a secondary condition as a causal one; the secondary condition would not occur without the existence of the primary condition. However, the causal relationship can be either direct or indirect. The common example of a direct etiological relationship is the development of pressure sores in persons who use wheelchairs and are limited in activity as a result of spinal cord injury. An example of an indirect relationship is that of a disabling condition that causes new stresses—uncertainty about the future, changes in living environments and social relationships, and frustrations from being unable to gain access to a building—that in turn can cause hypertension or other stress-related diseases. In addition, disabling conditions can magnify the influence of other existing risk factors. Continuation of smoking, heavy drinking, poor dietary habits, and other deleterious behaviors greatly increases the likelihood that a secondary condition will develop.

TABLE 7-1 Causes of Some Common Secondary Conditions

Secondary Condition	Causes
Decubitus ulcers	Inaccessibility to adequate health care, improper seating for those with the disuse syndrome, lack of continuous personal hygiene.
Genitourinary tract disorders	Inaccessibility to adequate health care, genetic disorders, alcohol and drug abuse, nutritional disorders, lack of personal hygiene, acute and chronic illness.
Cardiovascular disorders	Alcohol and drug abuse, tobacco use, nutritional disorders, stress, inaccessibility to adequate health care, acute and chronic illness, lack of physical fitness.
Stroke	Lack of physical fitness, nutritional disorders, tobacco use, stress, alcohol and drug abuse, inaccessibility to adequate health care (hypertension control).
Musculoskeletal problems	Lack of physical fitness, injuries, stress, genetic disorders, perinatal complications, acute and chronic illness, inaccessibility to adequate health care.
Arthritis	Speculated lack of physical fitness, nutritional disorders, stress and possibly genetic disorder.
Respiratory problems	Lack of physical fitness, acute and chronic illness, environmental quality problems, alcohol and drug problems, tobacco use, unsanitary living conditions, genetic disorders.
Hearing loss	Genetic disorders, acute and chronic illness, injuries, violence, environmental quality problems (noise pollution).
Speech and language problems	Genetic disorders, acute and chronic illness, injuries, environmental quality problems, neurological deficits (such as strokes), cancer and respiratory problems.
Vision problems	Genetic disorders, acute and chronic illness, injuries, violence, nutritional disorders, environmental quality problems, inaccessibility to adequate health care.
Emotional problems	Genetic disorders, stress, alcohol and drug abuse, deleterious child-rearing practices and familial-cultural beliefs; inaccessibility to adequate mental health care.
Skin disorders	Genetic disorders, acute and chronic illness, injuries (fires and burns), nutritional disorders, unsanitary living conditions, stress.

SOURCE: Adapted from Marge, 1988.

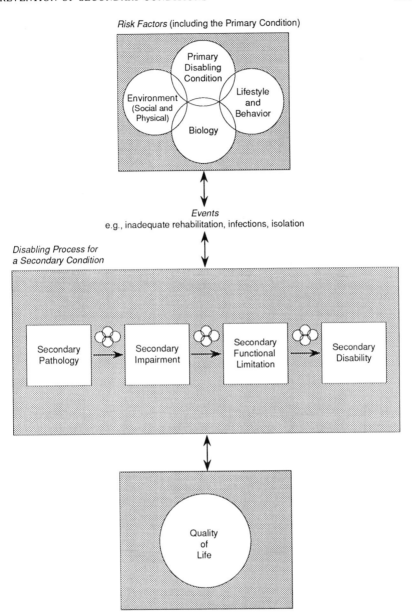

FIGURE 7-1 Model of secondary conditions. Note the addition of the "primary disabling condition" as an additional risk factor. By definition, a "primary condition" is a risk factor for the secondary condition. This model shows that a secondary condition can be anything from a pathology to a disability. It also allows for interaction between the primary and the secondary conditions.

It is important to note that the existing disabling condition and other risk factors work in combination, and that secondary conditions can have many consequences. The example of J.R., described in the first box, illustrates some of the feedback loops involved in the development of secondary conditions that influence the nature and severity of the condition's effects. J.R.'s experience clearly demonstrates the importance of the life course perspective on longitudinal health care, as well as the significant role played by nonmedical factors.

Surveillance and Epidemiological Understanding

Although clinical experience has generated a long list of secondary conditions that frequently occur in people with disabling conditions, epidemiological information on the incidence and prevalence of secondary conditions and on the underlying causative factors is sparse. This epidemiological blind spot is emblematic of existing data systems that do not contain information about the causes of the specific disabling conditions. Thus it is extremely difficult to determine to what extent a person's disability is the result of primary or of secondary conditions.

A partial exception is the National Health Interview Survey (NHIS), which asks respondents with disabling conditions to list the main cause of their disabling condition, as well as of other conditions that may be involved. In addition, the NHIS collects information on the onset of conditions in these people. But because this information on the timing of onset is very general, it is often impossible to determine the order in which the conditions occurred, and the distinction between primary and secondary conditions can rarely be made.

LaPlante (1989b) analyzed NHIS data to determine the frequency of co-occurrence for 22 conditions or groups of conditions. A variety of conditions were found to co-occur more frequently than expected, indicating a possible causal relationship. For example, the prevalence of hypertension and asthma among people with disabling conditions was 2.63 per 1,000 persons—more than four times the expected rate. LaPlante notes that NHIS data can also be used to ascertain the extent of activity limitation associated with co-occurring conditions, but adds that "understanding of the causal models underlying statistically dependent conditions must come from other sources of information."

The true magnitude of secondary conditions is not known, but several studies suggest that it is large. For example, about 40 percent of all people with activity limitation report multiple conditions as the cause of limitation. As discussed in a previous chapter, the prevalence of multiple conditions among people with activity limitation has been increasing. But, again, the factors contributing to this increase cannot be determined with existing data. This increase may include a rising rate of secondary conditions, but it

J.R. is a 29-year-old man who became quadriplegic from a spinal cord injury sustained after an automobile crash five years ago. He has function only at the level of C5 and above. Therefore, he has no effective use of his hands or his body below shoulder level. In addition, he has sensation in the skin only over the head, neck, upper shoulders, and outside arms. Following his initial injury he was hospitalized for 9 months, receiving comprehensive rehabilitative care. During the next 4+ years since his discharge from the rehabilitation hospital, several problems occurred that reduced his independence and his quality of life.

During the first two years after discharge, his bladder periodically became infected which led to two- to three-week periods of high temperatures, marked fatigability, and inability to function at his best level. These infections were caused by a catheter that was inserted during his stay in a nursing home immediately after his discharge from the rehabilitation hospital. However, living now with an attendant in an apartment and utilizing intermittent catheterization for control of his bladder, J.R. has had only one minor infection during the last two years.

While in the nursing home, J.R. developed pressure sores over the ischial tuberosities (from sitting in a chair that had no mechanism for pressure relief). At the time, he had difficulty in getting funding for a power recline chair and thus sat for long periods in a standard high-backed wheelchair with a standard cushion, which was not sufficient to keep him from developing ischial pressure sores. As a result of these pressure sores, he was admitted to an acute hospital for two weeks and subsequently referred back to the nursing home. For a period of eight weeks, he was not able to sit up in a chair but rather had to move from place to place on a cart in order to avoid pressure over the healing sores.

Because of his continued dependency in the nursing home and the unavailability of privacy or people of his own age in the institution, J.R. became depressed for approximately four months. During this period he contributed little to his own self-care, had no interest in developing either vocational or recreational activities, and tended to alienate those about him because of his passivity. He was so inactive for a while that he developed thrombophlebitis of the deep femoral veins. Treating this condition required surgery to place a device in his inferior vena cava that would prevent migration of clots to the lungs; otherwise, sudden death from pulmonary embolism might occur.

At the time of his discharge from the rehabilitation hospital, J.R. had spasticity that primarily involved the lower extremities but that did not substantially interfere with his activities. However, he subsequently developed increased tightness and episodes of "jumping" of the legs that made his balance in the wheelchair precarious and interfered with his sleep at night. More recently, with a regular program of stretching, control of his bowel and bladder functions, and adequate positioning when sitting up in his chair and when lying in bed, he has had little functional problem with the continued spasticity in his lower extremities.

Continued on next page

J.R. quickly depleted all of his financial resources and was dependent on Medicaid for payment of his health services for the first three and a half years after his injury. At two years after his injury, his medical expenses were supplemented through Medicare. He also was placed on Social Security six months after his injury because he had worked regularly prior to his injury.

Initially, J.R. was also dependent on public housing assistance (Section 8) and waited three and a half years for an appropriate apartment with adequate accessibility (resulting in the prolonged stay in the nursing home).

Prior to his injury, J.R. had been a drafting technician. After his injury, J.R. developed the capability of working in an adapted work station as a receptionist in an architectural firm. However, he found the income from this position to be too high to retain his eligibility for Social Security, Medicare, and Medicaid and yet not sufficient to cover the costs of his medical transportation and attendant care needs. As a result, he was unable to continue working even though he found significant satisfaction from it.

could also reflect an increase in independent conditions or be the result of other factors, such as increased access to health services and improved health awareness.

The paucity of data also limits the ability to accurately estimate the economic costs associated with secondary conditions and, therefore, the potential savings that can be achieved with effective interventions. Advocates of people with disabling conditions and clinicians who treat them generally agree that the associated costs are substantial, and that significant savings can be achieved with consistent, appropriate programs of medical care, rehabilitation, and social support.

An example is suggestive of the potential savings. The Committee on Trauma Research (National Research Council, 1985) reported that 35 percent to 40 percent of the estimated 200,000 people with spinal cord injury develop pressure sores of varying severity. Because the average cumulative cost per pressure sore is an estimated $58,000 (National Institute on Disability and Rehabilitation Research, 1990), the savings from preventing this avoidable secondary condition are likely to be large.

A disability surveillance system is needed to collect data on the incidence and prevalence of secondary conditions, including psychiatric conditions. These data are needed to improve understanding of risk factors associated with secondary conditions and to guide development of effective intervention strategies for preventing secondary conditions.

Mental Health Conditions

Potentially debilitating illness or injury elicits psychological and behavioral responses that are peculiar to each individual. Despite the diversity of responses, the stresses and other forces that persons with disabling conditions must confront are often quite similar. The two examples given in the second box are illustrative. The similarities between the two patients are striking; yet the first patient appears to be adapting positively, whereas the second patient exhibits symptoms of major depressive disorder. The second patient's psychological state underlies his failure to comply with his prescribed dietary and exercise regimen, which elevates the risk of developing a secondary condition.

The finding by Wells and colleagues (1989) that "depression and chronic medical conditions had unique and additive effects on patient dysfunctioning" is especially pertinent to the care of people with disabling conditions. Depression following the loss of function is common and usually treatable. Krueger (1981) describes depression as a normal and expected response. "If it does not occur, even transiently," Krueger advises, "an alarm should sound because its absence indicates the reality of the loss has not been emotionally recognized." Prolonged depression is not inherent, and in most patients it abates within weeks or months without intervention. Careful psychiatric monitoring can alert the physician to the danger of prolonged depression, permitting early intervention.

Krueger also points out that the more a person's disabling condition interferes with his or her work, recreation, self-esteem, or normal coping mechanisms, the more psychologically devastating the condition will be. While finding that there is no characteristic pattern of psychological response based on type of disabling condition, Gallagher and Stewart (1987) report that anger, depression, and anxiety increase with the severity of the disabling condition. Researchers (Gallagher and Stewart, 1987; Castelnuovo-Tedesco, 1981) also have found that the severity of the psychological response is inversely related to the age at which the disabling condition is acquired. In terms of psychological vulnerability, according to Castelnuovo-Tedesco, the least unfavorable time for a disabling condition to develop tends to be after stable adult integration has occurred.

A person's mental health prior to the onset of a disabling condition and other antecedent variables appears to influence the likelihood and intensity of psychological complications. Factors predictive of depression following physical illness or injury include a personal history of depression, a family history of depression, and a predisposition to depression based on a personal history of early parental loss or childhood trauma (Krueger, 1981).

Brodsky's (1987) examination of motivational issues in a population of people who sustained job-related injuries elucidated several nonmedical factors

Patient 1 is a 44-year-old white, Protestant, married physician who is the father of three teenage children and suffers an occlusion of the anterior descending coronary artery. After three weeks in the hospital, he returns home on a regimen of aspirin, a low-cholesterol diet, and a systematic exercise program. When his cardiologist sees him for a follow-up visit after two months, the patient has returned to his medical practice and reports that he has lost 7 lbs. In addition, the patient describes the resumption of his sexual life, his usual parenting activities, and leisure time pursuits. While still somewhat anxious about his prognosis, he requires no psychiatric intervention or psychotropic medication.

Patient 2 is another 44-year-old white, Protestant, married physician who is the father of three and who suffers an occlusion identical to that of Patient 1. After three weeks in the hospital, he also returns home on a regimen of aspirin, a low-cholesterol diet, and a systematic exercise program. However, when his cardiologist sees him for a follow-up visit, after two months, Patient 2 and his wife report that he constantly feels tired, stays in bed, avoids exercise including sex, and has made sporadic visits to his office but has not seen patients. On interview, the patient reports being terrified of a fatal recurrence of the myocardial infarction. In addition, he is having difficulty sleeping, eats sporadically but not in accord with his diet, can't enjoy sex and other pleasurable activities, and feels that his active life is over and that he is "no longer a man." Although there is no difference between the cardiac status of Patients 1 and 2, four months later Patient 2 is still unable to return to work and his family life is colored by his inability to resume his functions as an effective father and husband.

that play significant roles in the occurrence of work disabilities. One such factor is the degree to which an individual has been socialized for work and thus the degree to which personal worth and success are defined in the context of one's occupation. Similarly, level of educational attainment is also related to the risk of work disability. Brodsky maintains that with increasing educational attainment comes a greater belief in the intrinsic rewards of work, a greater likelihood of extrinsic rewards derived from work, and a more intellectually rewarding content of work.

Some of the workers in the Brodsky study who developed disability perceived themselves prior to injury as physically, emotionally, or intellectually inadequate, a perception underlain by a variety of factors including those related to age, job-personality fit, and family relationships. For these individuals, disability is a more likely outcome than for those who do not feel inadequate on the job.

The nature of the work performed also influences the outcome of work-related injury: low pay, boring and repetitive work, and heavy physical labor are associated with increased disability. Lack of on-the-job autonomy, adversarial employee-employer relationships, poor communication, and discrimination were all found by Brodsky to increase the chances that disability would result from work-related injury.

More research is needed to identify risk factors for secondary mental health conditions, clarify the role of these factors in contributing to additional disability, and develop effective interventions to prevent secondary psychiatric conditions. Research should include evaluations of the interactions and contributions of biological and psychodynamic factors such as perceptions of the significance and meaning of disability; the availability of familial, social, and cultural support; and perceived prospects for personally gratifying future activity.

COMPONENTS OF A COMPREHENSIVE
PREVENTION PROGRAM

People with disabling conditions and those who treat these conditions generally believe that the techniques used to minimize the physical, psychological, and social effects of primary disabling conditions also are beneficial in the prevention of secondary conditions. This consensus is largely the product of intuition rather than rigorous scientific evaluation of interventions. Nevertheless, since secondary conditions are often predictable, they also should be preventable.

There is a paucity of empirical evidence on the effectiveness of preventive approaches for at least two reasons. First, the lack of valid, reliable assessments for determining what works and what does not work extends to virtually all areas of health care, not just disability. Second, the widely held view that disabling conditions are unchanging, static (or worse, inevitably deteriorating) conditions has limited the amount of attention devoted to prevention of secondary conditions.

Limits to our knowledge mean that, at least in the short term, efforts to prevent secondary conditions will be developed largely on a trial-and-error basis. However, the committee believes that service providers and people with disabling conditions can increase the probability of success in preventing secondary conditions by adhering to some fundamental principles. For example, practices that promote general well-being and good health are as critical to people with disabling conditions as they are to those who are free of limitations. In fact, available evidence suggests that health-promoting behaviors may be more important to the population of people with disabling conditions, given their elevated risk for secondary conditions and, consequently, for negative effects on the quality of their lives. In addition, service providers also should strive to deliver services that are comprehensive and integrated. Obviously, the mix of services is contingent upon levels of available public, private, and personal resources. Nonetheless, the effectiveness of each element within a particular set of services is enhanced if the elements are comprehensive, well coordinated, and integrated from the perspective of the client.

In general, the prevention of secondary conditions in people with disabling conditions requires a comprehensive approach that includes at least the following components: (1) organization and delivery of services; (2) availability of appropriate assistive technologies, as well as adequate training in the use of these technologies; (3) adoption of health-promoting behaviors; (4) education; and (5) consideration of environmental factors. The following sections discuss these components as they relate to the development of effective intervention strategies for the prevention of secondary conditions.

Organization and Delivery of Services

Preceding chapters have discussed the incongruity that characterizes the current patchwork of public and private health care and social services for people with disabling conditions. Services are compartmentalized and poorly coordinated, whereas the needs of people with disabling conditions are overlapping and long term. Even if the full spectrum of needed services are available, it is unlikely that services will be well integrated and easily accessible. More than half of the respondents in a 1986 survey of Americans with disabling conditions said it was "somewhat hard," "very hard," or "almost impossible" to identify available services (Louis Harris and Associates, 1986).

Because of the service system's fragmented organization and its emphasis on acute conditions, many people with disabling conditions are underserved and little attention is focused on prevention. One consequence is the occurrence of avoidable secondary conditions that worsen a disabling condition and increase the need for services.

Observers of the U.S. health care system often note that form follows funding. That is, funding policies directly determine the makeup of available services. Current funding policies, however, do not reflect the needs of people with disabling conditions; therefore, available services often do not provide the appropriate types and levels of care. Programs for income maintenance, rehabilitation, health care, and independent living are governed by their own separate policies rather than by an encompassing, unified disability policy.

Funding for health care and social services should follow client needs. But the needs of people with disabling conditions are diverse, and their requirements for services are equally diverse. Although a range of services should be available, not every person with a disabling condition will require all of these services. Thus funding of the health care and social service system must permit flexibility at the community level. The community is the appropriate site for making decisions on what services an individual needs and how best to provide them. Independent living centers are discussed below as an example of effective community-based programs that assist people with disabling conditions.

Independent Living Centers

Independent living centers provide one model of how to address the multiple needs of people with disabling conditions. These community-based centers, which usually are staffed by persons with disabling conditions who live independently, offer a variety of services and act as resource and referral centers, achieving linkages among the disparate elements of the health care and social service system.

Services offered by independent living centers typically include the following:

• organizing and coordinating family support for people with disabling conditions;
• organizing coalitions among people with different types of disabling conditions;
• peer counseling;
• long-term monitoring and follow-up of referred clients;
• computerized information and referral system;
• health maintenance programs, often developed in conjunction with local rehabilitation centers;
• transportation;
• housing assistance; and
• advocacy, including participation in the development of policies that foster integration of people with disabling conditions into the community.

Collectively, these services and activities constitute a comprehensive, rational approach to the prevention of secondary conditions, addressing not only health concerns but also issues related to the quality of life. Indeed, the aim of the independent-living movement—to foster "control over one's life based on the choice of acceptable options that minimize reliance on others in making decisions and in performing everyday activities" (Texas Institute for Rehabilitation and Research, 1978)—is an appropriate goal for guiding the development, organization, and coordination of disability prevention programs.

Assistive Technologies

Assistive technologies are devices and techniques that can eliminate, ameliorate, or compensate for functional limitations. Essentially enabling tools, assistive technologies help people with disabling conditions interact more efficiently and more effectively with the social and physical elements of their environment. Assistive technologies encompass a broad range of devices. Some incorporate the most advanced offerings of high technology, but the great majority of assistive devices are "off-the-shelf" products that can be used with little or no modification. A microwave oven, for example, may allow a person who is limited in movement to cook, whereas an electric or gas stove may not. At the high end of the technology range (and still under development) are voice-activated robotic arms that can prepare a meal and assist individuals in performing a variety of basic activities such as feeding, tooth brushing, face washing, and hair combing.

By helping people to interact more fully with their environment, assistive technologies can improve or at least maintain functional capacity, and by fostering greater control over one's activities, assistive technologies foster autonomy, which often translates into a higher quality of life. In turn, these benefits spawn the additional advantage of reducing the risk of secondary conditions.

There are three categories of assistive technology: (1) personal technologies, such as tools used in grooming and other hygienic tasks, exercise, and skin protection; (2) activity-specific technologies such as writing and other communication aids and equipment that enable participation in recreational or work-related activities; and (3) environmental technologies, primarily those that ensure physical access (e.g., curb cuts and building ramps) and also those that offer opportunity for participation in societal affairs (e.g., closed-caption programming and specially adapted telephones that allow people to converse by typing and reading). Many assistive technologies directly or indirectly reduce the risk of injury. Grab bars and nonslip bathtubs, for example, greatly reduce the risk of injury in the bathroom, and curb cuts and ramps not only help people with disabling conditions but also assist those carrying heavy objects or pushing strollers.

Advances in electronics and the associated miniaturization of devices open the door to exciting opportunities for developing highly useful assistive technologies. Perhaps the most interesting avenues lie in the area of implantable devices that can substitute for damaged body parts. Yet despite the sizable benefits to be reaped by applying today's high technology to the needs of people with disabling conditions, many manufacturers of medical devices are scaling back their investments in research and development because of government regulations on the pricing of devices (National Academy of Engineering, 1988).

Although complex applications of cutting-edge technology attract most of the public's attention, the greatest benefits, at least in the short term, are likely to come from applying "low technology" to the needs of people with disabling conditions. Such simple devices as adaptive eating implements for people with manual limitations cost only a few dollars, but they can contribute significantly to personal independence. This is not to suggest that advanced technology is not appropriate for people with disabling conditions. In many instances, it can be. But the innovative adaptation of readily available commercial products has the advantage of costing less than the development of products solely for the population of people with disabling conditions.

Applying commercially available technology to the needs of people with disabling conditions would seem to be a relatively straightforward exercise in technology transfer. Unfortunately, a major impediment exists in the form of the reimbursement criteria of public and private insurers. Tailored to the treatment of acute conditions, reimbursement criteria emphasize curative medicine and rarely recognize the importance of maintaining health and improving functioning. Thus most assistive technologies, which are tools of preventive care, do not qualify for reimbursement.

Medicare, the public insurance program for the elderly and people with disabling conditions, uses a standard of "medical necessity" that has been adopted by most private insurers. Assessed by this standard, assistive technologies are likely to be dismissed as "not primarily medical in nature" or as "convenience items" (Table 7-2). Thus coverage is often denied for equipment that can reduce the risk of secondary conditions, especially those that arise from injuries.

Denial of reimbursement for technology that assists in the performance of daily activities and reduces the risk of secondary conditions is likely to result in long-term costs that exceed initial savings. For example, Medicare regards grab bars for bathrooms as convenience items, even though falls in the bathroom are a leading cause of hip fractures and other injuries among the elderly. The health care costs associated with hip fractures alone are large and growing. This shortsightedness is also reflected in the inadequate coverage that most insurers provide for long-term maintenance and replacement of the few assistive technologies they do fund.

The beneficial effects of assistive technologies in reducing and preventing disability and secondary conditions need to be recognized in determinations of medical insurance coverage, which should not be restricted on the basis of medical necessity or convenience. Similarly, the beneficial effects of personal assistance services and durable medical equipment need to be recognized for their effectiveness in preventing disability and secondary conditions.

Health Promotion

The concept and benefits of health promotion are the same for people with disabling conditions as for people without them, and both groups must

TABLE 7-2   Durable Medical Equipment that Assists in Preventing
Secondary Conditions and the Reasons Given for Denying Coverage Under
Medicare

Item	Reason for Denied Medical Coverage
Bathtub lifts	Convenience item; not primarily medical in nature
Auto lift	Convenience item; not primarily medical in nature
Nolan bath chair	Comfort or convenience item; hygienic equipment, not primarily medical in nature
Cheney safety bath lift	Convenience item; not primarily medical in nature
Raised toilet seats	Convenience item; hygienic equipment, not primarily medical in nature
Bathtub seats	Comfort or convenience item; hygienic equipment, not primarily medical in nature
Grab bars	Self-help device, not primarily medical in nature
Safety grab bars	Self-help device, not primarily medical in nature
Disposable sheets and bags	Nonreusable disposable supplies
Incontinence pads	Nonreusable supply; hygienic item
Patient lifts	Covered only if intermediary's physician determines patient's condition is such that periodic movement is necessary to effect improvement or to arrest or retard deterioration in patient's condition
Bed baths	Hygienic equipment

SOURCE: U.S. Health Care Financing Administration, 1983.

assume general responsibility for their physical, psychological, and social
well-being. However, disabling conditions often necessitate the development
of special skills and the availability of additional information and assistive
technology in order to assume this responsibility.

Disabling conditions require adjustments and adaptations in many spheres
of an individual's life. Changes in diet, for example, are often necessary
because of an altered metabolism or the influences of prescribed medications.
If the person has a progressive condition, nutritional requirements may have
to be reviewed regularly. Lifestyle behaviors must also be reviewed and
changed in accordance with the limitations imposed by the disabling condition.
Behaviors known to be deleterious, such as smoking or abuse of alcohol and
other drugs, should be eliminated. Training may be required in a number of
areas. Persons with sensory limitations must be instructed on observing
their bodies to detect irregularities and to accommodate biological needs. A
person with spinal cord injury, for example, must be taught to inspect his
legs—visually and by touch—to detect skin conditions.

A person with a disabling condition might need to be familiarized with alternative forms of exercise and recreation, schooled in the appropriate techniques, and provided with the necessary assistive technology. Training in coping skills and stress management is essential. For example, people with disabling conditions can benefit from learning communication techniques for responding to questions about their limitations and, if desired, for refocusing the discussion.

Nutrition, Exercise, and Medications

People with disabling conditions must be thoroughly advised of their nutritional needs. If the disabling condition reduces a person's level of activity, for example, then their caloric requirements are also likely to be reduced. Moreover, medications can suppress or increase appetite, alter nutritional balance, or diminish energy and motivation, reducing one's desire to cook. For example, use of anticonvulsant drugs has been shown to reduce serum levels of vitamin D and several B-complex vitamins (Whitney and Cataldo, 1983). Thus people with disabling conditions must be fully apprised not only of their nutritional needs but also of the name, dosage, timing of administration, purpose, side effects, and dietary restrictions for each medication they are taking. Development of an appropriate diet is likely to require the combined input of physician, nutritionist, and pharmacist (Marge, 1988).

Exercise is especially important for people with disabling conditions. Many disabling conditions limit the range of motion of joints, increasing the risk of contractures. Disabling conditions also may restrict mobility, thus reducing opportunities for strenuous physical exercise, which improves blood circulation. In addition, people with disabling conditions tend to gain weight as they age. This excess weight further restricts mobility, often results in fewer weight shifts to relieve pressure on the skin, and increases the risk of abrasions and bruises during transfers.

Regular exercise can have several risk-reducing benefits: it improves circulatory and pulmonary functioning, helps maintain normal blood pressure, decreases serum levels of cholesterol and low-density lipoproteins, helps prevent obesity, helps improve strength and endurance, and helps delay degenerative changes that can accompany aging (Brandon, 1985). Moreover, exercising extremities through their full range of motion and stretching all muscle groups affecting each joint help to prevent contractures.

People with physical limitations should engage in a program of aerobic exercise at least three times a week. Each session should include at least 15 minutes of repetitive, continuous exercise. Setting up such an exercise program can be a challenge, however. Options may be limited by lack of access to fitness centers or by the unavailability of required adaptive exercise equipment. The National Handicapped Sports and Recreation Association and several other organizations offer information on exercise and other health promotion activities for people with disabling conditions.

Education and Information

The definition of disability, as it is often used in U.S. society, is synonymous with dependency. The view that disabling conditions entail loss of control over one's affairs is pervasive not only among the general public but also among health care and social service professionals. The paternalistic attitudes that stem from this stereotypical view are antithetical to what should be the primary goal of prevention programs: to facilitate greater autonomy among people with disabling conditions. Education is the key to fostering a more realistic and more constructive understanding of the capabilities, rights, and needs of people with disabling conditions. Educational efforts should focus on three target populations: (1) the general public; (2) members of the social service and health care professions, especially physicians; and (3) people with disabling conditions, their families, advocates, and personal attendants.

Public Education

Many secondary conditions can be prevented with the aid of an appropriately informed public. Many advocates of people with disabling conditions and many care providers believe that if physical and attitudinal barriers to participation in society, including employment, are eliminated, then the estrangement, isolation, depression, and poverty that often accompany disabling conditions will decrease.

The committee recognizes that societal attitudes are slow to change, although the recently passed Americans with Disabilities Act can be an important catalyst. Moreover, to be effective, education programs must be the product of thoughtful and deliberate planning. This committee is not expert in the field of education, and therefore does not prescribe specific educational measures to foster integration of people with disabling conditions into the community. Rather, it recommends that education planners and others focus their efforts on conveying five basic messages:

1. People with disabling conditions constitute a large segment (14 percent) of the population.
2. Regardless of their current health status, most people are at risk of developing a disabling condition.
3. All rights of citizenship extend to the population with disabling conditions.
4. People with disabling conditions can be productive members of society.
5. People with disabling conditions can achieve a high quality of life.

Education of Health Care Professionals

Most schools of medicine, nursing, and allied health have not properly prepared health care professionals to address problems and issues related to disability and chronic disease. Medical schools, for example, rarely include rehabilitation as a standard clinical rotation, nor do they foster the interdisciplinary skills and the commitment to teamwork that are necessary to address the varied needs of people with disabling conditions.

The complexity of problems associated with chronic illness and disability demands that all health care professionals become familiar with the rehabilitation process and the importance of evaluating the entire social situation of the person with a disabling condition. In medical schools, the likely locus for this responsibility would be a department of physical and medical rehabilitation (PMR). Unfortunately, most medical schools do not have such a department, although the Graduate Medicine Education National Advisory Committee identified PMR as one of three medical specialties with personnel shortages. The shortage of PMR specialists underscores the importance of acquainting all future health care professionals with the needs of people with disabling conditions.

Specific accreditation criteria are needed for assessing whether medical schools provide adequate education on the prevention of disability and secondary conditions and on the rehabilitation of people with physical or mental disability. In addition, training in disability prevention and in rehabilitation should be included, as appropriate, in the education of medical specialists. Similarly, schools of nursing and allied health should include the prevention of physical and mental disability and of secondary conditions in their curricula.

Given the prevalence of disabling conditions in the general population and the demographic trends, ever larger numbers of practicing health care professionals will be called on to provide treatment, health maintenance, and related services to people with chronic disease or disabling conditions.

The continuing education of physicians and other health care professionals should include training on the risks of secondary conditions and on general methods of rehabilitation.

Education of People with Disability

Information, it has been said, is power. This adage certainly applies to people with disabling conditions, who should retain primary responsibility for decisions affecting their health and quality of life. The problem, however, is that people with disabling conditions need sound information on which to base their decisions. Often the information is not available; if it is, it frequently must be gathered from disparate, hard-to-identify sources.

In this "information age," one often hears that information overload is a problem—but this is not the case for people with disabling conditions. Numerous data bases on assistive technologies exist, for example, but most are small and they often contain incomplete or outdated information. Very few of these data bases achieve the desirable end of providing links among people with disabling conditions, health care professionals, and manufacturers of assistive technologies.

It would be naive to assume that comprehensive information networks—which might include information on community health and social services, assistive technologies, nutrition, and medications— can be developed overnight. But the tools do exist, and steps to achieve this goal could be undertaken incrementally. Independent living centers, many of which have developed data bases that provide at least some of the information people with disabling conditions need, offer a foundation on which to build comprehensive local information networks.

Technology, however, will never replace face-to-face interaction as a means for imparting necessary information and teaching important skills. If we expect people with disabling conditions to take primary responsibility for their well-being, then physicians and other service providers must advise their patients on how to maintain or improve their health status and reduce the risk of secondary conditions. Moreover, physicians must be prepared to counsel their patients and families on the strengths and limitations of alternative modalities of care, including potential impacts of these modalities on quality of life.

There is also an important ancillary role to be played by formal education programs on a variety of topics, including health promotion, assistive technologies, stress control, and home safety. These could be developed under the auspices of public health departments; departments of preventive medicine, geriatrics, or physical medicine and rehabilitation at local medical schools; independent living centers; local rehabilitation centers; foundations; and voluntary organizations.

Educational programs on topics related to the prevention of secondary conditions need to be expanded with emphasis placed on reaching people with disabling conditions, their families, advocates, and personal attendants.

Finally, persons with disabling conditions need to be taught skills that will help them live full, rewarding lives. Good organizational and time management skills can assist these people in compensating for their functional limitations, and training in these important skills is often necessary.

In addition, functional limitations often make it difficult, if not impossible, for adults with disabling conditions to return to their old jobs without training and modification of the work environment. Some will not be able to return to their previous occupation at all, necessitating training in a new skill or profession. Thus vocational training is often critical to ensuring one's return to the work force.

Environmental Considerations

The quality of life of a person with a disabling condition is closely linked to the person's social and physical environment, on both large and small scales. Because of the multifaceted nature of this relationship, trade-offs may be necessary. Someone who uses a wheelchair and lives in a northern state, for example, may be forced to limit his or her outdoor activities during the winter months because of icy conditions and low temperatures. A person who has the same limitation but lives in the South or Southwest will confront far fewer weather-related barriers. For many people, however, relocating to an area with a more benign climate is not financially feasible or even desirable. Moving may entail loss of friends and family contacts, loss of job, and other costs that outweigh climate-related advantages.

When the focus shifts to the individual's general surroundings, other important variables come into play, such as proximity to health services, work, stores, recreational establishments, and family and friends; accessibility to buildings and public transportation; availability of housing; and opportunities for employment. Not all of these variables are under the control of the individual. For example, social attitudes and public policy are the primary determinants of whether public buildings are accessible to people in wheelchairs or whether local employers are willing to invest in the workplace modifications that may be required by people with disabling conditions.

Distance to needed services, however, may be within the control of the individual. Generally, the greater the distance to services, the more dependent a person with a disabling condition is on the assistance of others. Thus a person who lives in an urban environment may be more autonomous in his or her personal affairs than someone who lives in a rural area and must depend on others for transportation and to make necessary purchases.

The home environment introduces new considerations that are primarily related to safety and to the performance of basic living activities. Financial resources and the reimbursement policies of public and private insurers are the primary determinants of whether the immediate living environment is adapted to the needs and capabilities of the person with a disabling condition. Many "off-the-shelf" assistive technologies can be instrumental in promoting greater autonomy. But, as discussed previously, these technologies often do not qualify for insurance coverage.

PROTOCOLS FOR THE PREVENTION OF
SECONDARY CONDITIONS

Although many secondary conditions can be prevented, interventions are often ineffective because they fail to address the multiple risk factors related to the pathophysiology and life situation of the person with a disabling condition. To be successful, interventions must be multifaceted and comprehensive. The most effective prevention programs are longitudinal in nature and embody a variety of strategies, devised and carried out by a multidisciplinary team.

Protocols would foster the integration and comprehensiveness essential to the prevention of secondary conditions. A protocol lists the evaluation, treatment, and service delivery strategies that apply to a specific type of disabling condition and to the characteristics of the person with the disabling condition. Developed prospectively from general information, protocols serve as generic guidelines that assure completeness in the development of individual treatment and service plans. Often, a protocol will list several options for each element in the individualized plan. Specific interventions are chosen in light of the special circumstances of the person with the disabling condition.

As frameworks on which to build individualized plans, protocols must reckon with variability. The pathological processes that underlie a secondary condition vary considerably; they can stabilize after an acute event, fluctuate in severity over time, or be progressive. Similarly, the amount of additional disability that can result encompasses a broad range, influencing, for example, the decision of whether to prescribe major medical treatment or to rely on compensatory assistive technology. Moreover, the interactive relationship between the risk of secondary conditions and social, economic, and environmental characteristics introduces more variability that must be anticipated in the development of protocols.

Currently, protocols to guide the development of effective prevention programs are few. As noted previously, a serious obstacle is the paucity of evaluative information on the effectiveness and outcomes of interventions for many secondary conditions.

Evaluative studies are needed to determine the effectiveness and costs of interventions for major secondary conditions. As part of this effort, consensus conferences should be conducted to review existing knowledge in those areas where research and clinical experience are sufficient to develop model protocols for the prevention of secondary conditions. As the primary sponsor of effectiveness and outcomes research, the Agency for Health Care Policy and Research would be the appropriate agency to assume leadership in initiating these activities.

The nature of these recommended initiatives will differ somewhat from the effectiveness and outcome research and the protocol development going on in other areas of health care. One important distinction is the especially significant role played by social and environmental risk factors in the occurrence of secondary conditions. Another is the emphasis of preventive interventions on improving quality of life. The remainder of this chapter focuses on the general components of protocols for the prevention of secondary conditions.

Definition of Disability Category

The initial step in protocol development is to determine the category of the disabling condition. Ordinarily, a diagnostic category reflects what is known about the pathologic process, including the etiology and the anatomic site of involvement. Individual cases within a given diagnostic category will vary widely in their course. Recognition of this variability at the outset helps alert care providers using the protocol to the importance of evaluating alternative interventions.

The protocol should also list secondary conditions associated with the category. Supporting informational elements include descriptions of the signs and symptoms of the pathologies, impairments, and functional limitations that can lead to a secondary condition and additional disability. For each secondary condition, the range of potential outcomes should be specified.

Specification of Health Maintenance and Medical Interventions

The importance of preventive measures should be recognized at the outset of treatment for a disabling condition, and major emphasis on these measures should be sustained throughout the life of the person with the condition. As discussed previously, the cornerstones of a healthy lifestyle for people with disabling conditions are the same as those for people without disabling conditions. They include regular exercise, appropriate nutrition, weight control, abstinence from smoking and illicit drugs, moderate consumption of alcohol, stress control, and adequate sleep.

Strategies for accomplishing these healthful behaviors often must be tailored to the particular needs and functional limitations of the person with a disabling condition. A person with restricted motion of the joints, for example, will require assistance in performing stretching exercises, and adaptive equipment may also be needed. Failure to accommodate these needs increases the risk of contractures, pressure sores, and other secondary conditions. When possible, protocols should spell out the risks of developing secondary conditions when specific health promotion and maintenance objectives are not fulfilled.

Medical interventions are often prescribed to minimize the effects of the existing disabling condition. The protocol should familiarize providers with the potential iatrogenic effects of medications and other interventions commonly prescribed for people with a specific category of disabling condition. Drug side effects, for example, may increase the risk of developing a secondary condition.

If the primary disabling condition or other existing factors pose a high risk of secondary conditions, the physician should consider medical interventions for reducing the risk. Changes in bladder functioning and emptying dynamics following spinal cord injury, for example, require intermittent catheterization or other bladder management techniques. A consequence of these interventions is often an elevated risk for urinary tract infections. Thus the protocol for the care of people with spinal cord injury should include alternative strategies for bladder management and for reducing the risk of urinary tract infection.

Specification of Rehabilitation Interventions

Rehabilitative measures intended to minimize the effects of disabling conditions must be an integral part of protocols for preventing secondary conditions. Protocols should list measures that focus on the primary disabling condition and, where appropriate, on secondary conditions that are directly or indirectly related to the primary disabling condition. For instance, weakness of an extremity is common after plexus injury that involves nerves in the extremities. The nerve damage then predisposes the affected individual to contractures of the joints and muscles of the involved extremity; the contractures are secondary to the original pathology. Ordinarily, the more remote a secondary condition is from the original pathology, the greater the likelihood of success in preventing its occurrence, assuming appropriate interventions are applied.

Rehabilitation should focus on permitting the person with a disabling condition to perform the normal roles of life, with or without assistance. Accomplishing this goal entails decisions that require reckoning with trade-offs and evaluating the improvement in functioning that can result from intervention in medical and nonmedical contexts.

The prospects for successful rehabilitation are also influenced by predisability personality traits, and these need to be taken into account in the development of a rehabilitation protocol. Krueger (1981) notes that people who tend to be overly conscientious and strive for independence have traits that bode well for rehabilitation. Tucker (1984) makes the important points that motivation is a critical determinant of rehabilitation success and that motivation is both an intrapersonal and interpersonal phenomenon:

> If a patient is consistently devalued, is not given support for progress, and receives a hopeless prognosis, he or she will give up and appear

unmotivated. Once such a derogatory label is applied, it is a signal that rehabilitation efforts will fail. But if the person is given positive feedback, the individual's motivation to strive will be enhanced. Potentially, a beneficial cycle or "recipe for motivation" can emerge.

If the potential for improvement is only marginal, then the impact on the person's lifestyle may be insignificant. Therefore, it may be more fruitful to reallocate resources from physical therapy to purchasing assistive technology and training the person to use that technology. The impact of assistive technology on the individual's quality of life may be far greater than the minor improvement in functioning achieved with extensive occupational and physical therapy.

Specification of Assistive Technologies

Appropriate assistive technology can significantly reduce the impact of disabling conditions on personal autonomy and participation in the everyday affairs of society. Selection of assistive technology should be done in collaboration with the person with the disabling condition, who should identify the tasks that are most significant to maintaining his or her lifestyle.

Assistive technologies offer two separate but related strategies for helping to ensure personal autonomy. Some devices are used by the individual to improve function. Other technologies involve modifying the environment so that the person can accomplish tasks that would not otherwise be possible.

Product quality and costs are major considerations in the selection of assistive technologies. Initial cost savings, however, should not be achieved at the expense of reliability and quality. Moreover, protocols must acknowledge the importance of training individuals in the use of assistive devices and of providing maintenance services.

Specification of Environmental Changes

Although several steps in the protocol are concerned with issues related to environmental surroundings, explicit consideration of potential modifications is essential. The primary goals of these modifications are to ensure safety and to facilitate performance of tasks important to the individual. Inspection of the home and general neighborhood will be necessary to determine what modifications are necessary and the feasibility of making needed changes.

Specification of Elements in the Social Support Network

People with disabling conditions often live an isolated existence, dependent on others to initiate social contact and even to arrange for needed services. Depression and neglect of self-care are two of several common consequences of isolation that increase the risk of developing a secondary condition. Protocols must consider the availability of informal and formal social support mechanisms that foster social interaction and assist in the identification and procurement of needed services.

Care providers should familiarize themselves with the individual's family situation and determine whether family members or friends are available to provide assistance as needed. They should also be familiar with available community resources. If an independent living center or other advocacy organization exists, providers should link the individual to these resources. Peer support is an especially critical component of efforts to prevent secondary conditions.

A support network should be developed not only for the person with a disabling condition but also for his or her family. The form that these networks should take cannot be specified in advance because of the considerable variability among families. For some, regular, informal get-togethers may be sufficient. For others, more formalized measures, such as support group sessions offered by hospitals or rehabilitation facilities, may be needed.

In conclusion, protocols help ensure that the total spectrum of needed interventions are incorporated into individualized treatment and service plans. Such guidance is useful to all health care and social service professionals who work with people with disabling conditions. It is especially valuable for the many care and service providers who have little knowledge of the often debilitating effects of secondary conditions.

Protocols will not substitute for good professional judgment in formulating effective treatment and service plans. As problem-solving aids, protocols help facilitate the development of treatment plans that are comprehensive and integrate the necessary elements of care. Moreover, professional efforts to develop needed protocols will systematically focus attention on those areas lacking interventions that have been evaluated for effectiveness. Such a systematic approach will highlight critical research needs and guide development of future prevention programs.

Table 7-3 summarizes much of the information presented in this chapter. It is included as a guide for those who are interested in what information about the prevention of secondary conditions is available, and what is not known and needed. The information is organized into four categories: services, education, research and surveillance, and coordination and oversight.

TABLE 7-3 Known vs. Needed Information About the Prevention of Secondary Conditions

Category	Known/Available	Unknown/Needed
Services	Assistive technology is capable of decreasing disability and is in a rapidly expanding era with new innovations on the horizon.	Where efficacious, assistive technology should be paid for as part of clinical care if it allows for life activities including work, social, recreation, and activities of daily living.
	Protocols aid in disability prevention and rehabilitation planning and in the identification of potential physical and psychiatric secondary conditions.	Protocols and screening instruments are needed to identify, prevent, and treat potential secondary complications, both physical and psychiatric. Psychiatric consultation should be available to all rehabilitation personnel for patient monitoring and treatment.
Education	Medical school and speciality training impart insufficient knowledge and skills in principles of physical medicine and rehabilitation and psychosocial rehabilitation.	Medical school and appropriate speciality training should include curricular material in PMR and psychiatric principles appropriate to identify potentially disabling complications of illness and injury: the curriculum also should include material on appropriate preventive interventions, including consultation and collaboration. Parallel training for nurses and allied health professionals is recommended. Model protocols should be useful for these training curricula.
	Allied health professionals and consumers lack knowledge of disability prevention.	Consumers and the public require education about the needs of those with disability.
	Rehabilitation personnel are often unaware of psychoeducational approaches and processes.	Students, trainees, and professionals in rehabilitation disciplines should be trained in identification of behavioral and major mental illnesses, and the appropriate interventions and/or consultations.

TABLE 7-3 *Continued*

Category	Known/Available	Unknown/Needed
	Practitioners are unable to maintain skills and knowledge at a level of current need to deal with disability prevention, particularly with secondary conditions.	Postgraduate education should include physical and psychosocial principles and identification of secondary conditions with appropriate referral.
	Medical schools often lack curricula and departments of rehabilitation.	The Liaison Committee on Medical Education of the American Association of Medical Colleges (AAMC) should develop more specific criteria for accreditation of medical schools regarding adequate exposure to rehabilitative principles and practice. The AAMC's Accreditation Council for Graduate Medical Education should also require training in primary, secondary, and tertiary disability prevention principles and treatment planning for appropriate medical speciality trainees.
	Assistive technology is a growing aid to rehabilitation and disability prevention.	Curricula in assistive technology should be included in training for PMR, undergraduate medical education, and allied health, nursing, and related disciplines.
Research and surveillance	Spinal cord injury (SCI) is the only condition for which there exists surveillance of secondary disabilities.	Disability surveillance systems should include incidence and prevalence of secondary conditions, including psychiatric complications.
	When depression occurs as a comorbid condition with SCI, there is a high comorbidity of depression and other psychiatric complications, as well as a high correlation with physical complications such as contractures and decubiti.	Research is needed to determine how intervention affects the prevention of secondary conditions, including psychiatric complications.

TABLE 7-3 *Continued*

Category	Known/Available	Unknown/Needed
	Protocols can be useful in effective treatment planning, especially for trainees and for professionals with less specific training.	Assessment is needed of the efficacy of protocols for treatment of primary disabling conditions and prevention of physical and psychiatric secondary disabilities.
	Assistive technology can prevent some secondary disability (e.g., motorized wheelchair mobility and access to work, social activity, and recreation).	Support is needed for further research and development of assistive technology and its effect on secondary disabling conditions.
Coordination and oversight	Responsibility for research, service, education, and funding is under multiple state and federal auspices.	An interagency council or forum is needed to serve as the coordinating body for the prevention activities of all federal agencies.
	The National Institute on Disability and Rehabilitation Research (NIDRR) and the Veterans Administration sponsor and conduct large programs in rehabilitation research that are focused on secondary and tertiary care. NIDRR also directs the Interagency Council on Disability Research.	The Centers for Disease Control (CDC) should provide leadership in setting the national agenda and direction in services, research, and surveillance in the prevention of disability.
	CDC's new Disabilities Prevention Program draws on its expertise in epidemiology, surveillance, and technology transfer in sponsoring prevention activities.	Improved coordination is needed with increased emphasis on multidisciplinary approaches to prevention.

8
A Comprehensive Approach to Disability Prevention: Obstacles and Opportunities

Disability prevention is already a stated national goal, enunciated in the numerous federal, state, and local laws and policies that promote independence and equality of opportunity for people with disabling conditions. During the last two decades, Congress has passed more than a dozen laws designed to increase the participation of people with disabling conditions in the day-to-day activities of society (Vachon, 1989-1990). Yet the prevalence of disabling conditions is growing, and with it, annual disability-related expenditures (federal, state, local, and private), which are approaching $200 billion (Chirikos, 1989). Numerous factors underlie these trends, many of which, such as the link between disabling conditions and low socioeconomic status, are poorly understood. Nonetheless, it is reasonable to ask whether the vast resources expended on disability are yielding a sufficient return. The answer must be an unequivocal no.

Similarly, one can ask whether enough resources are devoted to measures to arrest the continuing increase in the economic costs of disabling conditions. Again, the answer is no. From a strictly economic vantage point, the aggregate costs of disabling conditions, measured as the sum of reductions in household income, net of income transfer payments, and purchases of goods and services made necessary by disabling conditions, totaled an estimated $176.7 billion in 1980. Between 1960 and 1980, according to the analysis that yielded this estimate, annual economic losses attributable to disabling conditions increased at an average rate of 2.7 percent (Chirikos, 1989). These estimates, although necessarily rough because of the inadequacies of data available on the population with disabling conditions, indicate the magnitude of savings that can be achieved with more comprehensive approaches to primary, secondary, and tertiary prevention.

Among national goals, disability prevention is akin to an orphan whose care has been entrusted to many well-intentioned guardians. Neglect is not so much the issue as the potential for inconsistency, lack of continuity, and, to some degree, shortsightedness. Without coherence and coordination in the planning and provision of services, progress against this societal and public health problem will be impeded.

In its 1986 report *Toward Independence*, the National Council on the Handicapped (now the National Council on Disability) criticized the "complexities, inconsistencies, and fragmentation in the various federal laws that affect Americans with disabilities." In public hearings convened by the council, people with disabling conditions stated that "many programs do not mesh well with other available services, and that too often the service delivery system exhibits gaps, inconsistencies, and inequities" (National Council on the Handicapped, 1986).

These failings are not surprising, given the magnitude of the disability problem and the numerous public and private programs that have evolved to address it. At the federal level, about 50 programs spread across five cabinet-level departments offer services beneficial to people with disabling conditions. Coordination is not easily achieved in such a far-flung bureaucracy, and this difficulty is compounded by the formidable challenge of developing effective linkages among federal, state, and local agencies and between the public and private sectors. Failure to improve the fragmented collection of programs is a virtual guarantee that the large social and economic costs associated with disability will continue to grow.

Disability prevention requires an effective system of longitudinal care, an integrated service delivery network that is responsive to the health, social, housing, and personal care needs of people who have disabling conditions or who have a high risk of developing them. Many of the elements of the desired network are already in place but now operate in isolation rather than as complementary parts of an integrated whole. Achieving an integrated service delivery network that is easily negotiated by client populations will be difficult. As noted in earlier chapters, the lack of an adequate epidemiologic surveillance system for tracking the incidence and prevalence of disabling conditions in sufficient detail hampers planning, including identification of service delivery priorities.

The inadequacy of current surveillance efforts is but one of many impediments that limit the overall effectiveness of the hundreds of public and private programs related to disability. Rather than evaluate these individual programs, the committee describes some of the obstacles and opportunities that exist vis-à-vis an integrated national system of disability prevention. Many of the issues are not new, and some, such as inadequate access to health care for certain high-risk populations, are subsets of broader social concerns. Progress toward a comprehensive approach to disability prevention requires reckoning with the problems outlined below and capitalizing on opportunities.

DEMEDICALIZATION

The so-called medical model has influenced the development of most of the nation's disability-related programs. The model defines disabling conditions as principally the product of physical and mental impairments that constrain performance. Influenced by this view, health and social agencies provide a mix of services that, for the most part, categorize affected individuals as permanently ill and incapable of meeting their own needs. Therefore, the problems that disability-related programs seek to address are often viewed as inherent to the individual and as independent of society.

The independent-living and disability-rights movements blame adherence to the medical model for the creation of disability-related programs that foster dependence rather than personal autonomy. Members of these movements correctly argue that disability is the result of a dynamic process involving complex interactions among biological, behavioral, psychological, social, and environmental factors. Some have called for the "demedicalization" of disability in order to reflect the broader role of society. To do so in the extreme sense, however, would allow the pendulum to swing too far in the other direction.

An example illustrates the need for a more balanced approach to disability. The 1987 survey commissioned by the International Center for the Disabled (ICD) reported that two-thirds of the unemployed respondents, more than 8 million people, would like to be working (Taylor, 1989). Were the majority of these people not working because their disabling conditions prevented them from doing so, or were they not working because of hiring discrimination, transportation difficulties, or other societal barriers? Doubtless, these and other reasons account for why at least a portion of these respondents do not have jobs, but they probably do not account for the majority.

A follow-up survey of U.S. employers, also done for ICD, found that the biggest single obstacle to employment for people with disabling conditions is the lack of qualifications (Taylor, 1989). Thus the survey results indicate that education and training are important elements of efforts to help people with disabling conditions secure jobs. Such training and education programs must be designed with full recognition of the limitations imposed by one's physical or mental condition. Moreover, continued employment will often require medical interventions that help maintain the health of the worker who has a disabling condition.

Timely and appropriate medical intervention is an essential element of the committee's recommended approach to disability prevention—an integrated system of longitudinal care. However, the committee agrees with Caplan (1988), who has argued that "health care should not be the major preoccupation of public policy" related to disability. "[T]reating chronic illness and disability strictly as medical problems," Caplan has written, "'disenfranchises' a large segment of society by making them permanent objects of social beneficence, a status that few if any members of our society would wish to occupy."

Disability prevention requires a change in the perspective of physicians and other health care providers to broaden modern medicine's cure-oriented emphasis on acute illness. Often, people with disabling conditions cannot be cured, although this is not to say that they do not require acute care services. For these people, medical interventions are more appropriately viewed as playing an enabling, or empowering, role. The standard of successful treatment should be achieving a level of health and functioning that allows people with disabling conditions to manage their own affairs and to participate in society.

When viewed as a complementary element of disability prevention, health care can move in new directions. For example, treatment protocols, as recommended in the previous chapter, would consider not only medical needs but also necessary environmental modifications, the availability of family support, and other nonmedical variables. Thus health care should be viewed as only one component of an array of enabling interventions that have a common aim: whether social, environmental, or medical, the services provided to people with disabling conditions should seek to ensure a reasonable quality of life.

Similarly, attention to quality of life may point the way to new intervention strategies and better measures of rehabilitation outcomes. For example, significant recovery of intellectual capacity and motor function in people who have sustained severe brain injuries is generally considered to constitute successful rehabilitation. Yet a growing body of research indicates a high frequency of behavior disorders in this population, a problem rarely addressed in rehabilitation even though it is believed to be a major cause of job loss. A greater emphasis on measures of quality of life in evaluations of the effectiveness of rehabilitation might spawn greater awareness and understanding of the problem.

NATIONAL HEALTH PROMOTION AND DISEASE PREVENTION OBJECTIVES

The status and importance of public health and preventive medicine were enhanced significantly in 1979, when the Public Health Service promulgated 226 health promotion and disease prevention objectives to accomplish five national health goals by 1990 (U.S. Department of Health and Human Services, 1980a). Measured against 1977 benchmark statistics, these goals were to achieve the following: 35 percent fewer deaths among infants, 20 percent fewer deaths among healthy children between the ages of 1 and 14, 20 percent fewer deaths among adolescents and adults between the ages of 15 and 24, 25 percent fewer deaths among adults between the ages of 25 and 64, and 20 percent fewer sick days among adults age 65 and older.

Among the many benefits attributable to this effort are the focusing of attention on important health priorities and the mobilizing of resources to achieve specific aims. A mid-decade review (U.S. Department of Health and Human Services, 1986) reported that the nation was progressing toward achieving about two-thirds of the measurable objectives. (About one-fourth of the objectives cannot be measured.)

The goal of disability prevention was only indirectly represented in the 226 health objectives, which were divided among 15 target areas such as control of high blood pressure, immunization, infant health, accident prevention and injury control, nutrition, and physical fitness. This is not to say, however, that accomplishing the objectives would not translate into significant advances against some disabling conditions. A review of the objectives to determine their applicability to disability prevention deemed nearly 80 percent to be relevant to the prevention of primary disabling conditions. An even larger percentage were considered applicable to the prevention of secondary conditions. Nonetheless, the objectives were far from comprehensive, failing to address, for example, hearing and vision disorders, learning disabilities, mental health problems, and concerns related to the health and functioning of the elderly (Nova Research Company, 1988).

A common criticism of the health objectives was that they focused almost exclusively on mortality and failed to reflect the importance of reducing morbidity. Indeed, a reduction in mortality, such as traffic-related deaths, may mask an increase in disabilities resulting from injuries sustained in motor vehicle collisions. A related criticism was that the objectives neglected the incidence and prevalence of major chronic diseases and other conditions that can lead to disability.

In September 1990, the U.S. Public Health Service promulgated national health objectives for the year 2000 (U.S. Department of Health and Human Services, 1990). *Healthy People 2000*—the completed volume of the year 2000 health objectives (U.S. Department of Health and Human Services, 1990) embraces disability prevention more fully as a national health priority than did the objectives for the preceding decade. In effect, each priority area has a disability prevention component as a natural corollary. In addition, one priority area focuses specifically on "diabetes and chronic disabling conditions." The priority areas for *Healthy People 2000* are listed in Table 8-1.

Integration of disability prevention into the health objectives framework should be enhanced further by a three-year project, begun in 1989, to tailor the implementation of the objectives to the special needs of people with disabilities. Funded by the Public Health Service, this project is being carried out by the American Association of University Affiliated Programs.

Despite the marked improvements suggested by *Healthy People 2000*, the

TABLE 8-1   Year 2000 Health Objectives Priority Areas Assigned to Categories of Health Promotion, Health Protection, and Preventive Services

Health Promotion	Health Protection	Preventive Services
Physical activity and fitness	Unintentional injuries	Maternal and infant health
Nutrition	Occupational injuries	Heart disease and stroke
Tobacco	Environmental health	Cancer
Alcohol and other drugs	Food and drug safety	Other chronic and
Family planning	Oral health	disabling conditions
Mental health		HIV infection
Violent and abusive behavior		Sexually transmitted
Educational and community-		diseases
based programs		Immunization and
		infectious diseases
		Clinical preventive services

Note: Each of the 21 priority areas contains objectives in the following age-related categories: healthy babies, healthy children, healthy adolescents and youth, and healthy older people.

SOURCE: U.S. Department of Health and Human Services, 1990.

importance of secondary and tertiary prevention is not fully acknowledged. Many objectives fail to recognize that mortality is not the only outcome of disease and injury. In fact, many chronic conditions do not ordinarily lead to death, and their impacts are measured more appropriately by indicators of quality of life rather than by mortality. For example, one objective calls for reducing stroke-caused deaths to no more than 20 per 100,000 people. However, disability and other forms of morbidity are more common outcomes of stroke than death. Thus an appropriate, related health objective might be to reduce the rate of disability or activity limitation caused by stroke.

The establishment of a distinct set of national goals related to disability was proposed in 1986 in federal rehabilitation legislation, but the proposal did not pass (Vachon, 1989-1990). The goal of disability prevention would be advanced significantly if it were fully incorporated into the nation's health objectives.

CLINICAL PREVENTIVE SERVICES

An important information resource is the *Guide to Clinical Preventive Services* (U.S. Department of Health and Human Services, 1989a), a report that details more than 100 effective interventions to prevent 60 different illnesses and conditions. Although mortality is the measure used for evaluating the impact of the interventions, the means of intervention go beyond primary intervention to include regular screening (secondary prevention) and recommendations for early and persistent treatment (tertiary prevention). The report describes a key role for primary caregivers in screening for many conditions and immunizing for others. It also emphasizes strengthening the clinician's role in counseling patients to change unhealthful behaviors related to diet, smoking, exercise, injury, and sexually transmitted disease. Indeed, this approach should be furthered to encompass the many interventions needed to address the biological, environmental, and lifestyle factors that affect primary and secondary disabilities.

FEDERAL PROGRAMS AND POLICIES

In 1986 the federal government spent about $60 billion on programs directly benefiting people with disabling conditions. About $57 billion was allocated for income support and medical coverage (National Council on the Handicapped, 1986). The remainder was divided among research and a variety of service-related activities, especially in the areas of education, housing, and transportation. Some programs, such as Social Security Disability Insurance (SSDI)—the largest in terms of expenditures and number of clients— are designed to serve the entire population with disabling conditions, as- suming individuals meet eligibility requirements. Others, such as the De- partment of Education's deaf-blind centers, are tailored to people with specific types of disabling conditions. The department's special education programs offer educational and related services focused on children and youth with disabling conditions, serving about 4.5 million individuals from birth through age 21 (U.S. Department of Education, 1989a). Moreover, several programs, especially those that provide income compensation, are linked to specific occupations or groups of employees, such as railroad workers, coal miners, and longshoremen, or to past military service.

The complexities inherent in this bureaucratic compartmentalization are exacerbated by the considerable variety in the way programs are managed and administered. For example, SSDI and Medicare are managed at the federal level, although many administrative responsibilities are delegated to the states. In contrast, the Supplementary Security Income program, Med- icaid, and vocational rehabilitation programs are jointly funded but administered at the state level, while municipalities manage most housing and transportation programs. This diffusion of administrative responsibility and direction manifests in fragmentation at the service delivery end. Intended beneficiaries often do not obtain needed services because of confusing, restrictive eligibility requirements, lack of information, separation of complementary services, lack of comprehensive goals, and other reasons.

Examples given in the following sections illustrate how the failure to develop consistency among programs undermines progress in efforts to re- duce the prevalence of disability.

Social Security Disability Insurance and Rehabilitation

The National Council on Disability criticized federal programs for an "overemphasis on income support and an underemphasis on initiatives for equal opportunity, independence, prevention, and self-sufficiency" (National Council on the Handicapped, 1986). This imbalance and its attendant problems are most apparent in the SSDI program, which made payments totaling $15.9 billion to 3 million working-age people with disabling conditions in 1988 (Social Security Administration, 1989).

Originating in a 1956 amendment to the Social Security Act, SSDI payments are intended to compensate people who have a recent work history but are unable to engage in any "substantial gainful activity" because of a medically determined physical or mental impairment that is expected to result in death or persist for at least one year. In practice, SSDI requirements assume that people who establish their eligibility for aid have permanent disabling conditions and have sustained a lifelong loss of income-earning ability. Thus SSDI has been described by some as a retirement pension.

The original legislation endorsed the tandem goals of income maintenance and rehabilitation. For example, states were authorized to withhold or reduce cash benefits if a beneficiary refused rehabilitation without good cause. Moreover, the Social Security Administration directed the states to require that every applicant for disability benefits be interviewed by a rehabilitation counselor. This requirement was waived in 1959, however, for applicants who were bedridden, institutionalized, or mentally ill, or who had a worsening impairment (Berkowitz and Fox, 1989).

At best, rehabilitation and disability prevention rank as subordinate goals of SSDI, an example of the underemphasis on promoting autonomy. Having satisfied rigid criteria, SSDI beneficiaries then have the option of undergoing rehabilitation, assuming that they meet an additional set of requirements, including a demonstrated potential for work. However, this potential might be viewed as jeopardizing one's eligibility for compensation, serving as a deterrent to rehabilitation. Moreover, even for those desiring rehabilitation, therapy and training are often delayed until completion of the lengthy eligibility-determination process, which can exceed two years if appeals are involved. During this period, a person's condition may deteriorate, and with it, the chances for successful rehabilitation. Other incongruities arise when it is determined that applicants do not meet SSDI requirements and yet are classified as too impaired to satisfy Social Security Administration eligibility standards for rehabilitation services.

Rehabilitation is a small component of SSDI and the Social Security Administration's other disability-related programs, and the results have been equivocal. The Beneficiary Rehabilitation Program, begun in 1965, allocated money from the SSDI trust fund to reimburse states in full for rehabilitation services provided to SSDI recipients who satisfied certain criteria, including predicted length of employment following rehabilitation. A program aim was to save trust fund money by ultimately decreasing the number of SSDI claimants. Early indications of promising performance, which spurred an increase in funding from $40.5 million in 1970 to $102.6 million in 1976, were not confirmed by cost-benefit analyses. The program was discontinued in 1981. Rehabilitation provisions of Social Security Administration disability benefit programs include federal reimbursement to states for vocational rehabilitation services provided to recipients of federal disability benefits. Among other restrictions, this provision applies only if the beneficiary returns to work and remains employed for nine consecutive months (Institute of Medicine, 1987). This provision is little used, as is provision for a trial work period that allows earning without reducing SSDI benefits (though it does affect Supplemental Security Income payments).

The bulk of public funding for vocational rehabilitation is allocated through a joint funding arrangement. The federal government, through the Rehabilitation Services Administration of the Department of Education, pays for 80 percent of the services, and the states provide the remaining 20 percent. This partnership spent $1.7 billion on vocational rehabilitation in 1988, funding such services as job training, counseling, and placement; some medical care; the purchase of prosthetic devices; and college education. A recent assessment of the vocational rehabilitation system (Vachon, 1989-1990) notes that, despite the growing work-disabled population and annually increasing outlays, the 220,000 recipients of these services totaled 45 percent fewer than the number served in 1974. Based on a survey conducted for the ICD (Louis Harris and Associates, 1986), Vachon (1987) reports that 10 percent of the working-age population with disabling conditions used the services of the publicly funded program, and half of this group said their participation was of little or no value in securing a job.

Vachon notes a high level of dissatisfaction with federal-state programs, noting that, for example, some state workers' compensation agencies have discontinued using program services and have opted to purchase private rehabilitation services. Another criticism is indicative of the controversy surrounding the role of vocational rehabilitation and the conflicting views over the proper client population. Vachon criticizes the "federally mandated 'order of selection,' which requires the most severely disabled to be served first, even though these individuals are the least likely to find jobs." It must be noted, however, that the opposite criticism has been leveled at the rehabilitation efforts of the Social Security Administration; that is, the agency has been accused by some of practicing a form of triage, in which only those most likely to find work are deemed eligible for services.

Equally controversial is Vachon's claim that the program focuses too much on people with mental or behavioral disorders, who represent more than 40 percent of program clientele. "People with such conditions," according to Vachon, "are difficult to treat and represent a small fraction of the work-disabled." His claim of an imbalance is supported by LaPlante's (1989b) analysis of the disability risks of chronic impairments, which found that about 1 million people, or about 3 percent of the population with activity limitations, have a form of mental illness. However, the inference that people with a mental illness are not appropriate targets of public vocational rehabilitation services is likely to foster considerable disagreement. In fact, anecdotal evidence indicates that shrinking labor supplies have increased private-sector interest in employing people with mental impairments. Firms that have reportedly increased hiring of workers who are mentally retarded or who have other disabilities include Marriott, Pizza Hut, McDonald's, United Airlines, and the International Business Machines Corporation (Kilborn, 1989).

Disagreement over the targeting of rehabilitation services is emblematic of the ferment in the field, which in turn exacerbates conflicts and contradictions inherent in public programs and their guiding policies. Debate over these issues could be constructive if it leads to a set of complementary goals and a rational set of services.

The boundaries of this debate should be expanded to take the experiences of other nations into account. Though international comparisons are limited, the few that have been conducted draw attention to this country's fragmented approach to addressing the financial and rehabilitation needs of people with disabling conditions. A six-country comparison found that only the United States failed to provide a "continuum of care" that creates an "environment conducive to reintegration into the work force" (Beedon and Zeitzer, 1988).

In the United States, individuals are often required to prove—before receiving rehabilitative care—that their disabling condition prevents them from working. In the Netherlands, West Germany, Switzerland, Israel, and Austria, rehabilitation usually precedes decisions on permanent disability pensions. The flexibility of programs in these countries permits extension of temporary financial benefits to accommodate continuing rehabilitation aimed at improving or restoring the skills necessary for returning to work.

Also notable is the combination of employer incentives and employee benefits that the foreign nations use to foster the return of people with disabling conditions to the work force. Public funds pay for adapting the job site to the workers' needs, whereas in the United States, tax incentives are used to elicit employer cooperation. Some of the foreign nations have instituted measures that address the transportation needs of workers with disabling conditions. Sweden, for example, pays for adapting vehicles for work-related transportation, and West Germany provides an allowance to help pay the cost of traveling to work.

The United States should more carefully consider the approaches used in

Western European countries (e.g., the Netherlands, Sweden, England, and France), where disability prevention is viewed from a broad perspective that includes social and ethical implications and socioeconomic costs. Part of the European approach entails the formation of councils and task forces comprising people with disabilities, their families, personal attendants, and advocates, and the elderly. These organizations are then active in negotiating with the governments on issues that affect health care on a national basis. The trend is thus to involve the consumers to an equal degree with health care providers and the payer. An international task force to study social and medical guidelines for the development of services to prevent disability and secondary conditions would be helpful.

Access to Medical Care and Preventive Services

This nation is deeply embroiled in a complex debate over the adequacy of health care coverage. The hallmarks of the debate are the vast and rapidly increasing sums expended on health care—estimated to total about $600 billion in 1990—and the sizable portion of the population without adequate insurance. Estimates of the number of uninsured Americans range from 22 million to nearly 40 million; millions more are underinsured, facing the risk of significant out-of-pocket expenses when in need of services for which they receive no or partial reimbursement.

Although the magnitude of this problem exceeds the scope of the present study, the committee is compelled to elaborate on the consequences of barriers to adequate care for the population with disabling conditions and the population that has a high risk of developing them. Lack of access to health care fuels the prevalence of disabling conditions by limiting the availability of services for the prevention of the impairments that lead to functional limitation and, ultimately, to disability. However, this is only one aspect of the problem, albeit a critical one. People who have private or public insurance often are not covered for the types of services that can halt the progression to disability and the development of equally debilitating secondary complications. Both issues warrant further comment.

Insurance Status

The few surveys that have investigated at least some aspects of health care coverage for the population with disabling conditions and chronic diseases yield only a cursory assessment. A 1984 National Health Interview Survey estimated that about 11 percent of 22.2 million people who are limited in the performance of their major activity do not have insurance (Table 8-2). The same survey also found that a substantially higher proportion of the population with disabling conditions—nearly 60 percent—were more

TABLE 8-2 Health Insurance Status of Persons With and Without Limitation of Major Activity Due to Chronic Conditions, 1984

Insurance Status	Persons With Major Activity Limitation		Persons Without Major Activity Limitation	
	Number (millions)	Percent Distribution	Number (millions)	Percent Distribution
Private insurance	14.0	63.1	154.5	78.3
Public insurance				
Medicaid	3.2	14.4	10.0	5.1
Medicare	8.2	36.9	15.6	7.9
Military-VA	1.7	7.6	5.7	2.9
Uninsured	2.4	10.8	26.5	13.4
Total	22.2	100.0	197.3	100.0

SOURCE: Adapted from Griss, 1988.

likely to depend, at least in part, on public insurance programs than were those in better health, 16 percent of whom have public insurance.

For persons with a work disability, the Survey of Income and Program Participation (SIPP) shows that uninsured persons with a work disability range from 11.9 percent among those employed full time to a high of 21 percent among those employed part time. About half the uninsured with a work disability are not employed and not receiving Supplemental Security Income or SSDI (Griss, 1988).

Given higher-than-average levels of poverty and unemployment among people with disabling conditions, and given the fact that poverty and unemployment are strongly correlated with lack of health care coverage, the population with disabling conditions is especially at risk of not having financial access to medical services, despite its greater need for these services. According to a 1986 Robert Wood Johnson Foundation survey (1987), 12 percent of the poor reporting a serious or chronic illness did not have insurance, as compared with 4 percent of the nonpoor population with similar conditions. Also revealing is the same survey's findings on use of health care services. Nearly 16 percent of the population with a chronic illness, or 7.7 million people, did not make a visit to a physician's office during the preceding 12 months. Given that the average chronically ill person made eight such visits during the year, the large number who did not receive ambulatory care strongly suggests a problem in obtaining needed services, even for individuals with some type of insurance coverage. The availability of insurance does not necessarily translate into access to needed services.

Compounding this problem are current trends in approaches to financing health care, which may be at odds not only with the aim of increasing insurance coverage but also with the goal of increasing employment among people with disabling conditions. Two-thirds of the working-age population with disabling conditions are unemployed, depriving them of access to employer-provided insurance, the primary source of coverage in the United States. Although many of these people say they are able and willing to work, the desire of businesses to control spending for employee health care benefits is likely to raise another obstacle to finding a job. Since the passage of the Employee Retirement and Income Security Act in 1974, an increasing number of businesses are opting for self-insurance. As allowed under the act, in exchange for assuming all or part of the risk of paying for claims submitted by their workers, self-insured firms are exempted from state insurance regulations. These businesses, which are estimated to employ more than half of all U.S. workers, have an economic incentive to screen job applicants and to remove from consideration those with chronic and disabling conditions that might lead to high medical expenses (Rublee, 1986). Between 1981 and 1983, nearly 60 percent of new workers underwent preemployment and preplacement screening, as compared with 48 percent of the workers hired between 1972 and 1974 (Ratcliffe et al., 1986; Stone, 1989).

Employment, however, does not guarantee health care coverage. Of the estimated 31.1 million Americans who are uninsured, according to federal estimates, more than half—a total of 16.6 million Americans—have jobs. More than 40 percent of the people who are employed but uninsured work at businesses with fewer than 24 employees (Freudenheim, 1990).

The underwriting practices of private insurance companies pose problems for people who would like to acquire coverage on their own. In contrast to workers who are automatically eligible for group coverage under the health plans of employers, individuals must undergo insurer-required medical examinations. Commonly, insurers deny coverage to people with chronic or disabling conditions, or they classify these applicants as "substandard risks" and charge higher premiums. Individual insurance is already much more expensive than group insurance, and for many people, especially those who cannot work full time because of a disabling condition, substandard premiums make commercial policies unaffordable. Sometimes insurers accept people with chronic conditions, but with an exclusion that waives coverage for preexisting conditions (see Table 8-3).

Types of Health Care Services

As noted in the preceding discussion, insurance coverage does not necessarily translate into coverage for the types of health care services required by people with disabling conditions. Generally, coverage is limited to acute care and for the most part excludes services recognized as important ele-

TABLE 8-3 Risk Classification by Commercial Health Insurers: Common
Conditions Requiring a Higher Premium, Exclusion Waiver, or Denial

Higher Premium	Exclusion Waiver	Denial
Allergies	Cataracts	AIDS
Asthma	Gallstones	Ulcerative colitis
Back strain	Fibroid tumor (uterus)	Cirrhosis of liver
Hypertension (controlled)	Hernia (hiatal/inguinal)	Diabetes mellitus
Arthritis	Migraine headaches	Leukemia
Gout	Pelvic inflammatory disease	Schizophrenia
Glaucoma	Chronic otitis media (recent)	Hypertension (uncontrolled)
Obesity	Spine/back disorders	Emphysema
Psychoneurosis (mild)	Hemorrhoids	Stroke
Kidney stones	Knee impairment	Obesity (severe)
Emphysema (mild-moderate)	Asthma	Angina (severe)
Alcoholism/drug abuse	Allergies	Coronary artery disease
Heart murmur	Varicose veins	Epilepsy
Peptic ulcer	Sinusitis, chronic or severe	Lupus
Colitis	Fractures	Alcohol/drug abuse

SOURCE: U.S. Congressional Office of Technology Assessment, 1988a, 1988c.

ments of secondary and tertiary care. Most private policies, for example,
cover rehabilitation services only in acute care hospitals, usually for the
length of the hospital stay or, perhaps, a month or two afterward. However,
for many traumatic injuries and chronic conditions such as stroke and paralysis,
rehabilitation should begin only after the acute condition has stabilized and
hospitalization is no longer needed.

Common to Medicare, Medicaid, and private policies, another restriction
is the stipulation that reimbursement will continue only for as long as the
person receiving rehabilitation services continues to show improvement in
functional capacity. Yet for many people—for example, those with head
injuries or chronic heart conditions—improvement in functional capacity
may not be apparent until long after the start of therapy. This restriction
also ignores the rehabilitation goal of maintaining capacity and of halting or
slowing declines in function in people with degenerative conditions.

Two major obstacles to longitudinal care are the apparent bias of public
insurance for institutionalization instead of in-home care and the denial of
coverage for assistive technologies and services that are necessary for personal
autonomy. Five federal programs fund in-home attendant-care services, and

each state has one program offering these services. Nonetheless, an estimated 3 million people who require the help of others in performing personal and household tasks are not receiving attendant-care services (World Institute on Disability, 1987a). The Study Group on State Medicaid Strategies estimated that 60 percent to 80 percent of long-term care services are provided by friends, neighbors, and relatives without payment (Meltzer, 1988). Given the strict eligibility requirements under public programs and the high-cost private insurance policies that cover these services, this heavy reliance on family and friends reflects, in part, necessity rather than choice.

Although it is not unreasonable to expect family members to contribute to the care of relatives, this option is not available to many people with disabling conditions. Moreover, the additional responsibilities of the caregiver have not received adequate attention. For example, an increasing number of households are providing care for elderly family members. The caregivers usually are middle-aged women, many of whom also have jobs and have primary responsibility for attending to the needs of their own families. A study of 150 Philadelphia families in which married women were providing care for their widowed mothers reported that half of the daughters were working. Half of those who were not working had quit their jobs to care for their mothers, and a quarter of those who were still employed contemplated quitting (Lewin, 1989). As the demands of caring for a chronically ill elderly adult or a relative with a disabling condition increase, the likelihood of institutionalization also increases.

Many people who do not receive attendant-care services are likely to end up in nursing homes, incurring costs that may greatly exceed those for care in the home. Federal and state governments pay for much of this bill; public expenditures account for more than 40 percent of nursing home payments. Public expenditures for in-home care are considerably smaller but still substantial, totaling about $2 billion, according to the World Institute on Disability (1987b). On the basis of its national study, the World Institute on Disability concluded that public funds expended for attendant-care services could be used more efficiently, resulting in improved services for a greater number of people in need and at least delaying institutionalization and its higher costs.

Recognition of this problem is growing. The Medicare Catastrophic Coverage Act paid for 38 days of home care and 80 hours of respite care for people who assist Medicare recipients in their homes. Strong opposition to the surtax designed to help finance these and other benefits led to the repeal of the act in late 1989, 16 months after its initial passage. Still continuing is a separate demonstration program to evaluate the effectiveness of respite care for people who attend to relatives with disabling conditions. The program is jointly funded by the federal government and participating states. In New Jersey, for example, the program provides up to $2,400 annually for visits by attendants or health care workers (Lewin, 1989).

Related to issues concerning the availability and nature of long-term care are often incongruous insurance policy restrictions on assistive technologies, as discussed in the preceding chapter. Medicare, which has covered SSDI beneficiaries since 1972, pays for certain equipment required by people with disabling conditions, but its criteria for determining what is essential are dictated by an outmoded concept of "medical necessity." In many cases, assistive technologies instrumental to maintaining an independent lifestyle and often essential to preventing secondary conditions do not satisfy the criteria on the Medicare screening list for durable medical equipment. When the importance of, for example, augmentive communication devices or personal hygiene aids is not recognized, dependence is fostered, which can lead to institutionalization.

Timing is also an important but often neglected element of effective longitudinal care. Again Medicare, which provides health care coverage for 37 percent of the population with disabling conditions, serves as an example. All SSDI recipients are eligible for Medicare. However, their coverage does not begin until two years after their first SSDI payments, which start five months after acceptance into the program. Because the SSDI approval process can exceed two years, some people may be without health care coverage for more than four years, a significant delay during which further deterioration in health status can occur. Although more studies are needed, a growing body of research indicates that the earlier rehabilitation begins after a patient's condition has stabilized, the better the rehabilitative outcome will be.

For some people, the progression to disability and the associated loss of employment may end with the ironic result of obtaining care that, if available earlier, could have prevented the onset of the disability. Researchers from the American Foundation for the Blind evaluated access to care for the estimated 2 million people with low-vision conditions (Kirchner et al., 1985). They studied four categories of care: (1) evaluation, diagnosis, and prescription; (2) therapy and training in the use of vision aids; (3) reimbursement for vision aids; and (4) related rehabilitation services. People with Medicaid were more likely than those with commercial health insurance to be covered for at least some low-vision services. The researchers estimated, however, that about a third of elderly, visually limited persons who are eligible for Medicaid lived in states that did not provide coverage for services in any of the four categories. Only 20 percent of this population lived in states that provided coverage for all categories of care.

The results point to a classic contradiction applicable to virtually all disabling conditions. The widespread unavailability of coverage for comprehensive care means that many working-age people are not insured for needed services while they are employed. If they cannot afford to pay for needed services and their conditions deteriorate, they are in jeopardy of losing their jobs. If they do become unemployed, however, they may be eligible for vocational rehabilitation services that may have averted their job loss.

THE NEED FOR COORDINATION

A large, multifaceted public health and social issue like disability must be addressed on several fronts. Many public and private programs are now doing so, but largely independent of each other. Some structural reorganization might promote greater coherence and coordination of efforts, but wholesale restructuring of the bureaucracy to create a superagency that embraces all disability-related programs would probably not be a fruitful endeavor. Fragmentation, inconsistency, and redundancy of effort—criticisms now leveled at the current bureaucratic structure—would likely persist.

The challenge facing existing programs is to develop working relationships that foster synergy rather than a series of isolated efforts. Integration of efforts within and among the categories of surveillance, research, and services and across governmental boundaries should be one of the primary goals of disability-related programs. This observation is not new, nor is the need unique to disability-related programs. Greater coordination is the grail of most large public and private organizations.

The committee considered the possible overlap between the congressionally mandated responsibilities of the federal Interagency Committee on Disability Research (ICDR), which is under the leadership of the National Institute on Disability and Rehabilitation Research, and the role of the recently established Disabilities Prevention Program at the Centers for Disease Control. The primary difference between these two activities is that the ICDR does not focus on prevention. Thus, although tertiary prevention is an integral component of rehabilitation, disability prevention per se has not been a major theme of rehabilitation research, planning, or interagency coordination.

The size and complexity of disability issues and the comprehensiveness of the public health approach required to address the compelling national need necessitate a large, well-coordinated program of disability prevention. A summary description of some of the federal programs that focus on rehabilitation research and disability prevention follows.

Rehabilitation Research

The federal government's lead agency for research on rehabilitation (which corresponds to tertiary prevention) is the National Institute on Disability and Rehabilitation Research (NIDRR), housed in the Department of Education. With a budget of nearly $60 million in 1990, NIDRR supports a broad program of applied and clinical research that has the aim of advancing procedures, methods, and devices that can improve the lives of people with mentally and physically disabling conditions. An overriding goal of the agency is to foster developments that facilitate integration of people with disabling conditions into independent and semi-independent community life.

Approximately one third of NIDRR's budget is allocated for support of 40 research and training centers and 18 rehabilitation engineering centers, most of which are located at universities. Both types of centers have core specialties, and emphasis is on transferring useful research results to the service delivery system. Specialties of the multidisciplinary centers include functional electrical stimulation, musculoskeletal disorders, work-site modifications, deafness and communication disorders, blindness and low vision, mental illness, mental retardation, and developmental problems of newborns with disabilities and neuromuscular disorders. Separate from the centers is the NIDRR-supported network of 13 Model Spinal Cord Injury Care Systems, each providing an integrated set of services to patients with spinal cord injuries. The network includes the National Spinal Cord Injury Statistical Center, which collects and analyzes demographic data and information on methods of patient management, secondary complications, and rehabilitation outcomes.

NIDRR also supports demonstration projects intended to address specific rehabilitation needs and to communicate research-generated information to service providers and their clients. The institute supports investigator-initiated research projects; awards small grants for testing new concepts, prototype aids and devices, and training curricula; and funds a small research training program. In addition, NIDRR maintains a national data base for disseminating information on rehabilitation research.

As mandated by Congress, NIDRR has primary responsibility for coordinating rehabilitation research among federal agencies. The NIDRR director is the chairman of the Interagency Committee on Disability Research, which is charged with promoting communication and joint research activities among the committee's 27 member agencies. These agencies include categorical institutes of the National Institutes of Health and the Alcohol, Drug Abuse, and Mental Health Administration; the National Science Foundation; units of the departments of Veterans Affairs, Education, and Labor; and the National Aeronautics and Space Administration.

Collectively, these agencies carry out a varied program of rehabilitation research. In 1984 the National Institutes of Health tabulated 688 rehabilitation-related research projects, which received total funding of $78 million. Apart from these projects are basic studies that are helping to elucidate the biological underpinnings of impairment and disability.

The Department of Veterans Affairs, through its Rehabilitation Research and Development Service, also supports a large rehabilitation research program, allocating approximately $22 million in 1990 to fund more than 175 separate projects at 60 Veterans Administration (VA) medical centers. It also supports three rehabilitation research and development centers and an evaluation unit that assesses new prototype devices and techniques and seeks to promote commercial interest in promising concepts. Priority research areas include prosthetics and amputation, spinal cord injury, and sensory aids. Aging, physical fitness, and psychosocial rehabilitation are other areas of emphasis (U.S. Veterans Administration, 1988).

In addition, the VA Rehabilitation Research and Development Service has developed a data base on rehabilitation-related research conducted in the United States and other nations. The service's 1988 tabulation of ongoing research included 384 projects sponsored by 70 public and private organizations (U.S. Veterans Administration, 1988).

Disability Prevention

The Injury Control and Disabilities Prevention Programs of the CDC's Center for Environmental Health and Injury Control embrace all three supporting elements—surveillance, research, and services—of an integrated system of prevention and longitudinal care. Projects address issues relevant to primary, secondary, and tertiary prevention. Communication of research results is facilitated by the CDC's status as the chief federal agency for prevention, a role in which it has fostered working relationships with state and local governments.

Established in 1985 with the aim of reducing the annual toll of 140,000 injury-caused deaths and 70 million nonfatal injuries, the Injury Control Program supports intramural and extramural research in three main areas: prevention, acute care, and rehabilitation. With an annual budget of approximately $24 million, the program supports 35 research projects and seven injury prevention research centers. Some centers carry out broad programs of research, whereas others focus on types of injury, such as motor vehicle collisions and intentional injuries, or the needs of high-risk groups, such as children and the elderly. In addition, program staff members are involved in cooperative research and demonstration projects with several universities and state and county health departments. The staff also provides technical assistance to requesting state and local agencies. At the federal level, the program had primary responsibility for developing the Year 2000 National Health Objectives for reducing the incidence of intentional and unintentional injuries.

Responding to a recommendation made by the National Council on the Handicapped in *Toward Independence* (National Council on the Handicapped, 1986), Congress called for the creation of the Disabilities Prevention Program at the CDC. The program focuses on three areas: developmental disabilities, injuries to the head and spinal cord, and secondary conditions in people with physically disabling conditions. Like the Injury Control Program, the new initiative aims to help states and localities build their capacity for disability prevention, develop surveillance systems for high-priority disabling conditions, and use the results of epidemiological analyses to identify targets for intervention and guide development of prevention strategies. In 1988 the CDC program initiated cooperative projects in nine states. In five of these states, the aim is to develop plans for disability prevention efforts; in four others, projects will focus on the implementation and evaluation of disability prevention plans.

Four university-based projects, begun in 1989, constitute the beginning of an effort to develop data bases on secondary complications. Concentrating on such problems as urinary tract infections and decubitus ulcers in people with spinal cord injuries and late-developing complications in people with poliomyelitis, the epidemiologic studies are expected to yield more detailed understanding of the scope of such problems and to aid identification of cost-effective interventions.

The CDC programs are notable for their public health approach to disability prevention. However, complementary programs, which also embody an integration of efforts, are carried out under the aegis of other agencies. For example, the National Institute of Child Health and Human Development (NICHHD) supports a variety of longitudinal, multidisciplinary studies on the biological and behavioral factors involved in normal and abnormal growth and development, from gametogenesis through maturity. Early detection and intervention, as well as restoration of function in children with disabling conditions, are overriding goals of the institute-supported research. Similarly, a major focus of research sponsored by the National Institute on Aging (NIA) is preventing degeneration of physical and mental functions in the elderly. In addition, the need and potential for rehabilitation among the elderly are addressed in NIA's epidemiologic, behavioral, clinical, and basic research programs.

In November, 1990, a National Center for Medical Rehabilitation Research was established within the NICHHD. The mandate of the center includes the conduct and support of research and research training, the dissemination of health information, and other programs for rehabilitation of individuals with physical disabilities stemming from diseases or disorders.

Public- and Private-Sector Partnerships

This committee believes that disability poses one of the greatest challenges currently facing the public health system. Recognizing it as such makes disability prevention a federal, state, and local responsibility. Government involvement at all three levels is a necessary condition for progress, but by themselves, public-sector efforts are not sufficient. Also necessary is the participation of the private sector and of individuals, who must recognize their personal responsibility for ensuring good health.

A recent study by the Institute of Medicine found that, although pockets of excellence exist, the public health system as a whole is deteriorating, a casualty of declining resources and a growing list of health problems (Institute of Medicine, 1988a). Disability prevention, however, can build on the traditional strengths of the public health system, assuming needed investments in capacity are made. In addition, new, more expansive approaches are required to develop the integrated service delivery network that is needed. Housing, transportation, education, employment, medical, nutrition, and other types of services must be easily accessible to target populations. As noted earlier, some services exist, but often within isolated administrative compartments of the bureaucracy, and each category of services often has its own peculiar set of eligibility requirements, typically a composite product of federal, state, and local rule making. Moreover, lack of flexibility is a hallmark, sometimes resulting in services that are not commensurate with needs.

Homelessness, for example, can lead to chronic conditions that increase the risk of disability. If adequate medical services are available, the progression to disability may be reversed, and the chances for finding a job and affordable housing increased. Conversely, the health of a person with a chronic condition who cannot obtain needed medical services is likely to deteriorate, and with it the ability to work. The resulting reduced income may not be sufficient to meet rent or mortgage payments. If unable to find affordable housing, this person may end up on the street, exacerbating the health problem and thus decreasing the prospects for finding alternative employment. In this simple example, it is clear that the effectiveness of one set of services is greatly limited by the unavailability of the other.

The increasing prevalence of disabling conditions is a national problem that must be addressed at the local level. For its part, the federal government should provide leadership, financial support, and technical resources to states and localities. Although federal budget constraints are real, they do not preclude setting realistic goals for disability prevention, nor should immediate budgetary exigencies obscure the cost savings and increased productivity that will accrue to prevention measures.

In addition, states and communities must act on their own, for they too will reap the benefits of disability prevention. The gains attributable to prevention have motivated several states to expand eligibility for prenatal health services. For example, through its new Maternity Outreach and Management Services (MOMS) program, New Jersey intends to make prenatal care available to all pregnant women. Services are free for women with annual incomes of about $18,000 or less (150 percent above the poverty level). For uninsured women with incomes between $18,000 and about $30,000 (250 percent above the poverty level) the state will pay on a sliding-scale basis. Financed by the state's uncompensated care trust fund, which is supported by a surcharge on private insurance, MOMS provides comprehensive medical and nutrition services, including counseling and home visits, and arranges for the transportation of pregnant women to and from their physicians' offices, as needed.

About 7 percent of the babies born to uninsured women in New Jersey are low-birthweight infants. If the new program reduces this rate by one-third, the state estimates that it will save $4 million annually in the form of reduced inpatient care for newborns. In addition, the drop in the number of low-birthweight infants will yield long-term savings because of expected reductions in later-appearing health problems associated with low birthweight (Sullivan, 1989).

Demonstration projects are also under way in several agencies of the federal government in addition to those mentioned above. The federal Health Care Financing Administration, for example, supports demonstration projects that are investigating the utility of social health management organizations, which, by including social, transportation, health, and other services under the same administrative umbrella, offer greater flexibility in meeting the multiple needs of clients. In nine cities, the Robert Wood Johnson Foundation and the National Institute of Mental Health are supporting efforts to develop a coordinated set of mental health services that are easily accessible to those in need.

Experience shows that good intentions alone do not result in coordination and streamlining of services. For example, the Department of Education's Rehabilitation Services Administration (RSA) and the National Institute of Mental Health (NIMH) signed the 1978 NIMH-RSA Cooperative Agreement calling for the coordination of vocational rehabilitation and mental health services, and 40 states enlisted their participation. Despite this seemingly strong support, the agreement has yielded few perceptible changes in the delivery of services at the local level.

Less rigidity in the eligibility criteria of locally operated service delivery programs and greater local discretion in the use of federal and state funds, allowing resources to be transferred across service categories, appear to be needed. The mechanisms for achieving local flexibility and accountability are not readily apparent, however. Thus efforts should be focused on devising and evaluating new approaches to service delivery.

Moreover, local efforts would benefit greatly from input and contributions from the private sector and individual members of the community. Clearly, all of the interrelated issues subsumed under the heading of disability prevention, from the need for affordable, widely accessible health care services to shortcomings of worker training and education programs, are of great concern to the private sector. Businesses and other private organizations already support a sizable fraction of rehabilitation research, and a small but growing number of firms have fully embraced the goal of equal employment opportunity for people with disabling conditions. The challenge is to add to this gradually building momentum by developing mechanisms for effective linkages within and between the public and private sectors.

Public and Professional Education

It is axiomatic that a public health goal is also a societal goal. Success in preventing disability and reducing its financial and human costs hinges not only on the efforts of professionals and institutions but also on the awareness, attitudes, and actions of the general public. The attitudes and behaviors of the public and those of health care workers, social workers, and other professionals can either facilitate the participation in society of people with disabling conditions or pose formidable obstacles.

Thus, public education is an essential element of disability prevention. It is the best means to eliminate stereotypes that translate into the denial of opportunity to people with functional limitations, which may as a result become disabilities. For too long, public understanding of disability has been synonymous with sympathy for individuals with disabling conditions, fostering their dependence and removing them from society's mainstream. Educational efforts should improve understanding of what Caplan calls a "peculiar Catch-22 situation." People with disabling conditions, he has written, "want to carry out the roles and duties that they are capable of, but they must depend on society's recognition that they cannot and should not be expected to carry out *all* the usual roles" (Caplan, 1988).

This committee cannot prescribe educational methods, an area beyond its expertise. It can, however, identify several appropriate educational themes (as described in Chapter 7): (1) people with disabling conditions constitute a large minority, one-seventh of the U.S. population; (2) most people will develop conditions that increase the risk of disability; (3) disability is not inherent in an individual; (4) like all citizens, people with disabling conditions have a right to participate in society, and their physical or mental conditions do not prevent them from playing productive roles; and (5) people with disabling conditions can achieve a high quality of life.

These themes are also pertinent to the education of physicians, other health care workers, social workers, counselors, and other professionals who may provide services to people with disabling conditions. With the exception of medical schools with departments of physical medicine and rehabilitation, however, it is unlikely that the special needs of the large population of people with disabling conditions are addressed in a formal manner, if at all. Many medical schools do not offer courses on disability and rehabilitation.

Moreover, pressing personnel shortages limit the capacity of the health care system to provide essential services. Physical medicine and rehabilitation is one of the few medical specialities with a shortage of physicians (Bowman et al., 1983). Shortages also exist in physical therapy and occupational therapy, as well as in the allied health and nursing professions.

Implementation of effective longitudinal care (i.e., over the life course), as described by this committee, requires more than an adequate supply of personnel in key specialities. It also requires the participation of knowledgeable nonspecialists. Typically, health care services for those with disabling conditions are provided by family physicians, general internists, psychiatrists, psychologists, nurses, social workers, and other professionals. Few in these professions receive formal training in how to address the needs of the large client population. In addition, few medical and nonmedical professionals have experience in working collaboratively in multidisciplinary teams. Yet effective care often depends on the coordinated contributions of many such professionals.

The Sum of the Parts

Viewed collectively, the disability prevention effort addresses many important public health issues. However, the overall effort is lacking, especially with regard to issues related to secondary prevention that halts or slows the disabling process. In addition, mechanisms for coordinating research efforts and ensuring the transfer of results to service providers are inadequate. Moreover, existing disability research activities are largely confined to the medical and biological aspects of disability. Such research is essential, but it must be supplemented by studies that address social and environmental factors that strongly influence the disabling process and the ability of affected individuals to live independently.

Few examples exist of crosscutting, interdisciplinary research. In the biomedical area, for example, research is often splintered according to types of diseases or impairments. Given the multitude of conditions that can lead to disability, division of effort is to be expected, but whenever possible, commonalities, such as shared risk factors or vulnerable populations, should be explored and prevention strategies pursued from a multidisciplinary perspective.

Quality of life is a unifying theme that could be used to organize disability-related research and to forge ties within and among medical and nonmedical disciplines. Traditionally, biomedical research has focused on reducing mortality. In fact, studies have shown that funding levels for biomedical research agencies correspond strongly to the number of deaths attributable to diseases in their research domain (Mushkin and Dunlop, 1979). The most tangible benefit from this mortality-based emphasis is the steady decline in deaths caused by heart disease. But as noted elsewhere in this report, declining death rates and increasing life spans can have side effects that are masked in mortality statistics, namely, increasing morbidity and low quality of life among survivors.

Increasing emphasis on disease prevention and health promotion attests to growing recognition of the importance of quality of life as a standard for measuring the performance of the nation's health care system and its supporting research enterprise. This standard should be applied more broadly and operationalized in ways that go beyond monitoring the incidence and prevalence of disease, measures that reflect only the effectiveness of primary prevention and acute care. Quality of life can also be gauged in ways that measure how effective secondary and tertiary prevention measures are, for example, in promoting independence among people with disabling conditions or in reducing work absences among the population with disabling conditions.

Fully embracing quality of life as a national health standard can bridge artificial boundaries between disciplines and between social and medical services. If averting disease and maintaining functional capacity among people with disabling conditions are shared goals, then once-isolated efforts addressing medical, housing, educational, transportation, and other relevant issues are more easily integrated, increasing prospects for achieving the coordination and synergy now lacking in disability-related programs.

9

Recommendations

As described and discussed throughout the report, the social and environmental aspects of disability and disability prevention are of critical importance and help to define limitations in the role of medicine in disability prevention. Indeed, the major disability-related roles for the fields of public health and medicine involve the prevention, early detection, diagnosis, treatment, and rehabilitation of potentially disabling conditions. Once such a condition is identified, however, the means of disability prevention go beyond rehabilitative restoration of function to include important social and economic factors.

Increasing attention to and understanding of the broad range of issues related to disability in this country recently resulted in the Americans with Disabilities Act being signed into law by President Bush on July 26, 1990. That same impetus, amplified by the desire for accessible, affordable quality health care for all, led to the committee's finding that there is an urgent need for a well-organized, coordinated national disability prevention program. An agenda for such a program is presented on the next page. The agenda includes the program's stated goal and five strategies for its achievement: organization and coordination of the national program, surveillance, research, access to care and preventive services, and professional and public education. Recommendations are presented to support each strategy.

ORGANIZATION AND COORDINATION

Organization and coordination of a national disability prevention effort requires action on several levels. There are a number of disability-related programs in the federal government, but currently no one agency has been charged with leadership responsibilities that focus on prevention. The pri-

A NATIONAL AGENDA FOR THE PREVENTION OF DISABILITY

GOAL

To reduce the incidence and prevalence of disability in the United States, as well as the personal, social, and economic consequences of disability in order to improve the quality of life for individuals, families, and the population at large.

STRATEGIES

Organization and Coordination—Establish leadership and administrative responsibility for implementing and coordinating the National Agenda for the Prevention of Disability within a single unit of the federal government. Implementation of the agenda should be guided by a national advisory committee, and progress should be critically evaluated periodically. In addition to federal leadership, achieving the goals of the agenda will require the strong, sustained participation of the state, local, and private sectors.

Surveillance—Develop a conceptual framework and standard definitions of disability and related concepts as the basis for a national disability surveillance system. Such a system should be designed to (1) characterize the nature, extent, and consequences of disability and antecedent conditions in the U.S. population; (2) elucidate the causal pathways of specific types of disability; (3) identify promising means of prevention; and (4) monitor the progress of prevention efforts.

Research—Develop a comprehensive national research program on disability prevention. The research should emphasize longitudinal studies and should focus on preventive and therapeutic interventions. Special attention should be directed to the causal mechanisms whereby socioeconomic and psychosocial disadvantage lead to disability. Training young scientists for careers in research on disability prevention should become a high priority.

Access to Care and Preventive Services—Eliminate the barriers to access to care, especially for women and children, to permit more effective primary prevention and prevent progression of disability and the development of secondary conditions. Existing programs of proven effectiveness should be expanded, and new service programs should be introduced. Returning persons with disabling conditions to productive, remunerative work is a high priority.

Professional and Public Education—Educate health professionals in the prevention of disability. Foster a broad public understanding of the importance of eliminating social, attitudinal, and environmental barriers to the participation of people with functional limitations in society and to the fulfillment of their personal goals. Educate health professionals, people with disability, family members, and personal attendants in disability prevention and preventing the development of secondary conditions.

vate sector must also be involved if such an effort is to be successful. The committee's recommendations below suggest mechanisms to organize and coordinate a national disability prevention program and to provide input from the diverse groups affected by disability.

Leadership of the National Disability Prevention Program

The congressionally mandated role of the National Council on Disability (NCD) is to provide advice and make recommendations to the President and to Congress with respect to disability policy. In keeping with its charter, the council has been and should continue to be an effective leader in developing disability policy in such areas as education, health care services, and civil rights.

In 1986 the NCD identified the need for a national program for disability prevention and recommended to the President and Congress that such a program be established in the Centers for Disease Control (CDC). In 1988 CDC initiated the Disabilities Prevention Program to build capacity in disability prevention at the state and local levels, establish systems of surveillance for disabilities, use epidemiological approaches to identify risks and target interventions, and provide states with technical assistance. It is the only federal program that has been charged specifically with disability prevention. Its initial focus has been prevention of the more readily identifiable injuries, developmental disabilities, and secondary conditions.

The committee endorses the emerging federal leadership in disability prevention at CDC. The agency's traditional strengths—epidemiology, surveillance, technology transfer, disease prevention, and communication and coordination with state, local, and community-based public health activities—are consonant with the needs of a national program. Moreover, CDC has demonstrated its leadership in the development and effective implementation of interventions in numerous specific public health situations, in quality control for screening programs and their implementation, in the development of school and other public health curricula, and in the evaluation of public health service delivery programs.

Given the magnitude of the public health problem disability presents and the large number of various types of disability-related public and private programs, there is a need for expansion and coordination of disability prevention activities. The committee's recommendations, which appear below, have been formulated to address that need and provide a framework for future program development. The CDC Disabilities Prevention Program is a good first step in the development of such a framework. In addition, the informal relationship that currently exists between it and the National Council on Disability appears to be a mutually beneficial one that has strengthened federal disability prevention activity during its infancy. To the extent that such a relationship remains beneficial to developing a national program for disability prevention, it should continue.

RECOMMENDATION 1:   Develop leadership of a National Disability Prevention Program at CDC

To advance the goal and carry out the strategies of the national agenda, the committee recommends that the CDC Disabilities Prevention Program be expanded to serve as the focus of a National Disability Prevention Program (NDPP). In assuming the lead responsibility for implementing the national agenda for the prevention of disability over the life course, the NDPP should coordinate activities with other relevant agencies, emphasizing comprehensive surveillance, applied research, professional and public education, and preventive intervention with balanced attention to developmental disabilities, injuries, chronic diseases, and secondary conditions.

As the national program develops, with its emphasis on prevention of disability throughout the life course, it should focus on identifying and modifying the biological, behavioral, and environmental (physical and social) risk factors associated with potentially disabling conditions, as well as monitoring the incidence and prevalence of the conditions themselves. The program should be conducted in cooperation and in partnership with state health agencies and other public agencies. A major component of the program should be the development at the state level of a sharply increased capacity to prevent disability.

A disability prevention program of the scope and ambition envisioned by the committee will require much more than can be accomplished by governments acting alone. The active participation of all segments of society is required.

RECOMMENDATION 2:   Develop an enhanced role for the private sector

The NDPP should recognize the key role of the private sector in disability prevention, including advocacy groups, persons with disabilities, business and other employers, the insurance industry, academia, the media, voluntary agencies, and philanthropies. Indeed, the potential contributions of the private sector in achieving the program's goals cannot be emphasized too strongly. Its role encompasses the provision of employment opportunities, modification of the workplace, research in and development of assistive technology, provision of appropriate insurance, and development of a national awareness program.

One way to involve the private sector might be to establish an independent forum on disability policy for the promotion, coordination, and resolution of disability-related issues that would facilitate prevention. Addressing many of these issues requires the collaborative support and involvement of a broad array of scientists and informed leaders from both the private and public sectors. The purpose of the forum would be to improve policymaking through a continuing dialogue among individuals and groups that play a significant role in shaping policy and public opinion. Areas for consideration might include access to assistive technology and personal assistance services, gaps in health insurance coverage, family leave policies, and implementation issues related to the Americans with Disabilities Act.

Advisory Committee

As stated throughout the report, disability is a public health and social issue. Thus a national disability prevention program will be centrally dependent on public attitudes toward people with disabilities and on the way community activities are organized, which includes access to housing, public transportation, and the workplace. Equally important is the reduction of prejudice and discrimination toward people with disabilities. An agenda for disability prevention will require cooperation among all levels of government; the health, social services, and research professions; business; educational institutions; churches; and citizens' organizations throughout the country.

RECOMMENDATION 3:   **Establish a national advisory committee**
An advisory committee for the NDPP should be established to help ensure that its efforts are broadly representative of the diverse interests in the field. The advisory group should include persons with disabilities and their advocates; public health, medical, social service, and research professionals; and representatives of business, insurance, educational, and philanthropic organizations, including churches. The role of the advisory committee would be to advise CDC on priorities in disability prevention research and the nationwide implementation of prevention strategies, as well as to assess progress toward the goal of the national agenda for the prevention of disability. The advisory committee should be appointed by the Department of Health and Human Services and meet at least three times a year. In keeping with its role in regard to disability policy, the National Council on Disability should be a permanent member of this committee.

Interagency Coordination and Periodic Review

The fragmentation of disability-related activities and the lack of continuity of care are highly disruptive to preventive efforts. Part of the problem derives from the fact that essential services are funded and provided by various agencies and by different levels of government without a clear focus of authority and responsibility, leading to gaps in services. The lack of coordination of health and medically related rehabilitation activities and social services is a long-standing problem that is not easily rectified. Improvements will require energy and direction, a focus on prevention, and a clear strategy for coordination, cooperation, and integration among several federal programs as they are administered at the local level. These federal programs include those concerned with health care (Health Care Financing Administration), disability benefits (Social Security Administration and the Department of Veterans Affairs), vocational rehabilitation (Department of Education), community support (National Institute of Mental Health), and housing (Department of Housing and Urban Development). Thus responsibility for planning, coordination, and evaluation of these activities should be highly placed in the federal government (e.g., in the Office of the Secretary of the Department of Health and Human Services) to facilitate the type of coordinated leadership at the federal level necessary to ensure cooperation at the local level.

RECOMMENDATION 4:   **Establish a federal interagency council**
A standing Interagency Council on Disability Prevention should be established by the Secretary of Health and Human Services.   The interagency council should be charged with examining and developing conjoint activities in disability prevention and with identifying existing policies that inhibit disability prevention and rehabilitation.   More specifically, the interagency council should be convened semiannually to identify, examine, and foster enhanced disability prevention strategies by (1) recommending the elimination of conflicting public policies and coordinating and integrating programs, (2) developing new policy initiatives, (3) improving service delivery, and (4) setting research priorities.   The interagency council should have a permanent staff and issue public reports to the Secretary of Health and Human Services, Congress, and the National Council on Disability.

The members of the interagency council should be high-level administrators drawn from the major agencies involved in the various aspects of disability, which include the following: Centers for Disease Control; Health Care Financing Administration; Alcohol, Drug Abuse, and Mental Health Administration; National Institute on Disability and Rehabilitation Research; Health Resources and Services Administration (HRSA), including the Maternal and Child Health Bureau; Agency for Health Care Policy and Research; Social Security Administration; National Institutes of Health; Consumer Product Safety Commission; Bureau of the Census; and other agencies within the Departments of Health and Human Services, Housing and Urban Development, Education, Transportation, Labor, Defense, Veterans Affairs, and others as appropriate.

RECOMMENDATION 5:   Critically assess progress periodically
There should be periodic, independent review of national disability prevention objectives and progress toward their achievement with a biennial report prepared by the interagency council and presented to the Secretary of Health and Human Services, Congress, and the National Council on Disability.

SURVEILLANCE

Although information on the incidence and prevalence of disability is available, it is organized in so many different ways that accurate, useful analysis is impeded. Estimates of the prevalence of disability vary by more than 100 percent. One difficulty is the conceptual confusion surrounding disability and its antecedent conditions. Until there is a consistently applied, widely accepted definition of disability and related concepts, the focus for preventive action and rehabilitation will remain uncertain.

Conceptual Framework

Conceptual confusion regarding disability is not limited to the United States, as indicated by the World Health Organization's development of the International Classification of Impairments, Disabilities, and Handicaps. The WHO classification scheme, which seeks to establish uniformity in the use of important concepts, is an important step toward international comparative studies of disability. The committee, however, saw a need to develop its own system and in this report presents a conceptual framework and model derived from the works of Nagi and the WHO that differs from both primarily in that it incorporates risk factors and quality of life. What is needed now is international agreement on a logical, conceptual system that would result in comparable disability statistics across nations. Existing frameworks represent only the initial steps in a process of conceptual refinement and evaluation.

RECOMMENDATION 6:   Develop a conceptual framework and standard measures of disability
The CDC, which is responsible for surveillance of the nation's health, should design and implement a process for the development and review of conceptual frameworks, classifications, and measures of disability with respect to their utility for surveillance. This effort should involve components of the private sector that collect disability data, as well as federal agencies including the National Institutes of Health; Alcohol, Drug Abuse, and Mental Health Administration; National Council on Disability; Office of Human Development Services (a component of the Department of Health and Human Services); Agency for Health

Care Policy and Research; Health Care Financing Administration; Bureau of the Census; Department of Veterans Affairs; Social Security Administration; and HRSA's Maternal and Child Health Bureau. The objective should be consensus on definitions, measures, and a classification and coding system of disability and related concepts. These elements should then be adopted by all local, state, federal, and private agencies that gather data and assemble statistics on disability. Collaboration with the WHO and other international agencies should be encouraged in developing a classification system to obtain comparable disability data across nations.

A National Disability Surveillance System

Despite its significance as a public health and social issue, disability has received little attention from epidemiologists and statisticians; consequently, surveillance of disabling conditions is inadequate in many ways. When disability is a focus of attention, surveillance is more often concerned with counting the number of people affected than with investigating its causes and secondary conditions. Without knowledge of the conditions and circumstances that can lead to disability, the problem in its many manifestations cannot be fully understood, nor can effective prevention strategies be systematically developed.

Disability prevention will require expanded epidemiological studies and surveillance to identify risk factors, the magnitude of risk, and the degree to which risk can be controlled. Because disability is the product of a complex interaction among behavioral, biological, and environmental (social and physical) factors, epidemiological investigations must encompass a broad range of variables that influence the outcomes of mental and physical impairment. Current surveillance systems are condition specific, permitting identification, for example, of the risk factors associated with injuries. None of them, however, track the risk factors associated with the progression from pathology to impairment to functional limitation to disability. Nor is there sufficient research on the range of consequences associated with specific behaviors and circumstances.

Congenital and developmental conditions, injuries, and chronic diseases that limit human activity do not occur randomly within the general population. Epidemiological principles can be used to identify high-risk groups, to study the etiology, or causal pathways, of functional limitations and disabilities, and to evaluate preventive interventions. More specifically, epidemiology and surveillance could play an increased role in the prevention of disability by (1) accurately determining the dimensions of the populations of people with disabilities, (2) identifying the causes of disabilities, (3) guiding the development and selection of preventive interventions, and (4) evaluating the implementation of interventions.

RECOMMENDATION 7: Develop a national disability surveillance system

A national disability surveillance system should be developed to monitor over the life course the incidence and prevalence of (1) functional limitations and disabilities; (2) specific developmental disabilities, injuries, and diseases that cause functional limitations and disability; and (3) secondary conditions resulting from the primary disability. The system should also monitor causal phenomena, risk factors, functional status, and quality of life, and provide state-specific data for program planning and evaluation of interventions. This system should be developed in cooperation with a broad range of federal agencies and private organizations and be implemented as part of the National Disability Prevention Program.

National Surveys

Incidence rates are direct indicators of risk and are fundamental in developing causal understanding. They provide a measure of the rate at which a population develops a chronic condition, impairment, functional limitation, or disability, thereby yielding estimates of the probability or risk of these events. Most existing data on disability provide information on prevalence, not incidence. Prevalence rates are influenced by changes in incidence and by the duration of disability. For example, if the incidence of spinal cord injury were to remain constant but the life expectancy of the population and the duration of time with that disabling condition were increased (a function of recovery rate and mortality), then prevalence would increase. When rates for population groups are compared, only incidence data provide a clear picture of how risks differ among populations. Prevalence data, on the other hand, reflect not only these risks but also differences in rates of recovery and mortality. Thus populations with equal risks of developing disability may differ in prevalence because of differences in access to medical and rehabilitative care. Information on incidence is therefore critical to a causal understanding of disability. Data on duration are also useful to gauge rates of recovery and mortality. What causes disability and what determines its course can be understood only when incidence and duration are known. Similarly, data are required on the incidence and duration of pathology, impairment, and functional limitation.

The United States has never had a comprehensive survey that addresses disability specifically. (Canada and Great Britain both recently conducted disability surveys.) The National Health Interview Survey (NHIS) includes some disability-related questions but is limited in scope because it was designed to be a general-purpose survey of the health of the nation and not an efficient investigation of the causes and risks of disability. Such an investigation requires a comprehensive longitudinal survey that addresses each path of the model displayed in Figure 4 and in particular the biological, behavioral, and environmental determinants of transitions from pathology (or chronic disease) to impairment, functional limitation, and disability. The following recommendations should be especially useful in the evaluation of the implementation of the Americans with Disabilities Act.

RECOMMENDATION 8: Revise the National Health Interview Survey
The NHIS should be modified to include more items relevant to understanding disability. Core questions on mental disorders and other disabling conditions should be added to the survey to estimate the magnitude of these conditions in the general population and the extent to which they contribute to disability.

RECOMMENDATION 9: Conduct a comprehensive longitudinal survey of disability
A longitudinal survey is needed to collect data on the incidence and prevalence of functional limitation and disability (for the states and other geographic areas where feasible). The survey should include specific conditions and a variety of measures reflecting the personal and social impacts and the economic burden of disability in the United States. Because of the dynamic nature of disability, consideration should be given to following surveyed individuals over time. The post-1990 Census Disability Survey currently being designed by the Bureau of the Census should include these features. In addition, the disability section of the 1990 census should be evaluated with a view toward developing additional questions for the year 2000 decennial census.

Disability Index

A disability index comparable to the infant mortality rate and the mortality and morbidity rates for cancer, heart disease, and stroke could serve as an important indicator of societal well-being and help focus the attention of the public and policymakers on this major public health problem. Moreover, such an index would facilitate easy-to-understand assessments of the adequacy of the nation's response to the problem. Many indexes of disability have been proposed, but disagreement in the field over the adequacy and validity of underlying measures has prevented the adoption of widely accepted benchmarks; a major limitation is the inadequacy of the data base for examining alternative measures. As discussed in Chapter 3, an objective analysis is needed that will lead to the development of alternative indexes of disability risk and public health impact. These indexes could be developed and used by the National Disability Prevention Program to help set priorities for prevention efforts among all conditions.

RECOMMENDATION 10: Develop disability indexes

A disability index or group of indexes is needed to help establish priorities for disability prevention among conditions and to gauge and monitor the magnitude of disability as a public health issue. These indexes should include measures of independence, productive life expectancy (both paid and unpaid), and quality of life.

RESEARCH

A wide variety of disability risk factors are associated with the spectrum of diseases and injuries that can lead to disability. These risk factors affect not only the occurrence of the initial event but also the progression of pathologies to impairments, functional limitations, and disabilities. To the extent that risk factors can be eliminated or moderated, the incidence of initial disabling conditions and the progression toward disability can be limited. Much more needs to be known, however, and such knowledge can be acquired only through a broad range of research activities.

Coordinated Research Program

RECOMMENDATION 11: Develop a comprehensive research program

A coordinated, balanced program of research on the prevention of disability associated with developmental disabilities, injury, chronic disease, and secondary conditions should be an essential component of the National Disability Prevention Program. Emphasis should be placed on identifying biological, behavioral, and environmental (physical and social) risk factors over the life course that are associated with disability and secondary conditions and on developing effective intervention strategies. A continuing effort should be made to incorporate functional assessment and quality of life indicators into the research agenda and surveillance measures.

Longitudinal Studies

The process of developing a disabling condition, as well as the associated potential for secondary conditions, is complex and longitudinal. Yet most available data on disability are cross-sectional, making it impossible to accurately gauge the course of disability in relation to varying risk factors or the impact of timely interventions on the development of disability. There is thus a great need for longitudinal studies that effectively describe the course of disability and identify the most strategic points for effective intervention.

RECOMMENDATION 12: Emphasize longitudinal research

A research program of longitudinal studies should be developed to determine the course of conditions and impairments that lead to disability and to identify the strategic points of preventive intervention. The research should emphasize the prevention of secondary conditions, improved functional status, and improved quality of life. In addition, because rapid changes are occurring for people with disabling conditions in terms of health services, public attitudes, and opportunities for social participation, cohort studies are needed to assess the effects of these changes over the life course.

Relationship of Socioeconomic Status

Deeper understanding of the biological underpinnings of pathologies, impairments, and functional limitations is an obvious need, and this knowledge is being pursued in a variety of biomedical research programs, such as those sponsored by the National Institutes of Health and the Alcohol, Drug Abuse, and Mental Health Administration. Far less effort has been devoted to the influence of behavioral, physical and social environmental, and social factors on the development of disability. One transcendent problem, for example, is the high rate of disability among people of low socioeconomic status. Most studies of disability attempt to control statistically for socioeconomic status because it is a powerful risk factor. Moreover, because socioeconomic status has sometimes been considered to be incidental to research investigations, the relationship between disability and socioeconomic status has rarely been addressed directly.

RECOMMENDATION 13: Conduct research on socioeconomic and psychosocial disadvantage

Research should be conducted to elucidate the relationship between socioeconomic and psychosocial disadvantage and the disabling process. Research that links the social and biological determinants of disability should result in improved understanding of the complex interactions leading to disability, an understanding that would help in developing new prevention strategies.

Interventions

There is a clear need to incorporate existing knowledge more efficiently into disability prevention. A concomitant need is to ascertain the effectiveness of current approaches in the wide variety of situations in which disability occurs. All areas of prevention require critical evaluations of the effectiveness of the tools and methods used in the prevention of disability and secondary conditions.

The federal government spends about $60 billion annually for medical coverage and to supplement the incomes of people with disabilities; it spends a relatively small amount on research to identify practices and technologies that can prevent the initial occurrence of disability or limit complications among people with disabilities to help them lead more productive lives. Moreover, the federal funding agencies that support biomedical research have not made prevention a high priority, and there has been little effort devoted to developing research programs on the prevention of disability and secondary conditions.

RECOMMENDATION 14: Expand research on preventive and therapeutic interventions

Research on the costs, effectiveness, and outcomes of preventive and therapeutic interventions should be expanded. The expanded research program should also include acute care services, rehabilitative and habilitative services and technologies, and longitudinal programs of care and interventions to prevent secondary conditions. The National Institute on Disability and Rehabilitation Research, the Department of Veterans Affairs, the National Institutes of Health, the Alcohol, Drug Abuse, and Mental Health Administration, and the Agency for Health Care Policy and Research should join with CDC to develop cooperative and collaborative research programs in the biological, behavioral, and social sciences as they relate to disability prevention. These programs should also emphasize the translation of new findings into national prevention efforts that inform and educate people with disabilities, their families, personal attendants, and advocates, as well as clinical practitioners. Consideration should be given to approaches used in other countries (e.g., the Netherlands, Sweden, England, and France), where disability prevention is viewed from a broad perspective that includes social and ethical implications and socioeconomic costs.

Research Training

RECOMMENDATION 15: Upgrade training for research on disability prevention

CDC, in collaboration with the National Institute on Disability and Rehabilitation Research, should establish an interdisciplinary, university-based research training program (e.g., center grants, cooperative agreements, research training fellowships, career development awards) focused on disability prevention. Such a program should emphasize the epidemiology of disability and research training related to the recommendations and priorities cited in this report. Where appropriate, universities should collaborate with state and local health departments or other organizations concerned with disability prevention.

ACCESS TO CARE AND PREVENTIVE SERVICES

Many persons with disabilities are not covered by Medicare or Medicaid and have little access to private coverage because they either are unemployed or have been rejected for insurance because of their disabilities. Thus the problem of access to care is even greater for people with disabilities than for the general American population. Moreover, persons with disabilities and those at risk of disability are disproportionately poor, making it difficult for them to purchase insurance, make required copayments, or purchase essential services and equipment for their rehabilitation. In addition, poverty compounds the difficulties faced by those with disabilities in gaining recognition of their needs (which are often complicated by the social circumstances associated with poverty) and in developing satisfactory relationships with health providers.

Accessible, Affordable Quality Care

The committee recognizes that the problems of access to health care are deeply embedded in the organization of the U.S. health insurance system and its relationship to employment and other issues. The committee is also aware that resolution of many of the problems identified in this report will require a fundamental restructuring of the financing and organization of the nation's health services. This committee was not charged with addressing these larger issues; nevertheless, its members feel strongly that the gaps in the nation's present system contribute to an unnecessary burden of disability, loss of productivity, and lowered quality of life, and that the United States must make basic health services accessible to all.

Thirty to forty million Americans, including millions of mothers and children, do not have health care insurance or access to adequate health services. Even those Americans who have health care insurance are rarely covered for (and have access to) adequate preventive and long-term medical care, rehabilitation, and assistive technologies. These factors demonstrably contribute to the incidence, prevalence, and severity of primary and secondary disabling conditions and, tragically, avoidable disability.

Recently, the U.S. Bipartisan Commission on Comprehensive Health Care (the Pepper Commission) recommended a universal insurance plan that emphasizes preventive care and identifies children and pregnant women as the groups whose needs should be addressed first. In addition, the American Academy of Pediatrics (AAP) has developed a specific proposal to provide health insurance for all children and pregnant women. The AAP proposal presents several principles relative to ensuring access to health care, as well as estimates of program costs and a package of basic benefits. Many aspects of the proposal could have favorable effects on the cost of health care (e.g., prenatal care should lower expenditures for intensive care of newborns and subsequent disabling conditions).

The committee believes that a system that provided accessible, affordable quality health care for all would have an enormous beneficial effect on the prevention of disability. Yet the economic and political hurdles to that end are formidable, and a near-term solution is not in sight. A first step that has been proposed is to provide quality health care services for all mothers and children (up to age 18). These services have a high probability of preventing disability; however, assessing or evaluating their cost implications was not part of the charge to this committee.

RECOMMENDATION 16:   Provide comprehensive health services to all mothers and children

Preventing disability will require access by all Americans to quality health care.   An immediate step that could be taken would be to ensure the availability of comprehensive medical services to all children up to the age of 18 and to their mothers who are within 200 percent of the poverty level; in addition, every pregnant woman should be assured access to prenatal care.   When provided, these services should include continuous, comprehensive preventive and acute health services for every child who has, or is at risk of developing, a developmental disability.   In certain circumstances—for example, providing prenatal care for the prevention of low birthweight—the economic consequences have been shown to be favorable, but they need to be explored further in other areas of health care delivery.

Research on prenatal care has demonstrated that comprehensive obstetric care for pregnant women, beginning in the first trimester, reduces the risk of infant mortality and morbidity, including congenital and developmental disability.   Researchers also have documented that women who have the greatest risk of complications during pregnancy—teenagers and women who are poor— are also the least likely to obtain comprehensive prenatal care. Furthermore, in its 1985 report, *Preventing Low Birthweight,* the IOM showed conclusively that, for each dollar spent on providing prenatal care to low-income, poorly educated women, total expenditures for direct medical care of their low-birthweight infants were reduced by more than $3 during the first year of life.

RECOMMENDATION 17:   Provide effective family planning and prenatal services

Educational efforts should be undertaken to provide women in high-risk groups with the opportunity to learn the importance of family planning services and prenatal care. Access to prenatal diagnosis and associated services, including pregnancy termination, currently varies according to socioeconomic status. The committee respects the diversity of viewpoints relative to those services but believes they should be available to all pregnant women for their individual consideration as part of accessible, affordable quality care.

Even among privately or publicly insured people with disabilities, access to needed services is often a problem. Coverage may be limited by an arbitrarily defined "medical necessity" requirement that does not permit reimbursement for many types of preventive and rehabilitative services and assistive technologies. Insurance policies tend to mirror the acute care orientation of the U.S. medical system and generally fail to recognize the importance and value of longitudinal care and of secondary and tertiary prevention in slowing, halting, or reversing deterioration in function. The presumption, which has never been thoroughly evaluated, is that rehabilitative and attendant services, assistive technology, and other components of longitudinal care are too costly or not cost-effective.

Access to health care, particularly primary care, is a major problem for persons with disabilities. Many report that they have great difficulty finding a physician who is knowledgeable about their ongoing health care needs. They also have problems obtaining timely medical care and assistive technology that can help prevent minor health problems from becoming significant complications. National data indicate that, relative to the general population, persons with disabilities, regardless of age, have high rates of use of health care services such as hospital care.

The problem of access to care for persons with disabilities transcends the availability of insurance or a regular relationship with a health professional (although for many large gaps exist in both these areas). More important is that the person have access to appropriate care during the full course of a disabling condition. Such care should be provided in a way that prevents secondary conditions and maximizes the person's ability to function in everyday social roles. It must have continuity and not be restricted by arbitrary rules that limit services necessary for effective rehabilitation and participation in society. Persons with disabilities often face enormous impediments to obtaining the coordinated services they need to prevent secondary conditions and improve their opportunity for successful lives. Such impediments include (1) lack of support from insurance and other funding agencies, (2) lack of locally available services, and (3) absence of local coordinating mechanisms.

RECOMMENDATION 18: Develop new health service delivery strategies for people with disabilities

New health service delivery strategies should be developed that will facilitate access to services and meet the primary health care, health education, and health promotion needs of people with disabling conditions.

These strategies should include assistive technologies and attendant services that facilitate independent living.

Although persons with disabling conditions are not by definition sick, they ordinarily have a thinner margin of health that must be scrupulously maintained if they are to avert medical complications and new functional limitations. Accordingly, the programs of health maintenance and health promotion advocated for the general population are especially important to persons with disabilities. Unfortunately, some of the health promotion strategies commonly used among people without disabilities are not appropriate for people with disabilities (e.g., some aerobic exercises for those unable to use their lower limbs). Thus there is a need to develop and implement health education and health promotion strategies specifically targeted toward persons with disabling conditions.

RECOMMENDATION 19: Develop new health promotion models for people with disabilities
Health promotion activities for people with disabling conditions should be developed and evaluated as part of the process of establishing a normal balance of activity within an individual's life. Health promotion efforts should include recreational and avocational activities that correspond to the individual's interests and activity patterns prior to acquiring the disabling condition. Demonstration projects should be initiated to test (1) new health education and health promotion strategies using independent living centers and other innovative hospital and community-based organizations, and (2) the cost-effectiveness of assistive technologies that will enable people with disabling conditions to pursue health promotion strategies that would not otherwise be accessible to them.

Building Capacity

A network of services that include information and instruction regarding personal care and assistance in finding a job is an important aspect of a National Disability Prevention Program. Public and private providers of services will need to work together in order to implement prevention strategies and provide needed assistance and longitudinal care. Effective delivery of the spectrum of prevention services to people who have a high risk of developing a disability and to those who already have disabling conditions is a formidable challenge. Unfortunately, most communities fall short of this goal. A series of community-based demonstration and evaluation projects carried out in various geographic areas and sociopolitical environments would help refine definitions of need as well as identify fresh initiatives for prevention that could be adapted to different areas of the country.

RECOMMENDATION 20: Foster local capacity-building and demonstration projects

The NDPP should support capacity-building and demonstration programs for state and local organizations to prevent primary disabilities and secondary conditions. The community-based demonstrations (including Health Care Financing Administration demonstrations) should emphasize surveillance, interventions and assessment of their effectiveness, and the special needs of low socioeconomic status populations (e.g., prenatal care, access to and financing of preventive services, and health promotion and disability prevention education).

RECOMMENDATION 21: Continue effective prevention programs

Public health programs with proven efficacy in the prevention of disability should receive continued federal support. Those programs that show promise should be continued and evaluated further. Priorities for additional support and evaluation should include the following few examples:
- Head Start and comprehensive day care programs;
- state-based systems to provide family-centered, community-based, multidisciplinary services for children with or at risk of chronic and disabling conditions; and
- interventions to reduce adverse outcomes associated with alcohol and other drug use in pregnancy.

Access to Vocational Services

Vocational services are crucial to ensure that return-to-work goals are achieved. These services may include counseling and work readiness evaluations, job training, job placement, work-site modification, and postemployment services (e.g., Projects with Industry) to ensure satisfactory adjustment and assistance in sustaining employment.

RECOMMENDATION 22: Provide comprehensive vocational services

Vocational services aimed at reintegrating persons with disabilities into the community and enabling them to return to work should be made financially and geographically accessible.

PROFESSIONAL AND PUBLIC EDUCATION

The prevention of disability requires not only access to care and restructuring of services but also a radically different mind-set among many health and other professionals (e.g., psychologists, sociologists, educational specialists) and the general public. As the committee observes throughout its report, the attitudes and behavior of health professionals and the public could either facilitate effective coping and productive lives for persons with disabilities or erect obstacles in their path. For example, many secondary conditions are preventable, but health professionals often are not familiar with the intervention strategies that can be used, and many provide inappropriate care as a result.

Education of Professionals

The committee notes that the field of physical medicine and rehabilitation is one of only a few medical specialties with a shortage of physicians. This situation is not surprising because rehabilitation has had a low priority in medical schools and residency training programs, and many do not even offer courses on disability and rehabilitation. Similarly, personnel shortages exist in physical therapy, speech therapy, occupational therapy, and all allied health and nursing disciplines dealing with disability. Yet the problem goes well beyond these shortages. Even if the numbers of practitioners in these specialties were substantially increased, many problems would remain (e.g., there are few incentives for practicing the types of longitudinal care this committee advocates, and health professionals who follow these careers historically have had little recognition and prestige within their professional groups). In addition, longitudinal care, which has its own special appeal, is also "patient intensive" and requires complex teamwork, two factors that may outweigh its rewards in the minds of many health professionals.

Steps must be taken to ease the current shortage of knowledgeable physicians, allied health professionals, and others (e.g., psychologists, sociologists, educational specialists) working in disability prevention. In fact, all specialties should have a better understanding of the process of disability and appropriate modes of preventive intervention. The longitudinal care described in this report is sometimes provided by specialists in physical medicine and rehabilitation, but most typically it will be provided by general internists, family physicians, psychiatrists, psychologists, social workers, and others. Any long-term strategy must address the education of a broad range of these professionals as part of a national agenda for the prevention of disability.

RECOMMENDATION 23:   **Upgrade medical education and training of physicians**

Medical school curricula and pediatric, general internal medicine, geriatric, and family medicine residency training for medical professionals should include curricular material in physical medicine, rehabilitation, and mental health. In addition, such curricula should address physiatric principles and practices appropriate to the identification of potentially disabling conditions of acute illness and injury. Appropriate interventions, including consultation and collaboration with mental health and allied health professionals, social workers, and educational specialists, and the application of effective clinical protocols should also be included.

RECOMMENDATION 24:   Upgrade the training of allied professionals
Allied health, public health, and other professionals interested in disability issues (e.g., social workers, educational specialists) should be trained in the principles and practices of disability prevention, treatment planning, and rehabilitation, including psychosocial and vocational rehabilitation.

RECOMMENDATION 25:   Establish a program of grants for education and training
A program of grants to medical schools and teaching hospitals, as well as to allied health and other professional schools, emphasizing disability issues should be established for the development of educational programs in the prevention and management of disability and secondary conditions. Such grants should include components that support education, training, and social reintegration of people with disabilities as well as basic clinical training in the prevention of disability and secondary conditions.

Education of the General Public

Because disability is a function of social context, many potentially disabling conditions can be prevented with the help of an appropriately informed public. If full participation of all citizens in the society is encouraged and facilitated, the general public will have increased contact with people who possess disabilities. This type of interaction should help relieve the prejudice and ignorance often found among those who have little firsthand experience of disability and serve to diminish the estrangement, isolation, and depression often felt by persons with potential disabilities.

As part of a national agenda for the prevention of disability, a broad approach to public education is needed to communicate several important messages: (1) a great number of people (about 35 million) from all walks of life have potentially disabling conditions; (2) most disability is preventable; and (3) people with disabilities have rights, productive capacity, and the potential for a high quality of life.

RECOMMENDATION 26:   Provide more public education on the prevention of disability
The general public should be made aware that disability and premature death can be prevented by reducing the risks associated with these conditions. The public should also be educated regarding the civil rights of persons with disabilities, which are guaranteed by law, and the role rehabilitation

and environmental modifications can play in reducing disability and increasing functional ability and quality of life.

Education of Persons with Disabilities and Their Families, Personal Attendants, and Advocates

People with disabilities and their families, personal attendants, and advocates should be better informed about the principles of disability prevention. Such education would contribute significantly to the prevention of disability and secondary conditions—those brought about by poor self-care as well as those induced by a lack of needed social and other support services, architectural inaccessibility, unequal educational and employment opportunities, negative attitudes toward disability, changes in living environments, and greater exposure to disruptive, frustrating events.

Independent living centers, which are controlled and staffed by persons with disabilities, are designed to deal with the prevention of secondary conditions and to be a source of information on the practical aspects of daily living with a disability. Because these centers are usually staffed by persons with disabilities who are living independently, they offer advice based on first-hand experience of the motivation and ingenuity needed to pursue an independent lifestyle. Being able to share experiences with peers who are independent brings to light those coping mechanisms that aid in preventing secondary conditions. Independent living centers are also effective advocates for attitudinal and architectural changes in society that would improve accessibility, stimulate social interaction and productivity, and facilitate an active, quality lifestyle.

RECOMMENDATION 27: Provide more training opportunities for family members and personal attendants of people with disabling conditions

Persons with disabilities, their families, personal attendants, and advocates should have access to information and training relative to disability prevention with particular emphasis on the prevention of secondary conditions. Independent living centers and other community-based support groups provide a foundation for such training programs and offer a source of peer counseling.

References

Accardo, P. J., and A. J. Capute. 1979. The Pediatrician and the Developmentally Delayed Child: A Textbook on Mental Retardation. Baltimore, Md.: University Park Press.

Alan Guttmacher Institute. 1987. Medicaid, Family Planning and the FY 1988 Budget: Legislative Analysis. Washington, D.C.: Alan Guttmacher Institute.

American College of Physicians, Health and Public Policy Committee. 1988. Comprehensive functional assessment for elderly patients. Ann Intern Med 109(1):70-72.

American Medical Association, Committee on Medical Rating of Mental and Physical Impairment. 1958. Guides to the evaluation of permanent impairment. J Am Med Assoc 168(4):475-488.

Amler, R. W., and H. B. Dull, eds. 1984. Closing the Gap: The Burden of Unnecessary Illness. New York: Oxford University Press.

Annegers, J. F., J. D. Grabow, L. T. Kurland, and E. R. Laws. 1980. The incidence, causes and secular trends of head trauma in Olmstead County, Minnesota, 1935-1974. Neurology 30(9):912-919.

Bach-y-Rita, P., ed. 1989. Traumatic Brain Injury. Vol. 2 of Comprehensive Neurologic Rehabilitation. New York: Demos Publications.

Badley, E. M. 1987. The ICIDH: Format, application in different settings, and distinction between disability and handicap. Int Disabil Studies 9:3.

Barnett, W. S. 1985. Benefit cost analysis of the Perry Preschool Program and its policy implications. Educational Evaluation and Policy Analysis 7(4):333-342.

Beedon, L. E., and I. R. Zeitzer. 1988. Reemployment incentives distinguish foreign rehabilitation systems. Bus Health (Jan):58-59.

Bellinger, D., A. Leviton, C. Waternaux, H. Needleman, and M. Rabinowitz. 1987. Longitudinal analyses of prenatal and postnatal lead exposure and early cognitive development. N Engl J Med 316(17):1037-1043.

Belloc, N. B. 1973. Relationship of health practices and mortality. Prev Med 2(1):67-81.

Belman, A. L., M. H. Ultmann, D. Horovpian, B. Novick, A. J. Spiro, A. Rubinstein, D. Kurtzberg, and B. Cone-Wesson. 1985. Neurological complications in infants and children with acquired immune deficiency syndrome. Ann Neurol 18(5):560-566.

Berkman, L. F., and L. Breslow. 1983. Health and Ways of Living: The Alameda County Study. New York: Oxford University Press.

Berkowitz, E. D. 1987. Disabled Policy: America's Programs for the Handicapped. New York: Cambridge University Press.

Berkowitz, E. D., and D. Fox. 1989. The politics of Social Security expansion: Social Security disability insurance, 1935-1986. J Policy History 1(3):233-260.

Berkowitz, M., and C. Greene. 1989. Disability expenditures. Am Rehab 15(1):7-15,29.

Berkowitz, M., and J. Rubin. 1978. The Costs of Disability, 1967-1975. Economic Report to the President. Washington, D.C.: U.S. Government Printing Office.

Berrol, S. 1989. Cranial Nerve Dysfunction. In: Physical Medicine and Rehabilitation: Traumatic Brain Injury, L. J. Horn and D. N. Cope, eds. Philadelphia: Hanley and Belfus.

Blair, E., and F. J. Stanley. 1988. Intrapartum asphyxia: A rare cause of cerebral palsy. J Pediatr 112(4):515-519.

Bleiberg, J., D. N. Cope, and J. Spector. 1989. Cognitive assessment and therapy in traumatic brain injury. In: Physical Medicine and Rehabilitation: Traumatic Brain Injury, L. J. Horn and D. N. Cope, eds. Philadelphia: Hanley and Belfus.

Blomquist, H. K., K. H. Gustavson, G. Holmgren, I. Nordensen, and U. Palsson-Strae. 1983. Fragile X syndrome in mildly retarded children in a northern Swedish county: A prevalence study. Clin Genet 24(6):393-398.

Bontke, C. F. 1989. Medical complications related to traumatic brain injury. In: Physical Medicine and Rehabilitation: Traumatic Brain Injury, L. J. Horn and D. N. Cope, eds. Philadelphia: Hanley and Belfus.

Bornschein, R. L., J. Grote, T. Mitchell, P. A. Succop, K. N. Dietrich, K. M. Krafft, and P. B. Hammond. 1989. Effects of prenatal lead exposure on infant size at birth. In: Lead Exposure and Child Development: An International Assessment, M. A. Smith, L. D. Grant, and A. I. Sors, eds. Boston: Kluwer Academic.

Bowman, M. A., J. M. Katzoff, L. P. Garrisson, and J. Wills. 1983. Estimates of physician requirements for 1990 for the specialties of neurology, anesthesiology, nuclear medicine, pathology, physical medicine and rehabilitation, and radiology: A further application of the GEMNAC methodology. J Am Med Assoc 250(19):2623-2627.

Bracken, M. B., M. J. Shepard, W. F. Collins, T. R. Holford, W. Young, D. S. Baskin, H. M. Eisenberg, E. Flamm, L. Leo-Summers, J. Maroon, L. F. Marshall, L. P. Phanor, J. Piepmeier, V. K. H. Sonntag, F. C. Wagner, J. E. Wilberger, and H. R. Winn. 1990. A randomized, controlled trial of methylprednisolone or naloxone in the treatment of acute spinal cord injury. N Engl J Med 322(20):1405-1411.

Braddock, D., and R. Hemp. 1986. Governmental spending for mental retardation and developmental disabilities, 1977-1984. Hospital and Community Psychiatry 37:702-707.

Brandon, J. 1985. Health promotion and wellness in rehabilitation services. J Rehabil 51(4):54-58.

Brehm, H. P., and T. V. Rush. 1988. Disability analysis of longitudinal health data: Policy implications for Social Security disability insurance. J Aging Studies 2(4):379-399.

Breitmayer, B. J., and C. T. Ramey. 1986. Biological nonoptimality and quality of postnatal environment as codeterminants of intellectual development. Child Devel 57(5):1151-1165.

Brodsky, C. M. 1987. Factors influencing work-related disability. In: Psychiatric Disability: Clinical, Legal, and Administrative Dimensions, A. T. Meyerson and T. Fine, eds. Washington, D.C.: American Psychiatric Press.

Broman, S. H., P. Nichols, P. Shaughnessy, and W. Kennedy. 1987. Retardation in Young Children: A Developmental Study of Cognitive Deficit. Hillsdale, N.J.: L. Erlbaum Associates.

Brooks, N. 1984. Head injury and the family. In: Closed Head Injury: Psychological, Social and Family Consequences, N. Brooks, ed. New York: Oxford University Press.

Bruce, D. A. 1983. Outcome following head trauma in childhood. In: Pediatric Head Trauma, K. Shapiro, ed. New York: Futura Publishing.

Bureau of Maternal and Child Health and Resources Development. 1989. Maternal and Child Health Research Program. 2: Completed Projects. Washington, D.C.: Health Resources and Services Administration, U.S. Department of Health and Human Services.

Burk, R. D. 1967. The nature of disability. J Rehabil 33(6):10-35.

Butler, J. A., B. Starfield, and S. Stenmark. 1984. Child health policy. *In*: Child Development Research and Social Policy, H. W. Stevenson and A. E. Siegel, eds. Chicago: University of Chicago Press.

Calame, A., C. L. Fawer, V. Claeys, L. Arrazoala, S. Ducret, and L. Jaunin. 1986. Neurodevelopmental outcome and school performance of very-low-birthweight infants at 8 years of age. Eur J Pediatr 145(6):461-466.

Caplan, A. 1988. Is medical care the right prescription? *In*: The Economics and Ethics of Long-Term Care and Disability, S. Sullivan and M. E. Lewin, eds. Washington, D.C.: American Enterprise Institute for Public Policy Research.

Carbine, M. E., and G. E. Schwartz. 1987. Strategies for Managing Disability Costs. Washington, D.C.: Washington Business Group on Health.

Carroll, T. J. 1961. Blindness: What It Is, What It Does, and How to Live with It. Boston: Little, Brown.

Casey, R., S. Ludwig, and M. C. McCormick. 1986. Morbidity following minor head trauma in children. Pediatrics 78(3):497-502.

Castelnuovo-Tedesco, P. 1981. Psychological consequences of physical defects: A psychoanalytic perspective. Int Rev Psychoanalysis 8(2):145-154.

Centers for Disease Control. 1985. Preventing Lead Poisoning in Young Children. Atlanta, Ga.: U.S. Department of Health and Human Services.

Centers for Disease Control. 1988a. Comprehensive Plan for Epidemiologic Surveillance. Atlanta, Ga.: U.S. Department of Health and Human Services.

Centers for Disease Control. 1988b. Congenital Malformations Surveillance. January 1982-December 1985. Atlanta, Ga.: U.S. Department of Health and Human Services.

Centers for Disease Control. 1989a. Chronic disease reports: Deaths from diabetes—United States, 1986. MMWR 38(31):543-546.

Centers for Disease Control. 1989b. Comorbidity of chronic conditions and disability among older persons—United States, 1984. MMWR 38(46):788-791.

Centers for Disease Control. 1990a. Childhood Injuries in the United States. Atlanta, Ga.: Department of Health and Human Services.

Centers for Disease Control. 1990b. HIV/AIDS Surveillance Report—January. Rockville, Md.: National AIDS Information Clearinghouse.

Chavez, G. F., J. F. Cordero, and J. E. Becerra. 1988. Leading major congenital malformations among minority groups in the United States, 1981-1986. MMWR Surveillance Summaries 37(3):17-24.

Chernoff, R., and D. A. Lipschitz, eds. 1988. Health Promotion and Disease Prevention in the Elderly. New York: Raven Press.

Chirikos, T. N. 1986. Accounting for the historical rise in work-disability prevalence. Milbank Q 64(2):271-301.

Chirikos, T. N. 1989. Aggregate economic losses from disability in the United States: A preliminary assay. Milbank Mem Fund Q 67(Suppl. 2, Part 1):59-91.

Chollet, D. 1988. Public and private issues in financing health care for children. EBRI (Employee Benefit Research Institute) Issue Brief 79:1.

Cicchetti, D., and L. A. Sroufe. 1976. The relationship between affective and cognitive development in Down's syndrome infants. Child Devel 47:920-929.

Cohen, M. 1957. A Preface to Logic. New York: Meridian Books.

Colvez, A., and M. Blanchet. 1981. Disability trends in the United States population 1966-1976: Analysis of reported causes. Am J Pub Health 71(5):464-471.

Commission on Chronic Illness. 1957. Chronic Illness in the United States. Vol. 4, Chronic Illness in a Large City. Cambridge, Mass.: Harvard University Press.

Cooper, K. D., K. Tabaddor, W. A. Hauser, K Shulman, C. Feiner, and P. R. Factor. 1983. The epidemiology of head injury in the Bronx. Neuroepidemiol 2(1-2):70-88.

Cordero, J. F., G. P. Oakley, Jr., F. Greenberg, and L. M. James. 1981. Is Bendectin a teratogen? J Am Med Assoc 245(22):2307-2310.

Crimmins, M., Y. Saito, and D. Ingegneri. 1989. Changes in life expectancy and disability-free life expectancy in the United States. Population and Development Review 15(2):235-267.

Crocker, A. C. 1989. The causes of mental retardation. Pediatr Ann 18(10):623-626.

Crocker, A. C. 1986. Data collection for the evaluation of mental retardation prevention activities: The fateful forty-three. Developmental Evaluation Clinic, Childrens Hospital, Boston, Mass.

Cutler, A. T., R. Benezra-Obeiter, and S. J. Brink. 1986. Thyroid function in young children with Down syndrome. Am J Dis Child 140(5):479-483.

Dahle, A. J., and F. P. McCollister. 1986. Hearing and otologic disorders in children with Down syndrome. Am J Ment Defic 90(6):636-642.

Davidoff, G., P. Thomas, M. Johnson, S. Berent, M. Dijkers, and R. Doljanac. 1988. Closed head injury in acute traumatic spinal cord injury: Incidence and risk factors. Arch Phys Med Rehabil 69(10):869-872.

Davidson, J., J. M. Hyde, and P. W. Alberti. 1988. Epidemiology of hearing impairment in childhood. Scand Audiol 17(30):13-20.

Deaver, G. G., and M. E. Brown. 1945. Physical Demands of Daily Life. New York: Institute for the Crippled and Disabled.

DeGraw, C., D. Edell, B. Ellens, M. Hillemeier, J. Liebman, C. Perry, and J. S. Palfrey. 1988. Public Law 99-457: New opportunities to serve young children with special needs. J Pediatr 113(6):971-974.

DeJong, G., and R. Lifchez. 1983. Physical disability and public policy. Sci Am 248(6):40-49.

DeJong, P. 1987. Work capacity and the probability of entry into the Dutch disability insurance program. *In*: Disability Benefits: Factors Determining Applications and Awards, H. Emanuel, E. H. De Gier, and P. A. B. Kalker Konijn, eds. Greenwich, Conn.: JAI Press, Inc.

DeVivo, M. J. 1989. What is known about the costs of spinal cord injury? *In*: Proceedings of the National Consensus Conference on Catastrophic Illness and Injury. The Spinal Cord Injury Model: Lessons Learned and New Applications. Atlanta, Ga.: Shepard Center for Spinal Cord Injury.

Dikmen, S., A. McLean, and N. R. Temkin. 1986. Neuropsychological and psychosocial consequences of minor head injury. J Neurol Neurosurg Psychiatry 49(11):1227-1232.

Diller, L., and Y. Ben-Yishay. 1989. Assessment in traumatic brain injury. *In*: Traumatic Brain Injury, P. Bach-y-Rita, ed. Vol. 2, Comprehensive Neurologic Rehabilitation. New York: Demos Publications.

Ditunno, J. F., M. L. Sipski, E. A. Posuniak, Y. T. Chen, W. E. Staas, and G. J. Herbison. 1987. Wrist extensor recovery in traumatic quadriplegia. Arch Phys Med Rehabil 68(5, Part 1):287-290.

Ditunno, J. F., S. L. Stover, M. M. Freed, and J. H. Ahn. 1989a. A comparison of motor recovery of the upper extremities of C4 and C5 SCI patients. Abstracts Digest, American Spinal Injury Association, 15th Annual Scientific Meeting, Las Vegas, Nevada.

Ditunno, J. F., S. L. Stover, M. M. Freed, and J. H. Ahn. 1989b. Course and extent of motor recovery of the upper extremities in traumatic quadriplegia. Arch Phys Med Rehabil 70(A):52.

Dixon, T. P. 1989. Systems of care for the head-injured. *In*: Physical Medicine and Rehabilitation: Traumatic Brain Injury, L. J. Horn and D. N. Cope, eds. Philadelphia: Hanley and Belfus.

Duckworth, D. 1984. The need for a standard terminology and classification of disablement. *In*: Functional Assessment in Rehabilitation Medicine, C. V. Granger and G. E. Gresham, eds. Baltimore, Md.: Williams & Wilkins.

Dumars, K. W., T. W. Gawron, C. L. Pearce, and C. A. Foster. 1987. Prevention of developmental disabilities: A model for organizing clinical activities. Res Dev Disabil 8(4):507-520.

Dutton, D. B., and S. Levine. 1989. Socioeconomic status and health: Overview, methodological critique and reformation. *In*: Pathways to Health: The Role of Social Factors, J. Bunker, D. Gomby, and B. Kehrer, eds. Menlo Park, Calif.: Henry J. Kaiser Family Foundation.

Edmonds, L. D., and G. Windham. 1985. Trends in the incidence of neural tube defects in the United States. *In*: Alpha-Fetoprotein and Congenital Disorders, G. J. Mizejewski and I. H. Porter, eds. Orlando, Fla.: Academic Press.

Edna, T. H., and J. Cappelen. 1987. Return to work and social adjustment after traumatic head injury. Acta Neurochir 85(1-2):40-43.

Eisenberg, H. M. 1985. Outcome after head injury: General considerations. *In*: Central Nervous System Trauma Status Report, D. P. Becker and J. T. Povlishock, eds. Bethesda, Md.: National Institute of Neurological and Communicative Disorders and Stroke, National Institutes of Health.

Environmental Protection Agency. 1986. Air Quality Document for Lead, vol. 4. EPA Pub. No. EPA-600/8-83/028DF. Research Triangle Park, N.C.: Environmental Criteria and Assessment Office.

Erickson, J. D., J. Mulinare, P. W. McClain, T. G. Fitch, L. M. James, A. B. McClearn, and M. J. Adams. 1984. Vietnam veterans' risks for fathering babies with birth defects. J Am Med Assoc 252(7):903-912.

Erickson, P., E. A. Kendall, J. P. Anderson, and R. M. Kaplan. 1989. Using composite health status measures to assess the nation's health. Medical Care 27(3, Suppl.):S66-S76.

Fishburn, M. J., R. J. Marino, and J. F. Ditunno. 1990. Atelectasis and pneumonia in acute spinal cord injury. Arch Phys Med Rehabil 71(3):197-200.

Frankowski, R. F., J. F. Annegers, and S. Whitman. 1985. The descriptive epidemiology of head trauma in the United States. *In*: Central Nervous System Trauma Status Report, D. P. Becker and J. T. Povlishock, eds. Bethesda, Md.: National Institute of Neurological and Communicative Disorders and Stroke, National Institutes of Health.

Freudenheim, M. 1990. Insurers seek help for uninsured. New York Times, Jan. 11:D1,D7.

Frey, W. 1984. Functional assessment in the 80s: A conceptual enigma, a technical challenge. *In*: Functional Assessment in Rehabilitation, A. Halpern and M. J. Fuhrer, eds. Baltimore, Md.: Paul H. Brookes Publishing Co.

Friedman, J. M., and P. N. Howard-Peebles. 1986. Inheritance of Fragile X syndrome: An hypothesis. Am J Med Genet 23(1-2):701-713.

Fries, J. F. 1988. Aging, illness and health policy: Implications of the compression of morbidity. Perspectives in Biology and Medicine 31(3)407-428.

Fries, J. F., and L. M. Crapo. 1981. Vitality and Aging: Implications of the Rectangular Curve. San Francisco: W. H. Freeman.

Fries, J. F., P. Spitz, R. G. Kraines, and H. R. Holman. 1980. Measurement of patient outcome in arthritis. Arthritis Rheum 23(2):137-145.

Fries, J. F., L. W. Green, and S. Levine. 1989. Health promotion and the compression of morbidity. Lancet 1(8636):481-483.

Frigoletto, F. D., and G. A. Little, eds. 1988. Guidelines for Perinatal Care, 2nd ed. Elk Grove, Ill.: American Academy of Pediatrics; Washington, D.C.: American College of Obstetrics and Gynecology.

Froster-Iskenius, U., G. Felsch, C. Shirren, and E. Schwinger. 1983. Screening for Fragile X q in a population of mentally retarded males. Hum Genet 63(2):153-157.

Gallagher, R. M., and F. Stewart. 1987. Psychiatric rehabilitation and chronic physical illness. *In*: Psychiatric Disability: Clinical, Legal and Administrative Dimensions, A. T. Meyerson and T. Fine, eds. Washington, D.C.: American Psychiatric Press.

Gardner-Medwin, D., and P. Sharples. 1989. Some studies of the Duchenne and autosomal recessive types of muscular dystrophy. Brain Dev 11(2):91-97.

German, P. S., and L. P. Fried. 1989. Prevention and the elderly: Public health issues and strategies. Ann Rev Pub Health 10:319-332.

Goldman, H. H., and R. W. Manderscheid. 1987. Chronic mental disorder in the United States. *In*: Mental Health, United States 1987, R. W. Manderscheid and S. A. Barrett, eds. Washington, D.C.: U.S. Government Printing Office.

Goodman, R. M., and R. J. Gorlin. 1983. The Malformed Infant and Child. New York: Oxford University Press.

Gortmaker, S. L., and D. K. Walker. 1984. Monitoring child health in communities. *In:* Monitoring Child Health in the United States: Selected Issues and Policies, D. K. Walker and J. B. Richmond, eds. Cambridge, Mass.: Harvard University Press.

Grabow, J. D., K. D. Offord, and H. E. Reider. 1984. The cost of head trauma in Olmsted County, Minnesota, 1970-1974. Am J Pub Health 74(7):710-712.

Graitcer, P. L. 1987. The development of state and local injury surveillance systems. J Safe Res 18(4):191-198.

Granger, C. V. 1984. A conceptual model for functional assessment. *In:* Functional Assessment in Rehabilitation Medicine, C. V. Granger and G. E. Gresham, eds. Baltimore, Md.: Williams & Wilkins.

Grant, L. D., and J. M. Davis. 1989. Effects of low level lead exposure on paediatric neurobehavioral development: Current findings and future directions. *In:* Lead Exposure and Child Development: An International Assessment, M. A. Smith, L. D. Grant, and A. I. Sors, eds. Boston: Kluwer Academic.

Green, D., M. Y. Lee, V. Y. Ito, T. Cohn, J. Press, P. R. Filbrandt, W. C. VandenBerg, G. M. Yarkony, and P. R. Meyer. 1988. Fixed- vs adjusted-dose heparin in the prophylaxis of thromboembolism in spinal cord injury. J Am Med Assoc 260(9):1255-1258.

Gresham, G. E., and M. L. C. Labi. 1984. Functional assessment instruments currently available for documenting outcomes in rehabilitation medicine. *In:* Functional Assessment in Rehabilitation Medicine, C. V. Granger and G. E. Gresham, eds. Baltimore, Md.: Williams & Wilkins.

Griss, B. 1988. Measuring the health insurance needs of persons with disabilities and persons with chronic illness. Access to Health Care, vol. 1, nos. 1 and 2. Washington, D.C.: World Institute on Disability.

Guralnik, J. M., L. G. Branch, S. R. Cummings, and J. D. Curb. 1989a. Physical performance measures in aging research. J Gerontol 44(5):141-146.

Guralnik, J. M., A. Z. LaCroix, D. F. Everett, and M. G. Kovar. 1989b. Aging in the eighties: The prevalence of comorbidity and its association with disability. Advance Data from Vital and Health Statistics, No. 170. DHHS Pub. No. (PHS) 89-1250. Washington, D.C.: U.S. Public Health Service.

Haan, M. N., G. A. Kaplan, and S. L. Syme. 1989. *In:* Pathways to Health: The Role of Social Factors, J. Bunker, D. Gomby, and B. Kehrer, eds. Menlo Park, Calif.: Henry J. Kaiser Family Foundation.

Haas, J. F., D. N. Cope, and K. Hall. 1987. Premorbid prevalence of poor academic performance in severe head injury. J Neurol Neurosurg Psychiatr 50:52-56.

Haber, L. D. 1975. Disability concepts: Implications for program and policy development. *In:* Report of the First Switzer Memorial Seminar, 1974. Washington, D.C.: National Rehabilitation Association.

Haber, L. D. 1988. Identifying the disabled: Concepts and methods in the measurement of disability. Soc Secur Bull 51(5):11-28.

Haber, L. D. 1990. Issues in the definition of disability and the use of disability survey data. *In:* Disability Statistics, An Assessment: Report of a Workshop. Washington, D.C.: National Academy Press.

Hamburg, D. A. 1984. Foreword. *In:* Behavioral Health: A Handbook of Health Enhancement and Disease Prevention, J. D. Matarazzo, S. M. Weiss, J. A. Herd, N. E. Miller, and S. M. Weiss, eds. New York: John Wiley & Sons.

Hamilton, K. W. 1950. Counseling the Handicapped in the Rehabilitation Process. New York: Ronald Press Co.

Harding, C. M., J. Zubin, and J. S. Strauss. 1987. Chronicity in schizophrenia: Fact, partial fact, or artifact? Hosp Community Psychiatry 38(5):477-486.

Haveman, R., V. Halberstadt, and R. V. Burkhauser. 1984. Public Policy Toward Disabled

Workers: Cross-National Analyses of Economic Impacts. Ithaca, N.Y.: Cornell University Press.

Heiskanen, O., and M. Kaste. 1974. Late prognosis of severe brain injury in children. Develop Med Child Neurol 16:11-14.

Hempel, C. G. 1963. Typological methods in the social sciences. *In*: Philosophy of the Social Sciences, M. A. Natanson, ed. New York: Random House.

Herbst, D. S., and J. R. Miller. 1980. Nonspecific X-linked mental retardation. II: The frequency in British Columbia. Am J Med Genet 7(4):461-469.

Herman, W. H., S. M. Teutsch, and L. S. Geiss. 1987. Diabetes mellitus. *In*: Closing the Gap: The Burden of Unnecessary Illness, R. W. Amler and H. B. Dull, eds. New York: Oxford University Press.

Hermanson, B., G. S. Omenn, R. A. Kronmal, and B. J. Gersh. 1988. Beneficial 6-year outcome of smoking cessation in older men and women with coronary artery disease. N Engl J Med 319:1365-1369.

Hill, R. 1958. Generic features of families under stress. Social Casework 39:139-150.

Hook, E. B., and A. Lindsjo. 1978. Down syndrome in live births by single year maternal age interval in a Swedish study: Comparison with results from a New York State study. Am J Hum Genet 30:19-27.

Houk, V. N., and S. B. Thacker. 1989. The Centers for Disease Control program to prevent primary and secondary disabilities in the United States. Pub Health Rep 104:226-231.

Howards, I., H. P. Brehm, and S. Z. Nagi. 1980. Disability: From Social Problem to Federal Program. New York: Praeger.

Infant Health and Development Program. 1990. Enhancing the outcomes of low-birth-weight, premature infants: A multisite, randomized trial. J Am Med Assoc 263(22):3035-3042.

Ingram, T. T. S. 1984. A historical review of the definition and classification of the cerebral palsies. *In*: The Epidemiology of the Cerebral Palsies, F. Stanley and E. Alberman, eds. Spastics International Medical Publications. Philadelphia: J. B. Lippincott.

Institute of Medicine. 1978. Perspectives on Health Promotion and Disease Prevention in the United States. Washington, D.C.: National Academy Press.

Institute of Medicine. 1985. Preventing Low Birthweight. Washington, D.C.: National Academy Press.

Institute of Medicine. 1987. Pain and Disability: Clinical, Behavioral, and Public Policy Perspectives. Washington, D.C.: National Academy Press.

Institute of Medicine. 1988a. The Future of Public Health. Washington, D.C.: National Academy Press.

Institute of Medicine. 1988b. Homelessness, Health, and Human Needs. Washington, D.C.: National Academy Press.

Institute of Medicine. 1988c. Prenatal Care: Reaching Mothers, Reaching Infants. Washington, D.C.: National Academy Press.

Institute of Medicine. 1989a. Advances in the Assessment of Health Status. Overview and Report of a Conference. Washington, D.C.: National Academy Press.

Institute of Medicine. 1989b. Care of the Elderly Patient: Policy Issues and Research Opportunities. Washington, D.C.: National Academy Press.

Institute of Medicine. 1990a. Healthy People 2000: Citizens Chart the Course. Washington, D.C.: National Academy Press.

Institute of Medicine. 1990b. The Second Fifty Years: Promoting Health and Preventing Disability. Washington, D.C.: National Academy Press.

Jacobs, H. E. 1988. The Los Angeles head injury survey: Procedures and initial findings. Arch Phys Med Rehabil 69(6):425-431.

Jette, A. M. 1984. Concepts of health and methodological issues in functional assessment. *In*: Functional Assessment in Rehabilitation Medicine, C. V. Granger and G. E. Gresham, eds. Baltimore, Md.: Williams & Wilkins.

Johnson, W. G. 1987. Comment. *In*: Disability Benefits: Factors Determining Applications and Awards, H. Emanuel, E. H. De Gier, and P. A. B. Kalker Konijn, eds. Greenwich, Conn.: JAI Press, Inc.

Kalsbeek, D., R. L. McLaurin, B. S. Harris, and J. D. Miller. 1980. The national head and spinal cord injury survey: Major findings. J Neurosurg Supp 1:519-531.

Kaplan, A. 1964. The Conduct of Inquiry. San Francisco: Chandler Publishing Company.

Kaplan, G., and M. Haan. 1989. Is there a role for prevention among the elderly? Epidemiological evidence from the Alameda County study. *In*: Aging and Health Care, M. Ory and K. Bond, eds. New York: Routledge.

Katz, M. M., and S. B. Lyerly. 1963. Methods for measuring adjustment and social behavior in the community: Rationale, description, discriminative validity and scale development. Psychological Reports, 13.

Katz, S. 1983. Assessing self-maintenance: Activities of daily living, mobility, and instrumental activities of daily living. J Am Geriatr Soc 31(12):721-727.

Katz, S., and C. A. Akpom. 1976. A measure of primary sociobiological functions. J Health Serv 6(3):493-508.

Katz, S., L. G. Branch, M. H. Branson, J. A. Papsidero, J. C. Beck, and D. S. Greer. 1983. Active life expectancy. N Engl J Med 309(20):1218-1224.

Keil, J. E., P. C. Gazes, S. E. Sutherland, P. F. Rust, L. G. Branch, and H. A. Tyroler. 1989. Predictors of physical disability in elderly blacks and whites of the Charleston Heart Study. J Clin Epidemiol 42(6):521-529.

Kessler, H. H. 1970. Disability—Determination and Evaluation. Philadelphia: Lea & Febiger.

Kiesler, C. A., and A. E. Sibulkin. 1987. Mental Hospitalization: Myths and Facts About a National Crisis. Newbury Park, Calif.: Sage.

Kilborn, P. T. 1989. For the retarded, independence in real jobs. New York Times, Jan. 2:A1.

Kirchner, C., M. Borgatta, and B. O'Meara. 1985. Third-party financing of low vision services: A national study. Journal of Vision Rehabilitation Summer:2-4.

Klonoff, H., M. D. Low, and C. Clark. 1977. Head injuries in children: A prospective five year follow-up. J Neurol Neurosurg Psychiatr 40:1211-1219.

Kolbe, L. J. 1986. Increasing the impact of school health promotion programs: Emerging research perspectives. Health Educ 17(5):47-52.

Koos, E. L. 1954. The Health of Regionville. New York: Columbia University Press.

Kraus, J. F. 1985. Epidemiological aspects of acute spinal cord injury: A review of incidence, prevalence, causes and outcome. *In*: Central Nervous System Trauma Status Report, D. P. Becker and J. T. Povlishock, eds. Bethesda, Md.: National Institute of Neurological and Communicative Disorders and Stroke, National Institutes of Health.

Krueger, D. W. 1981. Emotional rehabilitation of the physical rehabilitation patient. Int J Psychiatry Med 11(2):183-191.

Krute, A., and M. E. Burdette. 1980. Prevalence of chronic disease, injury, and work disability. *In*: Disability Survey 72, Disabled and Nondisabled Adults, D. T. Ferron, ed. Research Report No. 56. SSA Pub. No. 13-11812. Washington, D.C.: U.S. Government Printing Office.

Kudrjavcev, T., B. S. Schoenberg, L. T. Kurland, and R. V. Groover. 1983. Cerebral palsy—trends in incidence and changes in concurrent neonatal mortality: Rochester, MN, 1950-1976. Neurology 33(11):1433-1438.

Lalonde, M. 1974. A New Perspective on the Health of Canadians: A Working Document. Ottawa: Information Canada.

Lambert, N., M. Windmiller, and L. Cole. 1975. AAMD Adaptive Behavior Scale. Washington, D.C.: American Association on Mental Deficiency.

Lange-Cosack, H., B. Wider, H. J. Schlesener, T. Grumme, and S. Kubicki. 1979. Prognosis of brain injuries in young children (one until five years of age). Neuropaediatrie 10(2):105-127.

LaPlante, M. P. 1988. Data on Disability from the National Health Interview Survey, 1983-

1985. An InfoUse Report. Washington, D.C.: National Institute on Disability and Rehabilitation Research.

LaPlante, M. P. 1989a. Disability in Basic Life Activities Across the Life Span. Disability Statistics Report 1. San Francisco: University of California, Institute for Health and Aging.

LaPlante, M. P. 1989b. Disability Risks of Chronic Illnesses and Impairments. Disability Statistics Report 2. San Francisco: University of California, Institute for Health and Aging.

Last, J. M., ed. 1988. Maxcy-Rosenau Public Health and Preventive Medicine, 12th ed. Norwalk, Conn.: Appleton-Century-Crofts.

Lawton, M. P. 1972. Assessing the competence of older people. *In*: Research, Planning and Action for the Elderly, D. Kent, R. Kastenbaum, and S. Sherwood, eds. New York: Behavioral Publications.

Lazar, I., R. Darlington, H. Murray, J. Royce, and A. Snipper. 1982. Lasting Effects of Early Education. Monograph on Soc Res Child Development. 47(2-3), Serial No. 195.

Lazarsfeld, P. F. 1972. Some remarks on typological procedures in social research. *In*: Continuities in the Language of Social Research, P. F. Lazarsfeld, A. K. Pasanella, and M. Rosenberg, eds. New York: Free Press.

Lee, P. R. 1985. Health promotion and disease prevention for children and the elderly. Health Serv Res 19(6, Part 2):783-792.

Lemert, E. M. 1951. Social Pathology. New York: McGraw-Hill.

Levin, H. S. 1985. Outcome after head injury: Neurobehavioral recovery. *In*: Central Nervous System Trauma Status Report, D. P. Becker and J. T. Povlishock, eds. Bethesda, Md.: National Institute of Neurological and Communicative Disorders and Stroke, National Institutes of Health.

Levin, H. S., and F. C. Goldstein. 1989. Neurobehavioral aspects of traumatic brain injury. *In*: Traumatic Brain Injury, P. Bach-y-Rita, ed. Vol. 2, Comprehensive Neurologic Rehabilitation. New York: Demos Publications.

Levin, H. S., A. L. Benton, and R. G. Grossman. 1982. Neurobehavioral Consequences of Closed Head Injury. New York: Oxford University Press.

Levine, S. 1987. The changing terrains in medical sociology: Emergent concern with quality of life. J Health Soc Behav 28(1):1-6.

Levine, S., and S. H. Croog. 1984. What constitutes quality of life? A conceptualization of the dimensions of life quality in healthy populations and patients with cardiovascular disease. *In*: Assessment of Quality of Life in Clinical Trials of Cardiovascular Therapies, N. K. Wenger, M. E. Mattson, C. D. Furberg, and J. Elinson, eds. New York: Le Jacq.

Lewin, T. 1989. Ailing parent: Women's burden grows. New York Times, Nov. 14:A1.

Louis Harris and Associates, Inc. 1986. The ICD Survey of Disabled Americans: Bringing Disabled Americans into the Mainstream. New York: International Center for the Disabled.

Luft, H. S. 1978. Poverty and Health: Economic Causes and Consequences of Health Problems. Cambridge, Mass.: Ballinger.

Macken, C. L. 1986. A profile of functionally impaired elderly persons living in the community. Health Care Financing Review 7(4):33-49.

MacKenzie, E. J., S. Shapiro, R. T. Smith, J. H. Siegel, M. Moody, and A. Pitt. 1987. Factors influencing return to work following hospitalization for traumatic injury. Am J Pub Health 77(3):329-334.

MacKenzie, E. J., S. L. Edelstein, and J. P. Flynn. 1990. Trends in hospitalized discharge rates for head injury in Maryland, 1979-1986. Am J Pub Health 80(2):217-219.

Maddox, G. L. 1985. Intervention strategies to enhance well-being in later life: The status and prospect of guided change. Health Serv Res 19(6, Part 2):1007-1032.

Maddox, G. L., and P. Lawton, eds. 1989. Diversity in Aging: Annual Review of Gerontology and Geriatrics, vol. 8. New York: Springer Publishing Co.

Manton, K. G. 1988. Planning long term care for heterogeneous older populations. *In*: Diversity in Aging: Annual Review of Gerontology and Geriatrics, vol. 8, G. L. Maddox and P. Lawton, eds. New York: Springer Publishing Company.

Manton, K. G. 1989. Epidemiological, demographic, and social correlates of disability among the elderly. Milbank Mem Fund Q 67(Suppl. 2, Part 1):13-58.

Marge, M. 1981. The prevention of human disabilities: Policies and practices for the 80's. *In*: International Aspects of Rehabilitation: Policy guidance for the 1980's, L. G. Perlman, ed. Alexandria, Va.: National Rehabilitation Association.

Marge, M. 1988. Health promotion for people with disabilities: Moving beyond rehabilitation. Am J Health Promotion 2(4):29-44.

Marsolais, E. B., and R. Kobetic. 1988. Development of practical stimulation system for restoring gait in a paralyzed patient. Clin Orthoped 233:64-74.

Masaki, M., M. Higurashi, K. Iijima, N. Ishikawa, F. Tanaka, T. Fujii, Y. Kuroki, I. Matsui, K. Iinuma, N. Matsuo, K. Takeshita, and S. Hashimoto. 1981. Mortality and survival for Down's syndrome in Japan. Am J Hum Genet 33(4):629-639.

Matarazzo, J. D. 1984. Behavioral health: A 1990 challenge for the health sciences professions. *In*: Behavioral Health: A Handbook of Health Enhancement and Disease Prevention, J. D. Matarazzo, S. M. Weiss, J. A. Herd, N. E. Miller, and S. M. Weiss, eds. New York: John Wiley & Sons.

Matarazzo, J. D., S. M. Weiss, J. A. Herd, N. E. Miller, and S. M. Weiss. 1984. Preface. *In*: Behavioral Health: A Handbook of Health Enhancement and Disease Prevention. New York: John Wiley & Sons.

Maulitz, R. C., ed. 1989. Unnatural Causes: The Three Leading Killer Diseases in America. New Brunswick, N.J.: Rutgers University Press.

Mausner, J. S., and A. K. Bahn, eds. 1985. Epidemiology: An Introductory Text. Philadelphia: W. B. Sanders.

McBride, E. D. 1963. Disability Evaluation and Principles of Treatment of Compensable Injuries, 6th ed. Philadelphia: J. B. Lippincott.

McDonald, K. C., and R. L. Valmassey. 1987. Cerebral palsy: A literature review. J Am Podiatr Med Assoc 77(9):471-483.

McKinlay, J. B., S. M. McKinlay, and R. Beaglehole. 1989. A review of the evidence concerning the impact of medical measures on recent mortality and morbidity in the United States. Int J Health Serv 19(2):181-208.

McMichael, A. J., G. V. Vimpani, E. F. Robertson, P. A. Baghurst, and P. D. Clark. 1986. The Port Pirie cohort study: Maternal blood lead and pregnancy outcome. J Epid Commun Health 40(1):18-25.

Mechanic, D. 1989. Toward the year 2000 in U.S. mental health policymaking and administration. *In*: Handbook of Mental Health Policy in the United States, D. A. Rochefort, ed. Westport, Conn.: Greenwood.

Mechanic, D., and L. H. Aiken. 1987. Improving the case of patients with chronic mental illness. N Engl J Med 317:1634-1638.

Meisels, S. J., and S. Provence. 1989. Screening and Assessment: Guidelines for Identifying Young Disabled and Developmentally Vulnerable Children and Their Families. Washington, D.C.: National Center for Clinical Infant Programs.

Meltzer, J. 1988. Financing long-term care: A major obstacle to reform. *In*: The Economics and Ethics of Long-Term Care and Disability, S. Sullivan and M. E. Lewin, eds. Washington, D.C.: American Enterprise Institute for Public Policy Research.

Melvin, J. L., and S. Z. Nagi. 1970. Factors in behavioral responses to impairments. Arch Phys Med Rehab 5l(9):552-557.

Merck Manual of Diagnosis and Therapy, 15th ed., R. Berkow, ed. 1987. Rahway, N.J.: Merck.

Merli, G. J., G. J. Herbison, J. F. Ditunno, H. H. Weitz, J. H. Henzes, C. H. Park, and M. M. Jaweed. 1988. Deep vein thrombosis: Prophylaxis in acute spinal cord injured patients. Arch Phys Med Rehabil 69(9):661-664.

Merton, R. K. 1957. Social Theory and Social Structure. Glencoe, Ill.: Free Press.

Milunsky, A., H. Jick, S. S. Jick, D. S. MacLaughlin, K. J. Rothman, and W. Willett. 1989. Multivitamin/folic acid supplementation in early pregnancy reduces the prevalence of neural tube defects. J Am Med Assoc 262(20):2847-2852.

Miniszek, N. A. 1983. Development of Alzheimer's disease in Down's syndrome individuals. Am J Ment Defic 87(4):377-385.

Montamat, S. C., B. J. Cusack, and R. E. Vestal. 1989. Management of drug therapy in the elderly. N Engl J Med 321(5):303-309.

Morris, J. N., S. Morris, and S. Sherwood. 1984. Assessment of informal and formal support systems in high risk elderly populations. In: Functional Assessment in Rehabilitation Medicine, C. V. Granger and G. E. Gresham, eds. Baltimore, Md.: Williams & Wilkins.

Mulinare, J., J. F. Cordero, J. D. Erickson, and R. J. Berry. 1988. Periconceptional use of multivitamins and the occurrence of neural tube defects. J Am Med Assoc 260(21):3141-3145.

Mushkin, S. J., and D. W. Dunlop, eds. 1979. Health—What Is It Worth: Measures of Health Benefits. New York: Pergamon Press.

Nagi, S. Z. 1964. A study in the evaluation of disability and rehabilitation potential: Concepts, methods, and procedures. American Journal of Public Health 54:1568-1579.

Nagi, S. Z. 1965. Some conceptual issues in disability and rehabilitation. In: Sociology and Rehabilitation, M. B. Sussman, ed. Washington, D.C.: American Sociological Association.

Nagi, S. Z. 1969. Disability and Rehabilitation. Columbus: Ohio State University Press.

Nagi, S. Z. 1970. Congruency in medical and self-assessment of disability. Industrial Medicine 38(3):27-36.

Nagi, S. Z. 1975. Disability Concepts and Prevalence. Presented at the First Mary Switzer Memorial Seminar, Cleveland, Ohio.

Nagi, S. Z. 1976. An epidemiology of disability among adults in the United States. Health and society. Milbank Mem Fund Q 54:439-467.

Nagi, S. Z., and R. I. Haller. 1982. Limitations in Function: Indicators and Measures. Columbus: Mershon Center, Ohio State University.

National Academy of Engineering. 1988. New Medical Devices: Invention, Development and Use. Washington, D.C.: National Academy Press.

National Center for Health Statistics. 1970-1988. Current Estimates from the National Health Interview Survey. Vital and Health Statistics, Series 10. Washington, D.C.: U.S. Government Printing Office.

National Center for Health Statistics. 1972. Current Estimates from the National Health Interview Survey. Vital and Health Statistics, Series 10. Washington, D.C.: U.S. Government Printing Office.

National Center for Health Statistics. 1974. Vital Statistics of the United States, 1970. Vol. 2, Mortality. Part A. Pub. No. (HRA) 75-1101. Rockville, Md.: Public Health Service.

National Center for Health Statistics. 1981a. Health Characteristics of Persons with Chronic Activity Limitation: United States, 1979. Vital and Health Statistics, Series 10, No. 137. DHHS Pub. No. (PHS) 82-1565. Hyattsville, Md.: U.S. Department of Health and Human Services.

National Center for Health Statistics. 1981b. Health, United States, 1980. DHHS Pub. No. (PHS) 81-1232. Hyattsville, Md.: National Center for Health Statistics.

National Center for Health Statistics. 1983. Procedures and Questionnaires of the National Medical Care Utilization and Expenditure Survey. National Medical Care Utilization and Expenditure Survey, Series A, Methodological Report No. 1. DHHS Pub. No. 83-20001. Washington, D.C.: U.S. Government Printing Office.

National Center for Health Statistics. 1986. Current Estimates from the National Health Interview Survey, United States, 1985. Vital and Health Statistics, Series 10, No. 160. Washington, D.C.: U.S. Government Printing Office.

National Center for Health Statistics. 1987a. Current Estimates from the National Health Interview

Survey, United States, 1986. Vital and Health Statistics, Series 10, No. 164. Washington, D.C.: U.S. Government Printing Office.

National Center for Health Statistics. 1987b. The Supplement on Aging to the 1984 National Health Interview Survey. Vital and Health Statistics, Series 1, No. 21. DHHS Pub. No. (PHS) 87-1323, U.S. Public Health Service. Washington, D.C.: U.S. Government Printing Office.

National Center for Health Statistics. 1988. Current Estimates from the National Health Interview Survey, United States, 1987. Vital and Health Statistics, Series 10, No. 166. DHHS Pub. No. (PHS) 88-1594. Washington, D.C.: U.S. Government Printing Office.

National Center for Health Statistics. 1989a. Current Estimates from the National Health Interview Survey, 1988. Vital and Health Statistics, Series 10, No. 173. DHHS Pub. No. (PHS) 89-1501. Washington, D.C.: U.S. Government Printing Office.

National Center for Health Statistics. 1989b. The National Nursing Home Survey, 1985 Summary for the United States. Vital and Health Statistics, Series 13, No. 97. DHHS Pub. No. (PHS) 89-1758. Washington, D.C.: U.S. Government Printing Office.

National Center for Health Statistics. 1990a. Health, United States, 1989. DHHS Pub. No. (PHS) 90-1232. Hyattsville, Md.: U.S. Public Health Service.

National Center for Health Statistics. 1990b. Questionnaires from the National Health Interview Survey, 1980-84. Vital and Health Statistics, Series 1, No. 24. DHHS Publication No. (PHS) 90-1302. Washington, D.C.: U.S. Government Printing Office.

National Center for Health Statistics. 1990c. Vital Statistics of the United States, 1987. Vol. 2, Mortality. Part A. Hyattsville, Md.: U.S. Public Health Service.

National Council on the Handicapped. 1986. Toward Independence: An Assessment of Federal Laws and Programs Affecting Persons with Disabilities, with Legislative Recommendations. A Report to the President and to the Congress of the United States. Washington, D.C.: U.S. Government Printing Office.

National Institute on Aging. 1989. Special Report on Aging. Washington, D.C.: U.S. Government Printing Office.

National Institute on Disability and Rehabilitation Research. 1988. Program Directory, Office of Special Education and Rehabilitation Services. Washington, D.C.: U.S. Department of Education.

National Institute on Disability and Rehabilitation Research. 1989. Chartbook on Disability in the United States. An InfoUse Report. Washington, D.C.: U.S. Government Printing Office.

National Institute on Disability and Rehabilitation Research. 1990. Proceedings of the National Consensus Conference on Catastrophic Illness and Injury. The Spinal Cord Injury Model: Lessons Learned and New Applications. Atlanta, Ga.: Shepherd Center for Spinal Cord Injury.

National Institutes of Health. 1989. Mental Retardation: 1988 Research Accomplishments. Washington, D.C.: U.S. Department of Health and Human Services.

National Research Council. 1982. Diet, Nutrition and Cancer. Washington, D.C.: National Academy Press.

National Research Council. 1985. Injury in America: A Continuing Public Health Problem. Washington, D.C.: National Academy Press.

National Research Council. 1987. Counting Injuries and Illnesses in the Workplace: Proposals for Better Systems, E. S. Pollack and D. G. Keimig, eds. Panel on Occupational Safety and Health Statistics and Committee on National Statistics. Washington, D.C.: National Academy Press.

National Research Council. 1989. Diet and Health: Implications for Reducing Chronic Disease Risk. Washington, D.C.: National Academy Press.

National Research Council. 1990. Disability Statistics: An Assessment. Report of a Workshop, D. B. Levine, M. Zitter, and L. Ingram, eds. Washington, D.C.: National Academy Press.

National Safety Council. 1989. Accident Facts. Chicago, Ill.: National Safety Council.

Needleman, H. L., A. Schell, D. Bellinger, A. Leviton, and E. N. Allred. 1990. Long term effects of exposure to low doses of lead in childhood: An eleven year follow-up report. New Engl J Med 322(2):83-88.

Nelson, E., B. Conger, R. Douglass, D. Gephart, J. Kirk, R. Page, A. Clark, K. Johnson, K. Stone, J. Wasson, and M. Zubkoff. 1983. Functional health status levels of primary care patients. J Am Med Assoc 249(24):3331-3338.

New York Heart Association. 1953. Nomenclature and Criteria for Diagnosis of Diseases of the Heart and Blood Vessels, 5th ed. New York: New York Heart Association.

Newacheck, P. W., and M. A. McManus. 1988. Financing health care for disabled children. Pediatrics 81(3):385-394.

Nickel, R. E., F. C. Bennet, and F. N. Lamson. 1982. School performance of children with birth weights of 1000 g or less. Am J Dis Child 136(2):105-110.

Nova Research Company. 1988. Analysis of the 1990 Health Objectives for the Nation for Applicability to Prevention of Disabilities. Report for the Office of Disease Prevention and Health Promotion of the U.S. Department of Health and Human Services. Bethesda, Md.: Nova Research Company.

Oddy, M., and M. Humphrey. 1980. Social recovery during the year following severe head injury. J Neurol Neurosurg Psychiatry 43(9):798-802.

Oddy, M., T. Coughlan, A. Tyerman, and D. Jenkins. 1985. Social adjustment after closed head injury: A further follow-up seven years after injury. J Neurol Neurosurg Psychiatry 48(6):564-568.

Omran, A. R. 1979. Changing patterns of health and disease during the process of national development. *In*: Health, Illness, and Medicine, G. L. Albrecht and P. C. Higgins, eds. Chicago: Rand McNally.

Orme, T. C., and J. Rimmer. 1981. Alcoholism and child abuse: A review. J Stud Alcohol 42(3):273-287.

Paneth, N., and J. Kiely. 1984. The frequency of cerebral palsy. *In*: The Epidemiology of the Cerebral Palsies, F. Stanley and E. Alberman, eds. Spastics International Medical Publications. Philadelphia: J. B. Lippincott.

Parsons, T. 1958. Definitions of health and illness in the light of American values and social structure. *In*: Patients, Physicians and Illness, E. G. Jaco, ed. Glencoe, Ill.: Free Press.

Patrick, D. L. 1984. Quality of life measures for assessing disablement. *In*: Assessment of Quality of Life in Clinical Trials of Cardiovascular Therapies, N. K. Wenger, M. E. Mattson, C. D. Furberg, and J. Elinson, eds. New York: LeJacq.

Patrick, D. L., and M. Bergner. 1990. Measurement of Health Status in the 1990s. Ann Rev Public Health 11:165-183.

Patrick, D. L., and P. Erickson. 1988. What constitutes quality of life? Concepts and dimensions. Qual Life Cardiovascular Care Autumn:103-127.

Patrick, D. L., and H. Peach, eds. 1989. Disablement in the Community. New York: Oxford University Press.

Peckham, P. H., M. W. Keith, G. B. Thrope, and V. L. Menger. 1986. Control of hand function in the tetraplegic by functional neuromuscular stimulation. 1986 Academy congress abstracts. Arch Phys Med Rehabil 67(9):669-670.

Pinsky, J. L., L. G. Branch, A. M. Jette, S. G. Haynes, M. Feinleib, J. C. Cornoni-Huntley, and K. R. Bailey. 1985. Framingham disabilities study: Relationship of disability to cardiovascular risk factors among persons free of diagnosed cardiovascular disease. Am J Epidemiol 122(4):644-656.

Ragnarsson, K. T. In press. Traumatic brain injury: Secondary and tertiary prevention. NY State J Med.

Ragnarsson, K. T., S. Pollack, W. O'Daniel, R. Edgar, J. Petrofsky, and M. S. Nash. 1988. Clinical evaluation of computerized functional electrical stimulation after spinal cord injury: A multicenter pilot study. Arch Phys Med Rehabil 69(9):672-677.

Ramey, C. T., and F. A. Campbell. 1984. Prevention education for high-risk children: Cognitive consequences of the Carolina Abcedarian project. Am J Ment Defic 88(5):515-523.

Ratcliffe, J. M., W. E. Halperin, T. M. Frazier, D. S. Sundin, L. Delaney, and R. W. Hornung. 1986. The prevalence of screening in industry: Report from the National Institute for Occupational Safety and Health national occupational hazard survey. J Occup Med 28(10):906-912.

Rice, D. P. 1989. Demographic realities and projections of an aging population. *In*: Health Care for an Aging Society, S. Andreopoulous and J. R. Hogness, eds. New York: Churchill Livingstone.

Rice, D. P., and M. P. LaPlante. 1988a. Chronic illness, disability and increasing longevity. *In*: The Economics and Ethics of Long-Term Care and Disability, S. Sullivan and M. E. Lewin, eds. Washington, D.C.: American Enterprise Institute for Public Policy Research.

Rice, D. P., and M. P. LaPlante. 1988b. Costs of Chronic Comorbidity. *In*: American Public Health Association Annual Meeting Program. Washington, D.C.: American Public Health Association.

Rice, D. P., E. J. MacKenzie, and Associates. 1989. Cost of Injury in the United States: A Report to Congress. San Francisco: Institute for Health & Aging, University of California, and Baltimore: Injury Prevention Center, Johns Hopkins University.

Riley, M. W., and J. W. Riley, eds. 1989. The Quality of Aging: Strategies for Intervention. Annals of the American Academy of Political and Social Sciences. Newbury Park, Calif.: Sage Publications.

Rimel, R. W., B. Giordani, J. T. Barth, T. J. Boll, and J. A. Jane. 1981. Disability caused by minor head injury. Neurosurg 9(3):221-228.

Rimel, R. W., B. Giordani, J. T. Barth, and J. A. Jane. 1982. Moderate head injury: Completing the clinical spectrum of brain trauma. J Neurosurg 11(3):344-351.

Robert Wood Johnson Foundation. 1987. Access to Health Care in the United States: Results of a 1986 Survey. Special Report No. 2. Princeton, N.J.: Robert Wood Johnson Foundation.

Rogers, A., R. G. Rogers, and L. G. Branch. 1989. A multistate analysis of active life expectancy. Public Health Rep 104(3):222-226.

Rogers, R. G., A. Rogers, and A. Belanger. 1989. Active life among the elderly in the United States: Multistate life-table estimates and population projections. Milbank Mem Fund Q 67(3-4):370-411.

Rowe, J. W., and R. L. Kahn. 1987. Human aging: Usual and unsuccessful. Science 237(3811):143-149.

Rublee, D. A. 1986. Self-funded health benefit plans: Trends, legal environment, and policy issues. J Am Med Assoc 255(6):787-789.

Sagan, L. A. 1987. The Health of Nations: True Cases of Sickness and Well-being. New York: Basic Books.

Sarbin, T. R., and V. L. Allen. 1968. Role theory. *In*: The Handbook of Social Psychology, vol. 1, 2nd ed., G. Linsey and E. Aronson, eds. Reading, Mass.: Addison-Wesley Publishing Company.

Scheff, T. J. 1967. Introduction. *In*: Mental Illness and Social Processes, T. J. Scheff, ed. New York: Harper & Row.

Schneider, E. L., and J. M. Guralnik. 1990. The aging of America: Impact on health care costs. J Am Med Assoc 263(17):2335-2340.

Schwartz, J., C. Angle, and H. Pitcher. 1986. Relationship between childhood blood lead levels and stature. Pediatrics 77(3):281-288.

Schweinhart, L. J., and D. P. Weikart. 1986. What do we know so far? A review of the Head Start synthesis project. Young Children 41(2):49-54.

Selye, H. 1956. The Stress of Life. New York: McGraw Hill.

Shelton, T. L., E. S. Jeppson, and B. H. Johnson. 1987. Family-Centered Care for Children with Special Health Care Needs. Washington, D.C.: Association for the Care of Children's Health.

Shonkoff, J. P. 1982. Biological and social factors contributing to mild mental retardation. *In*:

Placing Children in Special Education: A Strategy for Equity, K. A. Heller, W. H. Holtzman, and S. Messick, eds. Washington, D.C.: National Academy Press.

Sirrocco, A. 1987. The 1986 inventory of long-term care places: An overview of facilities for the mentally retarded. National Center for Health Statistics, Advance Data from Vital and Health Statistics, No. 143, September 30. Washington, D.C.: U.S. Government Printing Office.

Smith, D. W. 1976. Recognizable Patterns of Human Malformation, 2nd ed. Philadelphia: W. B. Saunders.

Smithells, R. W., N. C. Nevin, M. J. Seller, S. Shepard, R. Harris, A. P. Read, D. W. Fielding, S. Walker, C. J. Schorah, and J. Wild. 1983. Further experience of vitamin supplementation for prevention of neural tube defect recurrences. Lancet 1(8332):1027-1031.

Sniezek, J. E., J. F. Finklea, and P. L. Graitcer. 1989. Injury coding and hospital discharge data. J Am Med Assoc 262(16):2270-2272.

Social Security Administration. 1981. Disability Survey, 1972: Disabled and Nondisabled Adults. Research Report No. 56. Washington, D.C.: U.S. Government Printing Office.

Social Security Administration. 1982. 1978 Survey of Disability and Work. Data Book. Washington, D.C.: U.S. Government Printing Office.

Social Security Administration. 1989. Social Security Bulletin 52(12):3-91.

Srole, L., A. K. Fisher, et al. 1962. Mental Health in the Metropolis: The Midtown Manhattan Study. New York: McGraw-Hill Book Company, Inc.

Stein, L. I., and M. A. Test, eds. 1980a. Alternatives to mental hospital treatment. 1. Conceptual model, treatment program, and clinical evaluation. Arch Gen Psychiatr 37(4):392-397.

Stein, L. I., and M. A. Test, eds. 1980b. Alternatives to mental hospital treatment. 3. Social cost. Arch Gen Psychiatr 37(4):409-412.

Stein, L. I., and M. A. Test, eds. 1985. The Training in Community Living Model: A Decade of Experience. New Directions for Mental Health Services, No. 26. San Francisco: Jossey-Bass.

Stewart, A. L., R. D. Hays, and J. E. Ware. 1988. The MOS short-form general health survey: Reliability and validity in a patient population. Med Care 26(7):724-735.

Stewart, A. L., S. Greenfield, R. D. Hays, K. Wells, W. A. Rogers, S. D. Berry, E. A. McGlynn, and J. E. Ware. 1989. Functional status and well-being of patients with chronic conditions. J Am Med Assoc 262(7):907-913.

Stine, S. B., and W. V. Adams. 1989. Learning problems in neurofibromatosis patients. Clin Orthop 245:43-48.

Stone, D. A. 1989. At risk in the welfare state. Social Res 56(3):591-633.

Stone, R., G. L. Cafferata, and J. Sangl. 1987. Caregivers of the frail elderly: A national profile. Gerontol 27(5):616-631.

Stover, S. L., and P. R. Fine, eds. 1986. Spinal Cord Injury: The Facts and Figures. Birmingham: University of Alabama Press.

Streissguth, A. P., P. D. Sampson, and H. M. Barr. 1989. Neurobehavioral dose-response effects of prenatal alcohol exposure in humans from infancy to adulthood. Ann NY Acad Sci 562:145-158.

Sullivan, D. F. 1971. A single index of mortality and morbidity. HSMHA Health Reports 86(4):347-354.

Sullivan, H. S. 1953. The Interpersonal Theory of Psychiatry. New York: Norton.

Sullivan, J. F. 1989. New Jersey will offer care to all pregnant women. New York Times, Dec. 5:A16,B1,B8.

Sunshine, J. 1979. Disability: A Comprehensive Overview of Programs, Issues, and Options for Change. Office of Management and Budget Technology Paper. Washington, D.C.: Office of Management and Budget.

Sunshine, J. 1980. Disability: A Comprehensive Overview of Programs, Issues, and Options for Change. Prepared for the President's Commission on Pension Policy.

Susser, M. 1990. Disease, illness, sickness; impairment, disability and handicap. Psychol Med 20:471-473.

Susser, M. W., W. Watson, and K. Hopper. 1985. Sociology in Medicine. New York: Oxford University Press.

Susser, M. W., W. A. Hauser, J. L. Kiely, N. Paneth, and Z. Stein. 1985. Quantitative estimates of prenatal and perinatal risk factors for perinatal mortality, cerebral palsy, mental retardation and epilepsy. *In*: Prenatal and Perinatal Factors Associated with Brain Disorders, J. M. Freeman, ed. DHHS Pub. No. (NIH) 85-1149. Bethesda, Md.: National Institutes of Health.

Sutherland, G. R. 1982. Heritable fragile sites on the human chromosomes. 8. Preliminary population cytogenetic data on the folic-acid-sensitive fragile sites. Am J Hum Genet 34(3):452-458.

Switzer, M. E. 1965. Remarks. *In*: Sociology and Rehabilitation, M. B. Sussman, ed. Washington, D.C.: American Sociological Association.

Syme, S. L., and L. F. Berkman. 1976. Social class, susceptibility, and sickness. Am J Epidemiol 104(1):1-8.

Szaz, T. 1974. The Myth of Mental Illness: Foundations of a Theory of Personal Conduct, rev. ed. New York: Harper & Row.

Tangsrud, S. E., and S. Halvorsen. 1989. Child neuromuscular disease in southern Norway: The prevalence and incidence of Duchenne muscular dystrophy. Acta Pediatr Scand 78(1): 101-103.

Taylor, H. 1989. Foreword. *In*: Louis Harris and Associates, Inc., ICD Survey. 2: Employing Disabled Americans. New York: International Center for the Disabled.

Texas Institute for Rehabilitation and Research. 1978. ILRU Source Book: A Technical Assistance Manual on Independent Living. Independent Living Research Utilization. Houston, Tex.: Institute for Rehabilitation and Research.

Thacker, S. B., and R. L. Berkelman. 1988. Public health surveillance in the United States. Epidemiol Rev 10:164-190.

Trussell, R. E., and J. Elinson. 1959. Chronic Illness in a Rural Area. Cambridge, Mass.: Harvard University Press.

Tucker, S. J. 1984. Patient staff interaction with the spinal cord patient. *In*: Rehabilitation Psychology, D. W. Krueger, ed. Rockville, Md.: Aspen Systems Corporation.

U.S. Bureau of the Census. 1984. Projections of the Population of the United States, by Age, Sex, and Race: 1983-2080. Current Population Reports, Series P-25, No. 952. Washington, D.C.: U.S. Government Printing Office.

U.S. Bureau of the Census. 1988. United States Population Estimates, by Age, Sex, and Race: 1980 to 1987. Current Population Reports, Series P-25, No. 1022. Washington, D.C.: U.S. Government Printing Office.

U.S. Congress, Subcommittee on the Administration of the Social Security Laws. 1959. Disability Insurance Fact Book. Prepared for the Use of the Committee on Ways and Means. Washington, D.C.: U.S. Government Printing Office.

U.S. Congressional Office of Technology Assessment. 1988a. AIDS and Health Insurance: An OTA Survey. Washington, D.C.: U.S. Government Printing Office.

U.S. Congressional Office of Technology Assessment. 1988b. Healthy Children: Investing in the Future. OTA Pub. No. H-345. Washington, D.C.: U.S. Government Printing Office.

U.S. Congressional Office of Technology Assessment. 1988c. Medical Testing and Health Insurance. OTA Pub. No. H-384. Washington, D.C.: U.S. Government Printing Office.

U.S. Department of Education. 1989a. Dropout Rates in the United States. Annual Publication of the Office of Educational Research and Improvement. Washington, D.C.: U.S. Government Printing Office.

U.S. Department of Education. 1989b. Eleventh Annual Report to Congress on the Implementation of the Education of the Handicapped Act. Washington, D.C.: U.S. Government Printing Office.

U.S. Department of Health and Human Services. 1980a. Promoting Health, Preventing Disease: Objectives for the Nation. Washington, D.C.: U.S. Government Printing Office.

U.S. Department of Health and Human Services. 1980b. Summary Report of the Graduate Medical Education National Advisory Committee, Vol. 1. DHHS Pub. No. 81-651. Washington, D.C.: U.S. Department of Health and Human Services.

U.S. Department of Health and Human Services. 1986. The 1990 Health Objectives for the Nation: A Midcourse Review. Washington, D.C.: U.S. Government Printing Office.

U.S. Department of Health and Human Services. 1988a. The Nature and Extent of Lead Poisoning in Children in the United States: A Report to Congress. Agency for Toxic Substances and Disease Registry. Atlanta, Ga.: Public Health Service.

U.S. Department of Health and Human Services. 1988b. Surgeon General's Workshop: Health Promotion and Aging. Proceedings and Background Papers, F. G. Abdellah and S. R. Moore, eds. Washington, D.C.

U.S. Department of Health and Human Services. 1989a. Guide to Clinical Preventive Services: An Assessment of the Effectiveness of 169 Interventions. Preventive Services Task Force. Baltimore, Md.: Williams & Wilkins.

U.S. Department of Health and Human Services. 1989b. Promoting Health, Preventing Disease. Year 2000 Objectives for the Nation. Draft Report for Public Comment. Washington, D.C.: U.S. Government Printing Office.

U.S. Department of Health and Human Services. 1989c. The Surgeon General's Report on Nutrition and Health. Washington, D.C.: U.S. Government Printing Office.

U.S. Department of Health and Human Services. 1989d. Task 1: Population Profile of Disability Prepared by Mathematica Policy Research, Washington, D.C.

U.S. Department of Health and Human Services. 1990. Healthy People 2000: National Health Promotion and Disease Prevention Objectives. DHHS Pub. No. (PHS) 91-50212. Washington, D.C.: U.S. Government Printing Office.

U.S. Department of Health, Education, and Welfare. 1979. Healthy People: The Surgeon General's Report on Health Promotion and Disease Prevention. DHHS Pub. No. (PHS) 79-55071 Washington, D.C.: U.S. Government Printing Office.

U.S. General Accounting Office. 1988. Occupational Safety and Health: Assuring Accuracy in Employer Injury and Illness Records. Report to the Chairman, Subcommittee on Labor, Health and Human Services and Education, Committee on Appropriations. GAO/HRD-89-23. Washington, D.C.: U.S. Government Printing Office.

U.S. Health Care Financing Administration. 1983. Medical Coverage Issues Manual. HCFA Pub. No. 6. Washington, D.C.: U.S. Government Printing Office.

U.S. Health Resources and Services Administration. 1989. Child Health USA '89. Washington, D.C.: U.S. Government Printing Office.

U.S. Interagency Committee on Learning Disabilities. 1987. Learning Disabilities: A Report to the U.S. Congress. Washington, D.C.: Department of Health and Human Services.

U.S. Interagency Head Injury Task Force. 1989. Interagency Head Injury Task Force Report Bethesda, Md.: National Institute of Neurological and Communicative Disorders and Stroke, National Institutes of Health.

U.S. National Committee for Injury Prevention and Control. 1989. Injury Prevention: Meeting the Challenge. Supplement to the American Journal of Preventive Medicine, Vol. 5, No. 3 New York: Oxford University Press.

U.S. Public Health Service. 1989. Caring for Our Future: The Content of Prenatal Care. Washington, D.C.: U.S. Department of Health and Human Services.

U.S. Veterans Administration. 1988. Rehabilitation R&D Progress Reports, 1988. Vol. 25 Annual Supplement to the Journal of Rehabilitation Research and Development. Baltimore, Md.

Uomoto, J. M., and A. McLean. 1989. Care continuum in traumatic brain injury rehabilitation Rehabil Psychol 34(2):71-79.

Uzzell, B. P., T. W. Langfitt, and C. A. Dolinskas. 1987. Influence of injury severity on quality of survival after head injury. Surg Neurol 27(5)419-429.

Vachon, R. A. 1987. Inventing a future for individuals with work disabilities: The challenge of writing national disability policies. In: The Changing Nature of Work, Disability, and Society, D. E. Woods and D. Vandergoot, eds. New York: World Rehabilitation Fund.

Vachon, R. A. 1989-1990. Employing the disabled. Issues in Science and Technology 6(2):44-50. Washington, D.C.: National Academy Press.

Van Dyke, D. C., and C. A. Gahagan. 1988. Down syndrome: Cervical spine abnormalities and problems. Clin Pediatr 27(9):415-418.

Venier, L. H., and J. F. Ditunno. 1971. Heterotopic ossification in the paraplegic patient. Arch Phys Med Rehabil 52(10):475-479.

Verbrugge, L. M. 1984. Longer life but worsening health? Trends in health and mortality of middle-aged and older persons. Milbank Mem Fund Q 62(3):475-519.

Verbrugge, L. M., J. M. Lepkowski, and Y. Imanaka. 1989. Comorbidity and its impact on disability. Milbank Mem Fund Q 67(3-4):450-484.

Vimpani, G. V., P. A. Baghurst, N. R. Wigg, E. F. Robertson, A. J. McMichael, and R. R. Roberts. 1989. The Port Pirie cohort study—cumulative lead exposure and neurodevelopmental status at age two years: Do HOME scores and maternal IQ reduce apparent effects of lead on Bayley mental scores? In: Lead Exposure and Child Development: An International Assessment, M. A. Smith, L. D. Grant, and A. I. Sors, eds. Boston: Kluwer Academic.

Walker, D. K., J. S. Palfrey, J. A. Butler, and J. Singer. 1988. Use and sources of payment for health and community services for children with impaired mobility. Pub Health Rep 103(4):411-415.

Weddell, R., M. Oddy, and D. Jenkins. 1980. Social adjustment after rehabilitation: A two year follow-up of patients with severe head injury. Psychol Med 10(2):257-263.

Weintraub, A. H., and C. A. Opat. 1989. Motor and sensory dysfunction in the brain injured adult. In: Physical Medicine and Rehabilitation: Traumatic Brain Injury, L. J. Horn and D. N. Cope, eds. Philadelphia: Hanley and Belfus.

Welch, R. D., S. J. Lobley, S. B. O'Sullivan, and M. M. Freed. 1986. Functional independence in quadriplegia: Critical levels. Arch Phys Med Rehabil 67(4):235-240.

Wells, K., A. Stewart, R. Hays, A. Burnam, W. Rogers, M. Daniels, S. Berry, S. Greenfield, and J. Ware. 1989. The functioning and well-being of depressed patients: Results from the medical outcomes study. J Am Med Assoc 262(7)6:914-919.

Wenger, N. K., M. E. Mattson, C. D. Furberg, and J. Elinson, eds. 1984. Assessment of Quality of Life in Clinical Trials of Cardiovascular Therapies. New York: Le Jacq.

Whiteneck, G. G., C. Adler, R. E. Carter, D. P. Lammertse, S. Manley, R. Menter, K. A. Wagner, and C. Wilmot, eds. 1989. The Management of High Quadriplegia. New York: Demos Publications.

Whitman, S., R. Coonley-Hoganson, and B. T. Desai. 1984. Comparative head trauma experiences in two socioeconomically different Chicago area communities: A population study. Am J Epidemiol 119(4)570-580.

Whitney, E. N., and C. B. Cataldo. 1983. Understanding Normal and Clinical Nutrition. St. Paul, Minn.: West Publishing Company.

Wiener, J. M., R. J. Hanley, R. Clark, and J. F. Van Nostrand. 1990. Measuring the activities of daily living: Comparisons across national surveys. Journal of Gerontology: Social Sciences 45(6):5229-5237.

Williams, M. E., and N. M. Hadler. 1983. Sounding board. The illness as the focus of geriatric medicine. N Engl J Med 308(22):1357-1360.

Williamson, W. D., M. M. Desmond, L. P. Andrew, and R. N. Hicks. 1987. Visually impaired infants in the 1980s: A survey of etiologic factors and additional handicapping conditions in a school population. Clin Pediatr 26(5):241-244.

Wilson, R. W., and T. F. Drury. 1984. Interpreting trends in illness and disability: Health statistics and health status. Ann Rev Publ Health 5:83-106.

Wistar, C., and P. Vernon. 1986. The Prevalence of Disability in New York State. Report to the New York State Developmental Disabilities Planning Council. Albany: New York State Department of Health, Division of Planning, Policy and Resource Development, Bureau of Analysis and Program Evaluation.

Wolfe, B. L. 1987. The demand for disability transfers: Recent research and research needs. *In*: Disability Benefits: Factors Determining Applications and Awards, H. Emanuel, E. H. De Gier, and P. A. B. Kalker Konijn, eds. Greenwich, Conn.: JAI Press, Inc.

Wolfe, B. L., and R. Haveman. 1990. Trends in the prevalence of work disability from 1962 to 1984, and their correlates. Milbank Mem Fund Q 68(1):53-80.

World Health Organization. 1947. Constitution of the World Health Organization. New York: World Health Organization.

World Health Organization. 1980. International Classification of Impairments, Disabilities and Handicaps: A Manual of Classification Relating to the Consequences of Disease. Geneva: World Health Organization.

World Health Organization. 1984. The Uses of Epidemiology in the Study of the Elderly. Technical Report Series 706. Geneva: World Health Organization.

World Institute on Disability. 1987a. Attendant Services Network 1(2):1-4.

World Institute on Disability. 1987b. Attending to America: Personal Assistance for Independent Living. Berkeley, Calif.: World Institute on Disability.

Wright, B. A., ed. 1959. Psychology and Rehabilitation. Proceedings of the Institute on the Roles of Psychology and Psychologists in Rehabilitation, Princeton, N.J., February 3-7, 1958. Washington, D.C.: American Psychological Association.

Wrightson, P., and D. Gronwall. 1984. Time off work and symptoms after minor head injury. Injury 12(6):445-454.

Yarkony, G. M., and V. Sahgal. 1987. Contractures. A major complication of craniocerebral trauma. Clin Orthop 219:93-96.

Yarkony, G. M., E. Roth, L. Lovell, A. W. Heinemann, R. T. Katz, and Y. Wu. 1988. Rehabilitation outcomes in complete C5 quadriplegia. Am J Phys Med Rehabil 67(2):73-76.

Yelin, E., M. Nevitt, and W. Epstein. 1980. Toward an epidemiology of work disability. Milbank Mem Fund Q 58(3):386-415.

Young, J. S., P. E. Burns, A. M. Bower, and R. McCutchen. 1982. Spinal Cord Injury Statistics. Experience of the Regional Spinal Cord Injury Systems. Phoenix, Ariz.: Good Samaritan Medical Center.

Zigler, E., and R. Cascione. 1984. Mental retardation: An overview. *In*: Malformations of Development: Biological and Psychological Sources and Consequences, E. S. Gollin, ed. New York: Academic Press.

APPENDIXES

A

Disability Concepts Revisited: Implications for Prevention

Saad Z. Nagi*

The significance of disability as an individual and a societal concern cannot be overstated. Whether measured in prevalence or in social and economic consequences, the impacts are daunting. Although the questions they ask may be phrased somewhat differently, comprehensive disability surveys are fairly consistent in estimating that about 6.5 percent of noninstitutionalized Americans ages 18 through 64 are so severely disabled that they are not able to work (see, for example, Nagi, 1976; Social Security Administration, 1981, 1982). Estimates of the number of people who are limited in the amount or kind of work they can do, but who are not totally prevented from working, vary widely; on average, however, they constitute an additional 6.5 percent of the same sector of the population (Haber, 1990). These figures mean that about one in every eight adults in the United States in these age categories is disabled or limited in vocational pursuits. Furthermore, 1.8 percent of the noninstitutionalized civilian U.S. population 18 years of age and older need assistance in personal care; 3.5 percent need assistance in shopping, housework, and outdoor mobility; and 6.3 percent are limited in performing these activities of daily living but do manage to carry them out independently (Nagi, 1976).

Most societies, especially those of the industrialized world, have developed various types of programs of benefits and services. These programs provide another way of estimating the magnitude of the problem in terms of numbers of beneficiaries (Sunshine, 1980). During the early 1980s there were about 915 million beneficiaries of long-term disability programs in this country. (Some people may have been counted more than once, however, if they derived benefits from more than one program.) Social Security

---

*Ohio State University

Disability Insurance, Supplemental Security Income, and Veterans Compensation programs are the largest contributors to this total. These three programs alone account for nearly three-quarters of all beneficiaries of long-term disability benefits. The picture of temporary disability and workers' compensation is not as clear because of the continuous movement of beneficiaries into and out of these programs. These programs handle an estimated 2 million persons at any given point in time.

The economic dimension of disability is equally massive. Total expenditures for disability-related transfer payments and health care for the disabled reached $114.2 billion in 1975 (Berkowitz and Rubin, 1978), a hefty 7.5 percent of the gross national product (GNP). These expenditures have been rising at faster rates than the GNP. They were $69 billion in 1970 and only $39 billion in 1967, representing 6 percent and 4.9 percent of the GNP, respectively, in those two years. Regarding the sources of the $114.2 billion spent in 1975, $56.7 billion came from the federal government (including matching funds), $13.7 billion from state and local governments, and $43.7 billion from the private sector. Two factors influence these figures: numbers of beneficiaries and levels of benefits. As a percentage of governmental expenditures in the United States, income support for the disabled grew from 5.8 percent to 8 percent during 1968-1978 (Haveman et al., 1984). The annual rate of growth during that period was 6.3 percent in real terms. To place these estimates in a comparative perspective, the rates of growth in the percentage of governmental expenditures for income support for the disabled amounted to 0.5 percent in the United Kingdom, 5.3 percent in Germany, 12.1 percent in Sweden, and 18.6 percent in the Netherlands.

Society has evolved certain policies, programs, and professions that address the prevention of disability and the alleviation of its consequences. In the United States, which is a democratic, pluralistic society, these developments have been incremental and uneven, producing an unintegrated set of programs that are not unlike immiscible liquids that defy integration. Adapted from varying traditions (but mostly European in origin), the programs as a body are characterized by serious gaps and unnecessary overlaps.

In spite of the substantial prevalence and consequential effects of disability on individuals, families, and society, related conceptual and theoretical developments are of recent origin. The field is much in need of a theory to guide and advance research, to enhance understanding on the part of the professions and the public at large, and to better focus related policies and programs and improve their effectiveness. By theory I do not mean speculation but rather a set of interrelated concepts and empirically testable propositions that describe the phenomenon of disability and explain variance in its occurrence. Fundamental to the development of such a theory is a conceptual analysis to clarify the nature of disability and its dimensions. This paper addresses that objective.

CONCEPTUAL HISTORY

Early attempts at conceptualizing disability and its dimensions were prompted by influences from several sources. Three are particularly important: rehabilitation, chronic diseases, and compensation and insurance benefits. There have been important shifts in the concept and programs of rehabilitation from those espoused in the Vocational Rehabilitation Act of 1920. This act rejected calls for a comprehensive program that would include medical and surgical services and limited the concept of rehabilitation in the main to vocational training. The act was administered by state departments of education along with vocational education. There followed a move to the concept of comprehensive services, which allowed for "corrective" surgery, therapeutic treatments to reduce or eliminate disability, hospitalization, education, equipment, licenses, and tools (Switzer, 1965). State commissions for rehabilitation were established as separate agencies or placed under departments of public welfare. In 1953 the U.S. Department of Health, Education, and Welfare assumed responsibility for the reorganized Federal Security Agency, including the administration of vocational rehabilitation. Another milestone was the Vocational Rehabilitation Act of 1954, which adopted a formula for federal-state financing. The act permitted "the establishment of comprehensive rehabilitation facilities; the creation of specialized clinics of speech, hearing, cardiac, and other disorders; and the development of a variety of services that at one time would have seemed unattainable" (Switzer, 1965).

The 1943 and 1954 rehabilitation acts led to the infusion of funds into the field of rehabilitation, the spread of comprehensive centers, and the involvement of many disciplines—including medicine, education, social work, psychology, vocational counseling, occupational therapy, and nursing, among others. Inevitably, this broad professional grouping led to competition over resources and concerns over the protection of professional domains (e.g., Hamilton, 1950; Wright, 1959). (Indeed, the issue of domains continues to linger and is expressed in a variety of forms [Nagi, 1975].) These developments set the stage for attempts at conceptual distinctions to delineate the roles of the different professions and to explain their interrelationships. For example, Hamilton (1950) distinguishes between disability and handicap: disability is "a condition of impairment, physical or mental, having an objective aspect that can usually be described by a physician. It is essentially a medical thing"; a handicap is "the cumulative result of the obstacles which disability interposes between the individual and his maximum functional level." Hamilton goes on to say that "it is the handicap, not the disability, that gives impairment its welfare significance."

Several notable efforts during the 1950s contributed to advances in conceptualization and measurement of disability. During the first half of the decade, the Commission on Chronic Illness (1957) conducted two comprehensive surveys in Baltimore, Maryland, and Hunterdon County, New Jersey. One of the objectives was to obtain estimates for the "prevalence of illness and disability resulting from chronic disease by diagnosis, degree and duration of disability." Three kinds of measures of the disabling effects of chronic conditions were used in the evaluation: (1) limitations on the ability to perform 11 selected activities of daily living; (2) limitations on overall functional capacity; and (3) limitations on the ability to work, keep house, or attend school (i.e., the person's usual major activity). The second measure remains one of the best scales for independent living. The third measure of limitations in roles, referred to here as activities, is an approach that has been used for decades in the National Health Interview Survey (National Center for Health Statistics, 1987a).

Interest in functional assessments during the 1940s and 1950s spurred the development of measures of functional deficits—what Deaver and Brown (1945) called "activities of daily living" (ADL). A variety of instruments were constructed including differing combinations of items (for an informative review, see Gresham and Labi, 1984). A review of ADL scales led Hoberman and Associates to conclude in 1952 that "daily activity measurement will have passed adolescence only when functional tests are properly graded, scored, validated, and normed, and their all-round practicability and utility demonstrated." More than 30 years later, Frey (1984) declared, "it is safe to say that, with the exception of only a very few ADL scales, development in this area remains preadolescent." In addition to the work of the Commission on Chronic Illness noted above, other notable efforts in the area include those of Lawton (1972), Lambert and colleagues (1975), and Katz and co-workers (1963, 1983).

The decade of the 1950s was marked by mounting concerns over criteria and decisions regarding compensation and other disability benefits, which led to other conceptual attempts—for example, by the American Medical Association (AMA) Committee on Medical Rating of Mental and Physical Impairment (1958). The committee's work was in response to the needs of workers' compensation programs—which had been plagued by litigations—to develop standardized ratings legitimized by the professional and scientific standing of the AMA. The committee distinguished between impairment and disability by pointing out that "permanent impairment is a contributing factor to, but not necessarily an indication of, the extent of a patient's permanent disability." To the committee, "[c]ompetent evaluation of permanent impairment requires adequate and complete medical examination, accurate objective measurement of function and avoidance of subjective impressions and non-medical factors such as the patient's age, sex, or employability." Because the committee's domain was defined as that of impairment, disability was left without further clarification. What is important, however, is the reference to the functional dimension. Such a reference was also included in a report by the Criteria Committee of the New York Heart Association

(1953), which described a complete diagnosis as accounting for etiological, anatomical, physiological, functional, and therapeutic aspects. Individual clinicians also developed approaches to measuring functional losses (e.g., McBride, 1963; Kessler, 1970).

A CONCEPTUAL FRAMEWORK

As the 1950s drew to a close, the situation was one of differing conceptions of disability and related phenomena and no shared concepts; a number of terms were applied unsystematically and often interchangeably. The lack of clarity in conceptual constructs was reflected in problems with criteria for the evaluation of disability for compensation and other benefits. The various programs relied heavily on impairment schedules and lists for their decisions concerning disability in vocational roles and earning potentials. In a sense, this corresponds to the analogy of looking for a key in a place where there happens to be some light rather than where the key was dropped. In regard to workers' compensation programs, the AMA Committee on Medical Rating of Mental and Physical Impairment (1958) concluded that "impairment is, in fact, the sole or real criterion of permanent disability far more often than is readily acknowledged." In a similar vein, the Subcommittee on Social Security of the House Ways and Means Committee (1959) gave the following instructions:

> The Subcommittee recognizes the difficulties of developing and enunciating criteria for the weight to be given non-medical factors in the evaluation of disability and the extreme sensitivity of this area. But the Subcommittee believes that the time has come, if it is not well overdue, to make a determined effort to develop and refine these criteria and make them available to the evaluators and to the public in the form of published regulations.

The decade also witnessed provisions for research development in the 1954 Rehabilitation Act and in other programs, which introduced the research community more extensively to disability and rehabilitation issues.

In the early 1960s, as part of plans for a large-scale study of decision making in the Social Security Disability Insurance (SSDI) program and in rehabilitation services for SSDI applicants and beneficiaries, Nagi (1964, 1965, 1969) built on existing knowledge to construct a framework of four distinct but interrelated concepts: active pathology, impairment, functional limitation, and disability.

1. The state of *active pathology* may result from infection, trauma, metabolic imbalance, degenerative disease processes, or other etiology. Such a condition involves (a) interruption of or interference with normal processes, and (b) the simultaneous efforts of the organism to regain a normal

state. Pathology then is not merely the surrender to an abnormal state of affairs but also the fight for health (Selye, 1956). Obviously, deficiencies in immune systems and other coping mechanisms can render the fight for health ineffective. In modern health practices, the organism is aided by surgical intervention, medication, and other forms of therapy to help regain equilibrium. Some means may become necessary over extended periods of time or indefinitely, as in the case of certain types of chronic diseases.

2. The concept of *impairment* indicates a loss or abnormality of an anatomical, physiological, mental, or emotional nature. The concept comprises three distinct categories: (1) all conditions of pathology, which are by definition impairments because such conditions involve anatomical, physiological, mental, or emotional deviation; (2) residual losses or abnormalities that remain after the active state of pathology has been controlled or eliminated (e.g., healed amputations, residual paralysis); and (3) abnormalities not associated with pathology (e.g., congenital formations). Thus, although every pathology involves an impairment, not every impairment involves a pathology. Impairments vary along a number of dimensions that affect their influence on the nature and degree of disability. Important among these are the degree of visibility and disfigurement, stigma, the predictability of the course of the underlying pathology, the prognosis and prospects for recovery or stabilization, threat to life, the types and severity of limitations in function they impose, and the point of onset in the life cycle—congenital, early childhood, during the productive years, or later in life.

3. *Functional limitations* and impairments both involve function. The difference, however, is in the level at which the limitations are manifested. Functional limitation refers to manifestations at the level of the organism as a whole. Many tissues, for example, may have an altered structure or function without limiting the ability of the organism as a whole. A significant number of muscle fibers must become denervated before discernible weaknesses occur; the walls of blood vessels must undergo a great deal of alteration before appreciable changes in the flow within these vessels ensue. Virtually an infinite number of similar examples can be noted. One could speak of limitations in function at the levels of molecules, cells, tissues, organs, regions, systems, or the organism as a whole. Although limitations at a lower level of organization may not be reflected at higher levels, the reverse is not true. An individual who is unable to reach overhead because of tightness in the shoulder can be expected also to have abnormalities at the levels of tissues and cells that make up the shoulder. It is important to note that limitations in function at higher levels of organization may result from differing impairments and limitations in function at the lower levels. For example, inability to lift a heavy weight may be related to mechanical problems in the lumbosacral region, or it may be the result of diminished cardiac output or pulmonary ventilation (Melvin and Nagi, 1970). Func-

tional limitations are the most direct way through which impairments contribute to disability. However, as mentioned earlier, certain disfiguring or stigmatizing impairments can lead directly to disability without the involvement of a functional deficit at the level of the organism as a whole.

4. *Disability* refers to social rather than to organismic functioning. It is an inability or limitation in performing socially defined roles and tasks expected of an individual within a sociocultural and physical environment. These roles and tasks are organized in spheres of life activities such as those of the family or other interpersonal relations; work, employment, and other economic pursuits; and education, recreation, and self-care. Not all impairments or functional limitations precipitate disability, and similar patterns of disability may result from different types of impairments and limitations in function. Furthermore, identical types of impairments and similar functional limitations may result in different patterns of disability. Several other factors contribute to shaping the dimensions and severity of disability. These include (a) the individual's definition of the situation and reactions, which at times compound the limitations; (b) the definition of the situation by others, and their reactions and expectations—especially those who are significant in the lives of the person with the disabling condition (e.g., family members, friends and associates, employers and co-workers, and organizations and professions that provide services and benefits); and (c) characteristics of the environment and the degree to which it is free from, or encumbered with, physical and sociocultural barriers.

Further clarifications of some issues concerning this framework were made earlier (Nagi, 1975); others are added here in response to questions and misinterpretations arising in professional meetings or in print. First is the issue of its applicability to mental and emotional conditions. The question reflects the position that mental and emotional conditions are more socially grounded than those of an anatomical and physiological nature (e.g., Lemert, 1951; Sullivan, 1953; Scheff, 1967; Szaz, 1974) and therefore do not conform to the same characteristic patterns. Equally important is that, except for organically beset conditions, indicators of pathology, impairment, and functional limitations are, so far, not separable in regard to mental and emotional conditions. In these cases, pathology and impairment are inferred from manifestations at the level of functional limitations. In psychiatric terminology there is reference to "functional" versus "organic" disorders. It is important to note, however, that distinctions between indicators of functional limitations and those of disability can be established with sufficient clarity. Intelligence tests, scales of psychophysiological reactions, other psychometric tests, and clinical assessments have been used to identify functional limitations independent of whether, and to what extent, a person is limited in performing expected roles and tasks.

The second issue concerns distinctions between disability and other forms of inability. Consider, for example, work and employment, which are affected by a variety of factors other than those identified in this framework. Ability or inability to perform social roles, vocational in this example, depends on an interaction between a set of individual characteristics and factors of a situational or environmental nature. A change in the economic or technological environments may lead to unemployment totally unrelated to health conditions. By the same token, family roles may be disrupted or altered by divorce, separation, or other expressions of incompatibility rather than impairment and functional limitation. It is important to reiterate that this framework is rooted within the context of health.

Third is the observation that the term disability implies a change from prior higher levels of functioning and is not applicable to congenital and early childhood conditions. In this respect, distinctions have been made between congenital and "adventitious" inabilities (Carroll, 1961), the latter being *dis*ability in the strict sense of the word. In this framework, however, the concept of disability is used in a generic sense to include those arising from congenital and early childhood conditions as well as those occurring later in life. The comparative reference for the former is the level of functioning of cohorts rather than of prior levels once maintained.

A fourth issue concerns the lines of differentiation between functional limitations and disability and where such activities as those of daily living and use of transportation fit within the concepts of social roles and tasks. To Parsons (1958), "a role is the organized system of participation of an individual in a social system."

> Roles, looked at that way, constitute the primary focus of the articulation and hence interpenetration between personalities and social systems. Tasks on the other hand, are both more differentiated and more highly specified than roles, one role is capable of being analyzed into a plurality of different tasks. . . [it] is legitimate to consider the task to define the level at which the action of the individual articulates with the *physical* world. . . . A task, then, may be regarded as that subsystem of role which is defined by a definite set of physical operations which perform some function or functions in relation to a role.

Sarbin and Allen (1968) differentiate between role expectations and role enactment. "Role expectations are comprised of the rights and privileges, the duties and obligations of any occupant of a social position in relation to persons occupying other positions in the social structure. . . . Overt conduct, that is, what the person does and says in a particular setting is the first specification of the role enactment." Typically each person performs multiple roles not only because of occupying multiple social positions but also because each position involves a role-set (Merton, 1957). Thus the position of a medical student "entails not only the role of a student in relation to his teachers, but also to other students, nurses, physicians, social workers, medical technicians, etc."

The point to be made is that components of roles—expectations, acts, actions, and tasks—are learned, organized, and purposeful patterns of behavior and not isolated muscle responses (Sarbin and Allen, 1968). Some acts, actions, and tasks are role specific, whereas others are common to the enactment of more than one role. Activities of daily living are learned, organized, and purposeful patterns of behavior. They are part of the set of expectations inherent in family, vocational, and a variety of other roles. Severe limitations in performing these tasks often result in reciprocal role relationships of dependency/assistance, which at times become contractual. The same reasoning applies to driving, the use of public transportation, the use of means of communication, and similar tasks, each of which separately does not constitute a social role but is part of many roles. Limitations in performing these tasks are components of the concept of disability.

The fifth issue concerning the disability framework relates to another criterion for differentiating the concept of disability from those of functional limitations, impairment, and pathology. For this, it will be useful to consider differences between concepts of attributes and properties on the one hand and relational concepts on the other (Cohen, 1957). Concepts of attributes and properties refer to the individual characteristics of an object or a person, such as height, weight, or intelligence. Indicators of these concepts can all be found within the characteristics of the individual. Pathology, impairment, and functional limitations are concepts of attributes and properties. One need not go beyond examining a person to identify the presence and extent of physiological and anatomical losses or disorders, or to assess limitations in the functioning of the organism. In contrast, indicators of a relational concept cannot all be accounted for among the attributes of an individual. They include characteristics of other segments of the situation. Disability is a relational concept; its indicators include individuals' capacities and limitations, in relation to role and task expectations, and the environmental conditions within which they are to be performed.

The sixth and final issue is the question of whether disability, as conceptualized here, is limited to work. By now, it should be clear that the answer is no. Because of emphasis in public policy on concerns with dependence in economic and personal terms, and greater availability of support for studies of these dimensions, research developments were pushed largely in the direction of work disability and problems in independent living. However, the concept is inclusive of all socially defined roles and tasks. For heuristic purposes, Nagi (1969) applied a stress curve (Koos, 1954; Hill, 1958) to illustrate the processes of disability. As depicted in Figure A-1, the line between (a) and (b) represents the usual level of performance of an individual. The minor fluctuations are within the individual's margin of

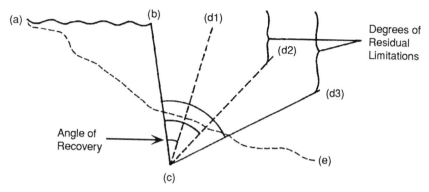

FIGURE A-1   Applying a stress curve to illustrate the processes of disability. Adapted from Nagi, 1969; used with permission of Ohio State University Press.

tolerance. The major emphasis during such periods is on primary prevention to maintain performance at that level. At point (*b*) a health condition occurs (disease or injury) that results in a deviation from normality that is beyond the individual's tolerance and coping abilities. The condition is in an acute stage, and the major emphasis is on treatment until the pathology is eliminated or controlled as represented by point (*c*). (Failure to control the pathology would, of course, result in death.) An important feature of the stress curve is the angle of recovery, that is, the angle formed by the two lines (*b*)-(*c*) and (*c*)-(*d*). In many cases the recovery is complete; in others a residual impairment may be precipitated. The angle of recovery implies a relationship between time and level of recovery. A smaller angle indicates shorter time and higher level of recovery, and vice versa. Once the condition has been stabilized after (*c*), the major emphasis shifts from treatment to restoration and rehabilitation.

This model is most appropriate for injuries and diseases that have identifiable onsets and for those that have stable residuals. Other models are better suited for describing the increasingly prevalent, gradually progressive chronic conditions that are forcing reassessments of approaches in all phases of health care. In the natural history of these pathologies and the limitations they precipitate, points (*b*) and (*c*) in Figure A-1 become less, if at all, identifiable. The residuals are hardly stabilized, and the prognosis is less certain. The dotted line (*a*)-(*e*) shows this pattern. The course of these conditions often involves acute episodes.

The same curve can be used to illustrate the different forms of functional limitations: physical, sensory, emotional, intellectual, and so on, as well as disabilities in the various roles and tasks (e.g., vocational, family, interpersonal and community relations, independent living). Such mapping requires meaningful concepts, valid and sensitive measures, and longitudinal data. It should yield information useful for studying the natural history of disability, accounting for factors that influence its course, identifying the types of services and benefits needed, and timing these services and benefits for optimal effectiveness.

A FRAMEWORK FROM THE WORLD HEALTH ORGANIZATION

In 1980 the World Health Organization (WHO) published a "manual of classification relating to the consequences of disease." In an introduction to this manual, Philip H. N. Wood points out that taxonomic approaches used in the development of the International Classification of Diseases were found unsatisfactory. "Separate classifications of impairments and handicaps were prepared" and "circulated widely in 1974." The following excerpts from the introductory remarks trace the steps that were to follow:

> . . . Responsibility for collating comments and developing definitive proposals was undertaken by Dr. Wood. These were submitted for consideration by the International Conference for the Ninth Revision of the International Classification of Diseases in October 1975. At this juncture the scheme incorporated a supplementary digit to identify disability, and the whole approach was acknowledged as being to a large extent experimental and exploratory. Having considered the classification, the Conference recommended its publication for trial purposes. In 1976, the Twenty-ninth World Health Assembly . . . approved the publication, for trial purposes, of the supplementary classification of impairments and handicaps as a supplement to, but not as an integral part of the International Classification of Diseases.

> The present manual, published under this authority, represents a considerable recasting of the detailed proposals submitted to the Ninth Revision Conference. (p. 13)

The conceptual scheme in the WHO publication (1980) is organized around four concepts: disease, impairment, disability, and handicap. In Wood's words, these four concepts are defined as follows:

> (i) *Something abnormal occurs within the individual*: this may be present at birth or acquired later. A chain of causal circumstances, the "etiology," gives rise to changes in the structure or functioning of the body, the "pathology". Pathological changes may or may not make themselves evident; when they do they are described as "manifestations", which in medical parlance, are usually distinguished as "symptoms and signs". These features are the components of the medical model of disease, . . .

> (ii) *Someone becomes aware of such an occurrence*: in other words, the pathological state is exteriorized. . . . In behavioural terms, the indi-

vidual has become or been made aware that he is unhealthy. His illness heralds recognition of *impairments*, abnormalities of the body structure and appearance, and of organ or system function, resulting from any cause. Impairments represent disturbances at the organ level. . . . *In the context of health experience, an impairment is any loss or abnormality of psychological, physiological, or anatomical structure or function.*

(iii) *The performance or behaviour of the individual may be altered* as a result of this awareness, either consequentially or cognitively. Common activities may become restricted, and in this way the experience is objectified. Also relevant are psychological responses to the presence of disease, part of so-called illness behaviour, and sickness phenomena, the patterning of illness manifested as behavior by the individual in response to the expectations others have of him when he is ill. These experiences represent *disabilities*, which reflect the consequences of impairments in terms of functional performance and activity by the individual. Disabilities represent disturbances at the level of the person. . . . *In the context of health experience, a disability is any restriction or lack (resulting from an impairment) of ability to perform an activity in the manner or within the range considered normal for a human being.*

(iv) *Either the awareness itself, or the altered behaviour or performance to which this gives rise,* may place the individual at a disadvantage relative to others, thus socializing the experience. This plane reflects the response of society to the individual's experience, be this expressed in attitudes, such as the engendering of stigma, or in behaviour, which may include specific instruments such as legislation. These experiences represent *handicap*, the disadvantages resulting from impairment and disability. . . . *In the context of health experience, a handicap is a disadvantage for a given individual, resulting from an impairment or a disability, that limits or prevents the fulfilment of a role that is normal (depending on age, sex, and social and cultural factors) for that individual.* (pp. 25-29)

The WHO publication includes a narrative section that outlines the history of the undertaking, the purposes, the conceptual framework, and the rationale for classification. It also includes the classifications themselves for impairments (Code I), disabilities (Code D), and handicaps (Code H).

ASSESSMENT OF FRAMEWORKS

The two frameworks outlined here—which are identified in the literature with Nagi and Wood—have been the subject of comparisons and analyses by several writers (e.g., Duckworth, 1984; Frey, 1984; Granger, 1984). These analyses are generally limited and frequently reveal that certain specifications are not clearly understood. The difference is not only in semantics nor simply that one framework is an extension of the other. There are also important substantive differences. It is often difficult to communicate conceptual constructs within the same discipline, let alone across varying disciplines and professional fields, which may account for some of the misinterpretations that have been plaguing this area.

The remainder of this paper assesses these frameworks in light of important criteria that govern conceptualization, classification, and theory construction. Kaplan (1964) suggests three sets of criteria for assessing frameworks: norms of coherence, norms of correspondence, and pragmatic norms. These criteria will be used as guides, and each framework will be examined individually rather than by a point-counterpoint discussion. Wood's scheme will be examined first. Table A-1 compares the Nagi and Wood taxonomies.

An important aspect of a framework's internal coherence is criteria that differentiate among concepts and categories. For Wood, a disease becomes an impairment when it is "exteriorized"; by that he means that "someone becomes aware of such an occurrence. . . . Most often the individual himself becomes aware of disease manifestations . . . deviations may be identified of which the 'patient' himself is unaware . . . as screening programs are extended. . . . Alternatively, a relative or someone else may draw attention to disease manifestations." By equating impairment with awareness, Wood is saying in effect that impairments do not exist independently of someone's recognition of them.

But what about asymptomatic disorders that have not been identified through screening or that go unnoticed by relatives and friends? Moreover, if "illness heralds recognition of impairments," what about impairments that are not associated with active pathology? Why does Wood's definition of impairment—"any loss or abnormality of psychological, physiological, or anatomical structure or function"—fail to make reference to awareness? It seems that this distinction confuses the conditions themselves with an awareness of their presence and the behavioral patterns evoked by such awareness.

Wood's criterion for differentiating between impairment and disability is "objectification," which he describes as "the process through which a functional limitation expresses itself as a reality in everyday life, the problem being made objective because the activities of the body are interfered with" (WHO, 1980:28). The term "objective" is the contrast of "subjective," and every concept has both objective and subjective aspects. For diseases and disorders, indicators of these two aspects are grouped as signs and symptoms, respectively. Similarly, impairments, functional limitations, and disabilities can all be considered from objective or subjective viewpoints. It is not clear that objectification is equated with an individual's awareness of a change in identity when disability takes form. An important question is what do objective and subjective distinctions and awareness have to do with differences between disease and impairment on the one hand and disability on the other? Again, criteria related to the conditions themselves and the levels of

TABLE A-1a Nagi Taxonomy of Disability

Element	Active Pathology	Impairment	Functional Limitation	Disability
Definitions	Interruption or interference with normal processes and efforts of the organism to regain normal state.	Anatomical, physiological, mental, or emotional abnormalities or loss	Limitation in performance at the level of the whole organism or or person.	Limitation in performance of socially defined roles and tasks within a sociocultural and physical environment.
Differentiating criteria	All conditions of active pathology constitute a subclass of impairments which in turn include two other subclasses: (1) residual loss and abnormality after active pathology has been arrested, and (2) congenital loss or abnormality not associated with active pathology. Impairment is a more inclusive concept.	Both impairment and functional limitation involve function; in impairment, reference is to the levels of tissues, organs, and systems; in functional limitation, reference is to the level of the organism or the person as a whole. Functional limitation refers to organismic performance; disability refers to social performance; disability is a relational concept, whereas the other three are concepts of attributes.		
Indicators	Symptoms and signs including observations; indicators are to be found in attributes of the individual.	Symptoms and signs including observations; indicators are to be found in attributes of the individual.	Limitations in the various activities of the organism such as walking, climbing, reaching, reasoning, seeing, hearing, etc.; indicators can be grouped into larger categories such as physical, mental, emotional, sensory, communication, etc.; indicators are to be found in attributes of the individual.	Limitations in performance of such roles and tasks as related to family, work, community, school, recreation, self-care, etc.; indicators are to be found in the relations on the one hand, and the conditions in the sociocultural and physical environment on the other.

TABLE A-1b Wood Taxonomy of Disability

Element	Disease	Impairment	Disability	Handicap
Definitions	Something abnormal within the individual; etiology gives rise to change in structure and functioning of the body.	Any loss or abnormality of psychological, physiological, or anatomical structure or function at the organ level.	Any restriction or lack of ability to perform an activity in the manner considered normal for a human being.	A disadvantage resulting from an impairment or a disability that limits or prevents the fulfillment of a role that is normal depending on age, sex, and sociocultural factors.
Differentiating criteria	A disease becomes an impairment when "exteriorized," that is, when someone becomes aware of it; impairment is more inclusive than disease because it does not necessarily indicate that disease is present.		Impairment becomes disability when the problem is made "objective because activities of the body are interfered with"; disability refers to performance of the organ or mechanism. Handicap is differentiated from disability in that the former is "socialized"; it involves "valuation," which is usually to the disadvantage of the individual; handicap is relative to other people.	
Indicators	Symptoms and signs.	Symptoms, signs, and awareness of the individual.	A wide range of categories including awareness, family and occupational roles, communication, personal care, locomotor, body disposition, dexterity, situational, skull, and other restrictions.	A variety of categories including orientation, physical independence, mobility, occupation, social integration, and economic self-sufficiency.

organization at which they are manifested are confused with awareness and behavioral patterns. Confusion in these verbal definitions of the concepts spills over into the operationalization of the classification system.

Disability turns into handicap as it becomes "socialized" in that "(i) some value is attached to departure from a structural, functional, or performance norm, either by the individual himself or by his peers in a group to which he relates; (ii) the valuation is dependent on cultural norms . . .; [and] (iii) . . . the valuation is usually to the disadvantage of the affected individual" (WHO, 1980:29). In these distinctions, Wood fails to differentiate between limitations in social performance and the causes for these limitations, that is, between the "what" and the "why." A concept is concerned with the what—a person is unable to work or is limited in performing a family role. Valuations, stereotyping, discrimination, service and benefits programs, labor market conditions, technological developments, architectural barriers, and other factors in the sociocultural and physical environment are causal influences that can facilitate or inhibit the optimal social performance of which a person is capable. These factors are part of why social performance becomes limited. The relationships between the "what" and the "why" are *empirical*, in that they are subsumed under testable propositions, rather than *definitional*, in the sense of being subsumed under a concept.

Wood is correct in stating that "it is a fundamental principle . . . that classification is subordinate to a purpose." However, as Hempel (1963) points out, "classification in empirical science, is subject to the requirement of fruitfulness. The characteristics which serve to define the different types should not merely provide neat pigeonholes to accommodate all the individual cases in the domain of inquiry, but should lend themselves to sound generalizations." These points are clarified further by Kaplan (1964):

> What makes a concept significant is that the classification it institutes is one into which things fall, as it were, of themselves. It carves at the joints. . . . [A] significant concept so groups or divides its subject matter that it can enter into many and important true propositions about the subject matter other than those which state the classification itself. Traditionally, such a concept was said to identify a "natural" class rather than an "artificial" one. Its naturalness consists in this, that the attributes it chooses as the basis of classification are significantly related to the attributes conceptualized elsewhere in our thinking. Things are grouped together because they resemble one another. A natural grouping is one which allows the discovery of many more, and more important, resemblances than those originally recognized. Every classification serves some purpose or other. . . . [I]t is artificial when we cannot do more with it than we first intended. The purpose of scientific classification is to facilitate the fulfillment of any purpose whatever, to disclose the relationships that must be taken into account no matter what.

There are no meaningful resemblances that would justify grouping under the same concept "family role disability" and "occupational role disability" on one hand and "foot control disability" and "crouching disability" on the other. How can "family role disability" and "occupational role disability" be assessed in the absence of expectations and what Wood refers to as valuations? The enunciation of the categories that make up codes in these areas is in itself a statement of expectations and valuations. These and numerous other examples demonstrate serious problems with the concept of disability as outlined in the WHO framework. Ambivalence is acknowledged about "functional limitations," which were regarded in an earlier draft "as being elements of disability" and were later assimilated with impairments. As part of the impairment grouping, functional limitations are conceptualized at the organ level rather than at the level of the whole organism. In addition, disability includes a mix of social and organismic performance. Thus the framework lacks a coherent and clearly delineated concept of performance at the level of the organism. This represents a major gap because functional limitations conceptualized at this level represent the most crucial link between impairment and social performance.

The definition of "handicap" leads the reader to expect major, if not exclusive, emphasis on factors in the sociocultural and physical environment—stereotyping, prejudice, discrimination, employment opportunities, and other kinds of barriers. The closest category to this conception is "social integration," but even there the emphasis is still on the individual's impairment and limitations. In some other categories, classification becomes exclusively that of severity of impairment and limitation in function—for example, restrictions in mobility to one's neighborhood, dwelling, room, or chair. Finally, the categories included under the handicap rubric significantly overlap with some of those under disability, such as in the case of family and occupational roles.

Some of the categories included under the handicap concept actually represent summaries of items included under other concepts. Every concept has an "attribute space" (Lazarsfeld, 1972), which comprises its dimensions and indicators or manifestations. When a number of indicators of a particular concept are combined in a typology or a larger category—which is by necessity more abstract—the newly created typology or larger category remains within the attribute space of the same concept. Consider, for example, several categories under "orientation handicap," which is no more than an attempt to combine a number of functional limitations, impairments, and diseases. Furthermore, the attempt to combine several limitations, their severities, compensatory aids, and the help of others is a recipe for a cumbersome classification. The elements of compensatory aids and help from others could have been handled in simpler ways without loss of information or precision. Simplicity without loss is an important norm of coherence.

Another important norm of coherence concerns the way a conceptual scheme is integrated into existing knowledge. This criterion need not be applied in a conservative manner that shuts out real breakthroughs. A new framework may be consistent with existing one(s), it may be different in part, or it may be altogether different. The test of integration serves at least two purposes: (1) it adds to the cumulative process that advances the development of knowledge, and (2) it can help avoid compartmentalization, duplication of effort, and, worse, confusion. Wood's conceptual framework and classification scheme fail to meet this requirement. Such statements as "the confusion . . . stems largely from the lack of a coherent scheme or conceptual framework" and that the purposes of surveys and studies in determining eligibility for benefits in the United States have been "to identify categories or groups of people fulfilling predetermined criteria; words of this type have, therefore, been concerned more with assignment than with evaluation" do not reflect the status of knowledge at that time. Frameworks existed prior to his initiative, and studies and surveys conducted during and since the 1950s have paid considerable attention to measurement (e.g., Commission on Chronic Illness, 1957; Trussel and Elinson, 1959; Srole et al., 1962; Nagi, 1969). By the mid-1970s, there was much more in the literature, especially in the United States, than can be justifiably dismissed in a short paragraph. A systematic review would probably have helped Wood's scheme by building on existing foundations, avoiding many of the problems identified above, and fitting the results into a fairly well-developed body of knowledge.

So far this discussion has focused on conceptualization and classification, definitional distinctions, resemblances among items and categories grouped under particular concepts, and the ways in which the whole framework does or does not fit within existing knowledge. Also of importance are norms of correspondence that refer to how a framework "fits the facts." "Science is fundamentally governed by the reality principle" (Kaplan, 1964). These norms apply to the results of empirical research based on concepts defined and operationalized in the manner outlined in the framework. Such research may be aimed at identifying the antecedents or consequences of the various concepts in the framework. Through the process of inquiry and verification, the adequacy of concepts, classifications, and propositions are put to the tests of correspondence. It is too early to assess Wood's framework in view of these criteria. The application of pragmatic norms would be similarly premature; these pertain to the working of a framework—what it can do to advance scientific developments and guide actions. It is important to note, however, that the problems in coherence identified above do not bode well for the framework to adequately fulfill correspondence or pragmatic criteria.

Claims of support by individuals, associations, or other organizations do not confer validity. "It must be kept in mind that the validation of theory— or of any other scientific belief—is not a matter of any official decision, the deliverance of a solemn judgement" (Kaplan, 1964). It is only through inquiry and evidence that frameworks can prove their worth. The developmental history of this framework, as cited by Wood, raises serious questions about the role of WHO's committees. If the present manual, published by WHO, "represents a *considerable recasting* [emphasis added] of the detailed proposals submitted to the Ninth Revision Conference," one has to wonder about the ability of the Conference to approve frameworks of concepts and terminology that meet Kaplan's criteria for classification. An unfortunate outcome is reintroducing confusion in concepts and terminology just as researchers, government agencies, and policy analysts have started to make significant gains toward shared concepts and common frames of reference.

Attempts to meet norms of coherence in Nagi's framework are embodied in the review of conceptual history, from which the framework evolved, as well as in the conceptual distinctions and clarifications presented in earlier sections of this paper. The literature review places this framework within existing knowledge, and the criteria of differentiation among concepts reveal the logic of its internal structure. A repetition of this discussion here would be unnecessary. Suffice it to say that this framework is consistent with conceptual and definitional discussions that have appeared during the last quarter of a century, including those by economists, historians, physicians, political scientists, and sociologists (e.g., Burk, 1967; Howards et al., 1980; Berkowitz, 1987; DeJong, 1987; Johnson, 1987; Haber, 1988, 1990). It is consistent with concepts used in major national surveys (e.g., Social Security Administration, 1981, 1982) and definitions of work disability by the U.S. Bureau of the Census.

Inquiries clarify concepts and theoretical frameworks through successive approximations that involve cycles of operationalization, empirical testing, and further specification. The evolution of this framework has been and continues to be subject to this process of improving correspondence among theory, concepts, and facts. Neither time nor space would allow for a comprehensive survey of studies and results that derived conceptual orientation from this framework.

B

Dissent and Response

Appendix B consists of two parts. Part 1 is a dissenting statement prepared by committee member Deborah Stone. Part 2 is a response to that statement by the other 22 members of the committee.

PART 1: DISSENT FROM THE REPORT
OF THE COMMITTEE

Deborah A. Stone

I dissent from the majority report for two reasons. First, I think the general quality of the report is poor. It purports to be a comprehensive agenda for disability prevention when in fact it suggests only a narrow approach to the problem. The "Summary and Recommendations" is a bland consensus document whose primary goal is to avoid controversy. The recommendations are mostly ritual calls for more leadership, professional training, data collection, research, and public education. They neglect more concrete and direct social policies that could prevent and mitigate disabilities. Moreover, many of the report's major recommendations are not supported by empirical evidence and were not the product of any serious investigation by the committee.

Second, the process of studying the problem and drafting the report did not meet the institution's standards of scientific objectivity and freedom from political pressures. The sponsors and funders of the study asked the committee to prepare a broad agenda for disability prevention; however, they structured the task and exercised influence over the committee and staff so as to produce a report that would bolster their own political agendas.

Critique of the Report

The agenda suggested in the majority report is composed primarily of vague slogans (e.g., "enhance the role of the private sector," "critically assess progress") and calls for more research, training, education, data collection, and coordination. Only 7 of the 27 recommendations (nos. 16 through 22) would provide services directly to people who could benefit from them, or would directly prevent disability. The remaining recommendations call for more bureaucracy, more training programs, and more jobs for educated, middle-class, mostly nondisabled people.

The report fails to set an agenda or even to suggest how policymakers might go about setting one. It merely provides a long list of things that could be done, without any indication of the relative importance of the various disabilities or the relative effectiveness of the various prevention measures, or any discussion of how policymakers ought to think about evaluating these questions. The "conceptual model" of disability developed in the report (a model that has been around since 1969) is useless as a policy tool. It provides no guidance for setting priorities among the items in the "wish list" of new research, data collection, training, and services that the committee recommends, nor does it suggest any criteria for setting priorities among the many types of disabilities discussed in the report.

Although the report pays lip service in many places to social, cultural, physical, and legal barriers as causes of disability, there is no analysis of any of these factors in the report. Important topics that are neglected in the report include the following:

1. *Handicap discrimination* is now a major legal field, with federal and state statutes, a sizable body of case law, and scholarly studies of the nature and impact of discrimination as well as the usefulness and limitations of civil rights remedies. The report makes brief mention of the Americans with Disabilities Act but provides no analysis of how and to what extent job market barriers prevent people with impairments from working. Apart from recommendation 26, which calls only for educating the public about the civil rights of the disabled, not one of the recommendations deals with discrimination, or with defining, enforcing, or funding the enforcement of civil rights.

2. Although many statements in the body of the report recognize the importance of *access to medical care* in preventing disability, the only recommendation to deal with this problem (no. 16) calls for comprehensive health services for mothers and children. A recommendation for universal health insurance that had been in earlier drafts was dropped from the final report. No recommendation deals with access to health insurance for people with chronic disease and disabilities, despite the acknowledged severity of this problem in Chapter 8.

3. The report makes no assessment of major national efforts in *adapting buildings and public transit* for accessibility. (Four sentences in Chapter 4 assert that adaptive devices and environmental modifications are useful and essential components of a prevention program.)

4. There is no analysis of *occupational causes of disability*, although they are known to be important factors in injury and some chronic disease. The major national effort to prevent occupationally caused disabilities (the Occupational Health and Safety Act, in place since 1973) is ignored in the report.

5. There is also a major national effort to prevent what might be called *secondary learning disabilities*, in the form of the Education for All Handicapped Children's Act and the early intervention program added in the 1986 amendments to that law. The aim of these programs is to ensure that children with physical, developmental, and emotional deficits receive whatever services are necessary for them to derive maximum benefit from their education and to prevent their being handicapped later on in social, intellectual, and vocational skills. These two programs merit half a page in Chapter 4. The report neither evaluates the experience of these programs nor considers how to make better use of them to prevent disability.

6. Within the area of *injury control*, automobile safety programs, various methods to curtail drunk-driving, and gun control measures are extremely important aspects of disability prevention. Although the report mentions these measures, it does not examine the large empirical literatures relevant to them. Nor does the report simply recommend that programs be instituted in these areas, although, as I show below, the committee makes recommendations for major national programs in other, less controversial areas (research, education, and training) without examining the empirical evidence of need or effectiveness.

7. The report neglects (except for some cursory mentions with intense obfuscation) *prenatal genetic testing, mass screening for genetic defects, and abortion* of affected fetuses. I take up this topic in more detail below because it is the issue that most clearly revealed the politicization of the committee's deliberative process.

Bland as the recommendations are, there is still a puzzling disparity between the body of the report and its recommendations. Most of the report is concerned with epidemiological and clinical information of the sort that would be useful in designing primary prevention programs (i.e., preventing disability before it happens). Most of the recommendations, on the other hand, are aimed not at primary prevention but at developing the "infrastructure" for a prevention policy—that is, data bases, research programs, training programs to develop manpower, government leadership programs, and coordinating agencies.

The decision to focus the recommendations on infrastructure instead of primary prevention appears to be a post hoc rationalization introduced half-way through the study process to relieve the committee of contentious debates about specific policies of primary prevention—for example, prenatal testing and abortion, gun control, national health insurance, and drug abuse programs. I say this because almost all of the recommendations that concern infrastructure are totally undocumented, and an examination of the body of the report shows that the committee spent no time collecting and analyzing information about infrastructural components. For example:

- *Recommendation 2* calls for an "enhanced role for the private sector," including advocacy groups, the media, voluntary agencies, philanthropies, and business. Nowhere does the report describe or analyze the current role of media, voluntary agencies, or philanthropies. Advocacy groups are mentioned a few times, notably the National Council on Disability, which cosponsored this study, but there is certainly no analysis in the report of the number, range of activities, or effectiveness of advocacy groups in preventing disability. The report mentions a few private employment programs for people with disabilities as good examples, but there is no inquiry into the scope of these programs, how many people they employ, whether they are cost-effective, and whether they have lasting effects.
- *Recommendation 15* calls for establishing a major, university-based training program for disability research. The report itself provides no information or analysis of the nature and scope of existing disability research and training programs.
- *Recommendations 23 and 24* call for upgrading medical education and training of physicians and allied professionals, but the committee made no inventory of existing training programs and curricula and the report provides no documentation that there is anything wrong with them. In several chapters, there are categorical statements to the effect that there is a shortage of personnel or programs, but no data are provided.

These recommendations (and others calling for more research and grants) easily found their way into the report's conclusions, not because they emerged from reasoned inquiry but because they offend no one. One might even say they benefit primarily the people who wrote them. In response to a previous draft of this dissent, a staff member replied:

> Indeed, the Committee did not undertake a systematic review of all the disability research training programs. Rather, among the Committee members there are several who are major figures in disability research training in the U.S. Their testimony on this subject was thought by the Committee to be well informed and adequate.

This attitude is emblematic of what was wrong with the whole committee process. Instead of engaging in genuine empirical inquiry, the committee accepted as evidence the informal opinions of its own members about a question in which they have a personal and institutional stake.

Critique of the Process

Many of the inadequacies and omissions detailed above can be explained by the process of study and deliberation that produced this report. The study was cosponsored by the Centers for Disease Control (CDC) and the National Council on Disability; funding came exclusively from CDC. I believe this sponsorship constrained the committee in some very concrete ways and led to a biased report.

The sponsors commissioned a report that would "develop a national agenda for prevention of disabilities." However, the Statement of Task they provided (see part 2 of this appendix) defined a limited set of approaches to disability prevention for the committee to consider. Moreover, it *specified in advance of the committee's deliberations what some of the recommendations should be.*

The statement of task set the structure of the report from the beginning by requiring a focus on data collection of the kind CDC already does. Three of the five tasks (nos. 1, 3, and 4) involved assessing traditional epidemiological information about the incidence, prevalence, and costs of disability. Two tasks (nos. 3 and 5) specifically asked the committee to "develop recommendations for" establishing a national surveillance system and applied research programs, and for a "strong, effective, coordinated effort for prevention of disability." One task (no. 2) asked for specific case studies of prevention activities in injury, chronic disease, and developmental disabilities, and two tasks (nos. 1 and 3) asked for a study of so-called secondary disability, or the additional disabilities that are sometimes caused by another disability. In addition, although CDC did not state this as part of the task, it really wanted the injury case study to focus on spinal cord and traumatic brain injuries, for which it already had a surveillance program, and it so informed the committee.

Thus, the committee was not free to examine the complex, multifaceted problem of disability and come to its own conclusions about which problems and approaches ought to have priority in the report. Indeed, a preliminary table of contents for the final report, based on the statement of task, was developed by the Institute of Medicine (IOM) staff and distributed at the first committee meeting. Also at that meeting, the committee was immediately divided into working groups corresponding to the chapter outline. Although it chose later to add the chapters on the conceptual model of disability and chronic disease, the committee never changed the structure of the final report from the original outline prepared before it had had any discussion.

The first recommendation of the report is that the CDC "assume the lead responsibility for implementing the national agenda for the prevention of disability." Yet, as is evident in the body of the report, the committee never considered the relative merits and disadvantages of locating a national prevention program in the CDC as compared with other agencies. For example, it did not discuss the implications of locating leadership for a disability prevention program in the Office of the Surgeon General (traditionally thought to be the chief disease prevention agency) or of locating it in a health agency as opposed to a Labor Department agency (e.g., the Occupational Safety and Health Administration) or a Justice Department agency (e.g., the Office of Civil Rights). Arguably, these and other agencies have as much experience with disability prevention as the CDC—albeit in nonmedical models of disability prevention. To my knowledge, the CDC never asked explicitly to be cast in the lead role, but the fact that the committee did so unreflectively, with no research into the question, suggests that the committee was operating under the strong influence of its sponsor.

Beyond the design of the task, the CDC constrained the committee in more immediate ways as well. CDC representatives attended the committee's meetings and occasionally indicated their satisfaction or dissatisfaction with the direction of the discussion. Committee members were told explicitly in one meeting that the CDC wanted a report they could "wave on the Hill" to demonstrate their need for larger appropriations.

Early in the course of the study, I was concerned that the emerging report neglected the whole topic of prenatal diagnosis and abortion. I made a presentation to the committee documenting the importance of access to contraception, prenatal diagnosis, abortion, and prenatal care in the prevention of developmental disabilities. During the discussion of my presentation, a representative of the CDC told the committee, "We don't want a report that is controversial."

Nevertheless, with the encouragement of staff, I drafted a piece about these issues for the report. Besides being read by the entire committee, the piece went back and forth between me and the staff for substantive editing. During one of these exchanges, I discovered that these drafts were being "blind copied" to the CDC. When I made this charge in an earlier draft of this dissent, the IOM staff produced a memorandum about the abortion draft on which the sponsors of the report were blind copied. The staff maintain that only an "informational" memorandum and not drafts of the abortion section were passed to the sponsors. I, of course, cannot prove exactly what pieces of paper were circulated to sponsors, but clearly some communication between committee staff and sponsors was concealed from committee members. Moreover, the staff indicated to me in phone conversations during the course of the study that the sponsors were "concerned" about my draft and wanted it "toned down," suggesting that committee staff were engaging in discussions about the content of the report with the sponsors. Regardless of how much was actually blind copied to the sponsors, one must ask *why there was any blind copying at all* during the course of this study. Is there any place for secrecy, for concealing communications between staff and sponsors, in a genuinely scientific deliberative process?

The topic of abortion *is* controversial, and was especially so during the period of this study, but it is nevertheless highly relevant to the report and to a prevention agenda. Genetic testing, prenatal diagnosis, and abortion of affected fetuses are already being widely used to prevent the birth of children with severe disabilities. Given the rapid pace of development of genetic technology, and the gap between our ability to detect serious diseases and to cure them, this trend will continue. As welcome as these techniques are to many parents and public health advocates, they are very objectionable to some in the disability rights community, as well as to people who oppose abortion on any grounds. Prenatal genetic testing, mass screening for genetic defects, and abortion of affected fetuses have been major topics of debate in both the scientific and popular press, and they will continue to be important topics in the 1990s.

These controversies should be acknowledged and discussed, not ignored, in an agenda for disability prevention. A genuinely deliberative and scientific research effort would have sought *more* information and discussion rather than suppressing the whole topic. In my draft, I documented extensively the connection between access to prenatal care, prenatal testing, and abortion on the one hand and reduction of disabilities on the other. But instead of building on this draft, the committee and the Institute of Medicine suppressed it. There are a few brief mentions of the topic, almost hidden in the report, in such phrases as "genetic screening and counseling and associated services," or "pregnancy termination." Yet there is not so much as a single full paragraph devoted to this topic, although recommendation 17 expresses the committee's "belief" that "prenatal diagnosis and associated services, including pregnancy termination" should be available to all women. Unfortunately, this recommendation, like so many others, is not supported by any analysis in the body of the report.

It is hard to say exactly why the topic of abortion was virtually omitted from the report. Many committee members were acutely uncomfortable with the extensive discussion of abortion. Some of them, as well as one of the sponsors (the National Council on Disability), were strongly opposed to the idea that prenatal testing and abortion might be used to prevent the birth of people with disabilities. Others were opposed to discussing abortion in this report because the topic is so controversial that it might deflect attention away from the rest of the report. One committee member strongly opposed use of the word "abortion" in the report and wanted the term "pregnancy termination" substituted instead. And of course the other sponsor, the CDC, made it plain during a committee meeting (if not in private meetings with committee staff) that it did not want anything controversial in the report.

I believe that the Institute of Medicine, as a scientific advisory body, should inform policymaking bodies about the scientific aspects of controversies and leave the ultimate political decisions to appropriate political bodies. Because this committee was so concerned about avoiding controversy, the report fails to educate policymakers and the general public about the most basic *scientific* aspects of the abortion and disability controversy.

This point is important beyond the Committee on a National Agenda for the Prevention of Disabilities. If a study committee of the National Academy of Sciences is prohibited from reporting, is afraid to report, or is pressured out of reporting on relevant but highly controversial aspects of a scientific and social problem, it and the Academy lose their integrity as scientific bodies.

PART 2: THE COMMITTEE'S RESPONSE TO THE DISSENT BY DEBORAH STONE

The preceding dissent to the report of the Committee on a National Agenda for the Prevention of Disabilities focuses on two matters: (1) the quality of the committee's report and (2) the possibility that inappropriate influence by the sponsors of the study could have constrained the committee's ability to act independently. In regard to the first matter, the report itself stands as the committee's response to Dr. Stone's critique. We believe that the study that this report documents fulfills the charge given to the committee by the Institute of Medicine and that the report has the potential for making substantial contributions to the field of disability prevention. We do, however, address below two specific points relative to the report's quality that were raised by Dr. Stone.

As to the second matter, we, the remaining 22 members of the committee, believe that Dr. Stone's criticisms of the committee process lack an informed basis—she is unable to judge what transpired during the committee's tenure because she did not participate in its deliberations. She attended only two of the six meetings of the full committee—the first and part of the third—and none of the additional six subcommittee working group meetings. At the third meeting (July 31, 1989), Dr. Stone presented a paper that she had written on her proposal for a national agenda for disability prevention. A large portion of her paper concentrated on calls to keep abortion legal, require Medicaid programs to pay for abortion, implement gun control policies, and establish some form of national health insurance. Her covering note stated, "I'm sure not everyone will agree with my views, and *it may be that I will want to write a minority report to accompany the main committee report*" (emphasis added). Although we were led to believe that she would continue to participate in the committee process, and help address the issues raised in her paper, Dr. Stone attended no other committee or working group meetings. In an effort to accommodate her schedule and focus on her concerns (primarily the abortion issue), the committee even set up a special working group meeting, but at the last minute Dr. Stone was unable to attend.

The committee process Dr. Stone criticizes so strongly is a slow, often arduous consensus-building exercise in which a group of experts study an issue as outlined in the statement of task, or charge, provided to them by the Institute of Medicine. Their findings, conclusions, and recommendations are then gathered together and presented in a report, which is subject to independent critical review by an anonymous group of authorities in the field at issue, appointed by the Institute of Medicine and the National Research Council. Such scrutiny is required before a report is approved for release to ensure that the committee has addressed its charge appropriately and substantiated its conclusions and recommendations.

The committee process is notable for the extent of its discussions, debates, and even arguments about available evidence and the conclusions to be drawn from it. Committee members are selected to bring varying points of view and so contribute to a broad perspective on the problem at hand. But in the consensus-building process, these views are often shaped, and—in the best sense—"influenced," not by sponsors, who take no part in the often heated give-and-take of committee deliberations, but by the ideas and opinions of other experts who bring their combined knowledge and understanding to bear. Dr. Stone's lack of participation in this process appears to have led to her misconception of the role played by study sponsors and her view of their ability to constrain the committee's conclusions and eventual recommendations. In the case of our committee, although sponsor representatives attended some meetings, they participated only as resources; when appropriate, they were excused from meetings so that the committee could discuss issues in their absence. Moreover, sponsor representatives did not attend working group meetings, during which most of the recommendation formulation work was carried out. The character, organization, and substance of the report clearly reflect the work of committee members alone; in addressing the committee's Statement of Task (see box) we made decisions about the content and organization of the report and how each point should be presented. The process was fair, and members' participation was broad and vigorous. No other committee member besides Dr. Stone, whose experiential basis for judgment must be considered extremely narrow, experienced feelings of constraint or pressure from the sponsors.

Much of Dr. Stone's critique of the process stems from her displeasure with the committee's handling of the abortion issue and the revisions that were made to the paper she submitted. She implies that the Centers for

---

STATEMENT OF TASK

The National Academy of Sciences/Institute of Medicine, through the Division of Health Promotion and Disease Prevention, will conduct a twenty-two month study to develop a national agenda for the prevention of disabilities. The study is to consider prevention and intervention strategies, emphasizing applied research in the development and evaluation of preventative interventions, rather than basic research. In conducting the study, the IOM shall:

(1) Assess and evaluate the public health significance of primary and secondary disability in the U.S., and the current status of activities designed to prevent them. Consideration should be given to incidence, prevalence, and cost.

(2) Review current and projected prevention activities in injury, developmental disability, and chronic disease, including intervention and prevention strategies used in other countries. Consider how these, or other activities, might assist in attaining the health objectives for the year 2000 and beyond.

(3) Identify critical gaps in the existing knowledge about the incidence, prevalence and cost of disability in America. Develop recommendations for the establishment of surveillance systems and applied research programs designed to prevent primary and secondary disability.

(4) Evaluate the need for a framework for setting priorities for disability prevention programs based on incidence, prevalence, preventability, and economic cost to society, and consider the role of the federal government and other sectors in implementing disability prevention activities.

(5) Recommend a system for the development of a strong, effective, and coordinated effort for the prevention of disability. Consider whether a national coalition should be formed.

Disease Control (CDC), one of the sponsors of the study, was somehow involved in revising her paper and removing "abortion" from the report—but she concedes also that she has no evidence for such a charge. Indeed, as Dr. Stone notes, some committee members expressed concern about the political realities of recommendations on the subject of abortion and the potential for their affecting the impact of the entire report. What Dr. Stone does not comment on, because she was not present for most of it, was the intense discussion of this issue among committee members at several points and the process leading to the consensus that was finally achieved, merging broad and opposing views (see recommendation 17 of the report, which calls for providing access to effective family planning and prenatal services, including pregnancy termination). CDC never exerted any pressure to remove material from the report or to influence the findings of the committee. As for the blind-copied correspondence Dr. Stone mentions, we consider this merely an expeditious method for informing the sponsor of the status and progress of the committee's deliberations—not an attempt to conceal information. The information conveyed in that correspondence was routine and nonconfidential, and in no way violated the confidentiality of committee deliberations or led to constraints in its independence of action.

Dr. Stone raises two other troubling points that we believe should not go unaddressed. First, with respect to her allegation that recommendation 1 in the report was made "unreflectively," we must once again note that Dr. Stone did not participate in the discussions that led to this recommendation and therefore has no knowledge on which to base this judgment. In addition, the committee was asked not to assess the disability-related programs of all federal government agencies but instead to "recommend a system for the development of a strong, effective, and coordinated effort for the prevention of disability." In executing this part of our charge, we came to realize that, far from showing preference for a sponsor, we had developed something of a bias against recommending CDC leadership in order to avoid any appearance of unwarranted preference. Objective consideration, however, of the merits of CDC leadership (its demonstrated strength and success in prevention activities through epidemiology, surveillance, and technology transfer, and its emphasis— unlike most other federal disability-related programs—on prevention rather than service delivery or rehabilitation research) led to the committee's recommendation that the existing Disabilities Prevention Program at CDC be expanded to serve as the focus of a National Disability Prevention Program.

In arriving at this judgment the committee called on the expertise and knowledge of its members to compare administrative structures and operations of some of the federal agencies that might accommodate a National Disability Prevention Program. Among our ranks are a former U.S. surgeon general and assistant secretary for health, a former director of the National Center for Health Statistics, and two former directors of what is now the National Institute on Disability and Rehabilitation Research. As is common in considering the organization, coordination, and development of federal programs, the committee relied on these experts to provide first-hand experience in these areas and supplement the limited documentation available in the public domain.

A second point Dr. Stone raises regarding the quality of the report is that of the strategy developed by the committee to formulate the national agenda on disability. As background to this matter, it is important to understand that most of Dr. Stone's substantive comments and recommendations focus on primary prevention—for example, prenatal testing and abortion, gun control, and national health insurance. The committee, however, decided to take a different approach. As the preface of the report notes,

> [t]his report goes beyond the traditional medical model to consider and address the needs of people with disabling conditions after those conditions exist and after they have been "treated" and "rehabilitated." Prevention of the initial condition (primary prevention) is certainly important, but the emphasis in this report is on developing interventions that can prevent pathology from becoming impairment, impairment from becoming functional limitation, functional limitation from becoming disability, and any of these conditions from causing secondary conditions. Theoretically, each stage presents an opportunity to intervene and prevent the progression toward disability. Thus, the report sets forth a model developed by its authoring body, the Committee on a National Agenda for the Prevention of Disabilities, that describes disability not as a static endpoint but as a component of a process.

One impetus for the committee's decision on its approach came from the sheer size of the charge it had to address. We decided that perhaps the best contribution we could make was to, first, describe the significance and magnitude of disability as a public health issue; second, describe a conceptual framework for consideration of disability prevention, taking into account quality of life and the strong emphasis the committee wanted to give to the social and other risk factors so essential to the causes of disability; and, third, develop recommendations that would serve as an infrastructure for a national program for prevention. By infrastructure, we mean the leadership, coordination, surveillance, research, personnel development, and public support needed for such a program, which would provide a framework for a long-term, comprehensive, and coordinated effort involving specific interventions. Thus, we did not formulate exhaustive lists of interventions for each area of disability addressed in the report (although the "focus chapters" on developmental disability, injury, chronic disease, and secondary conditions do present information on various types of intervention strategies, including some primary prevention, and their development status or proven effectiveness). Indeed, it is the report's focus on secondary and tertiary prevention that helps to set it apart from many other efforts in the field and, we believe, constitutes a major contribution to disability prevention for those individuals who already have potentially disabling conditions.

It is regrettable that Dr. Stone chose not to continue active participation in the committee and contribute more fully to its work. Many of the points she raised in her July 1989 paper appear in the report; see, for example, the recommendations on access to care in Chapter 9. Her views undoubtedly would have been better served, however, by fuller participation in the collegial deliberative endeavor that is the hallmark of this institution's consensus-building committee process.

C

Committee Biographies

ALVIN R. TARLOV (Chair) received his bachelor's degree from Dartmouth College and his medical degree from the University of Chicago. Following his internship and residency in internal medicine, he spent five years in hematologic research, partly at the University of Chicago and partly in the Department of Biological Chemistry at Harvard Medical School. In 1968, Dr. Tarlov became professor and chairman of the Department of Medicine at the University of Chicago, a post he held for thirteen years. In 1975, he began a five-year term as chairman of the Task Force on Manpower Needs of the Association of Professors of Medicine, and in 1978, he was appointed chairman of the Graduate Medical Education National Advisory Committee to advise the Secretary of Health, Education, and Welfare on desirable numbers, distributions, and geographic placements of physicians in each specialty. The committee's final report which was issued on September 30, 1980, is the standard reference on physician manpower needs in the United States.

Dr. Tarlov is a former Markle Foundation Scholar and Research Career Development Awardee of the National Institutes of Health. He has served as secretary-treasurer and president of the Association of Professors of Medicine and as chairman of the Federated Council of Internal Medicine. He is a member of the Association of American Physicians and of the Institute of Medicine. He is also a member of the U.S. General Accounting Office Research and Education Advisory Panel and is a Master of the American College of Physicians. In January 1984, he became president of the Henry J. Kaiser Family Foundation in Menlo Park, California, and guided the foundation to a national leadership role in health promotion and disease prevention, until assuming his current positions in October 1990 as Director, Division of Health Improvement, The Health Institute, New England Medical Center; professor of medicine, Tufts University

School of Medicine; and professor of health promotion at Harvard School of Public Health, Boston, Massachusetts.

HENRY A. ANDERSON is chief of Environmental and Chronic Disease Epidemiology for the Wisconsin Department of Health and Social Services, as well as adjunct professor of preventive medicine at the University of Wisconsin Medical School with a joint appointment in the Institute for Environmental Studies. He received his M.D. from the University of Wisconsin Medical School, Madison, and is a diplomate of the American Board of Preventive Medicine with an occupational medicine subspecialty. He is also a fellow of the American College of Epidemiology. Dr. Anderson currently serves on the Board of Scientific Councilors for the Agency for Toxic Substances and Disease Registries and the Surveillance Subcommittee of the National Institute of Occupational Safety and Health Board of Scientific Councilors. His major research interests include the epidemiology of chronic disease, chronic disease surveillance systems, workers' compensation and occupational disease and injury, risk communication, and behavior modification.

PETER W. AXELSON is president of Beneficial Designs, Inc., and a consultant to the rehabilitation community on all aspects of rehabilitation equipment design including testing, marketing, production and documentation of adaptive equipment for people with disabilities. He began his education at the U.S. Air Force Academy, but after a climbing accident which resulted in paralysis from the waist down, he was honorably discharged and continued his studies at Stanford University, where he earned an M.S. in mechanical engineering and design. Following graduation he worked as a rehabilitation engineer at the Palo Alto Veterans Administration's Rehabilitation Engineering Research and Development Center.

Mr. Axelson has written numerous articles and is a member of the board of the Rehabilitation Engineering Society of North America (RESNA). His work in the design and development of rehabilitation equipment gained the Silver Medal of the British Royal Society of the Arts for his encouragement of arts, manufacture, and commerce in the area of special products. On behalf of the Paralyzed Veterans of America, he also participates in the development of wheelchair standards as chairperson of the American National Standards Institute/Rehabilitation Engineering Society of North America (ANSI/RESNA) Wheelchair Standards Committee, and as the U.S. delegate to the International Standards Organization (ISO).

HENRY B. BETTS is currently medical director and chief executive officer of the Rehabilitation Institute of Chicago, and Magnuson Professor and chairman of the Department of Rehabilitation Medicine, Northwestern University Medical School. He received his bachelor's degree from Princeton Univer-

342

sity in 1950 and went on to medical studies, earning his M.D. from the University of Virginia. Following a residency at the New York University Medical Center's Institute of Physical Medicine and Rehabilitation, he spent two years in the U.S. Navy and two years as a teaching fellow at New York University. He then joined the Rehabilitation Institute of Chicago, rising to the post he holds today.

Dr. Betts is a member of several professional associations, including the American Academy of Physical Medicine and Rehabilitation, the American Congress of Rehabilitation Medicine (past president), the American Medical Association, and the American Spinal Cord Injury Association. He has served on panels and committees of the National Institutes of Health and the National Academy of Sciences and has authored or co-authored more than 25 publications in the field of rehabilitation medicine. He was recently honored for 25 years of service as leader of the Rehabilitation Institute.

ALLEN C. CROCKER is the director of the Developmental Evaluation Center and senior associate in medicine at the Children's Hospital in Boston. He holds a joint appointment as associate professor of pediatrics at Harvard Medical School and associate professor of maternal and child health at Harvard School of Public Health. His research interests involve the etiology of mental retardation, systems of care for persons with developmental disabilities, and prevention. He has co-edited two books and has had substantial involvement with planning and evaluation projects for the prevention of developmental disabilities, both nationally and in the programs of various states.

GERBEN DeJONG is director of research at the National Rehabilitation Hospital in Washington, D.C., and professor of the Department of Community and Family Medicine at Georgetown University's School of Medicine. Earlier, he was a senior research associate and associate professor in the Department of Rehabilitation Medicine at Tufts University School of Medicine in Boston.

Dr. DeJong's academic training is in economics and public policy studies. His main research interests are disability and health outcome measurement, health care utilization, disability policy, epidemiology, national health care policy, and medical ethics. He is the author of more than 100 papers on health, disability, and income policy issues but is perhaps best known for his seminal work on disability policy and the independent living movement. His works have appeared in such diverse publications as *Business and Health, Scientific American, Stroke*, and the *Journal of Health, Politics, Policy, and Law*. In 1985, he received the Licht Award for Excellence in Scientific Writing from the American Congress of Rehabilitation Medicine.

JOHN F. DITUNNO, JR., is director of the National Rehabilitation and Research Center in Spinal Cord Injury (Neural Recovery and Functional

Enhancement) and director of the Regional Spinal Cord Injury Model System Center at Thomas Jefferson University. His major research interests are motor recovery and functional prognosis and medical complications (e.g., deep vein thrombosis and pulmonary emboli prevention, atelectasis and pneumonia) in spinal cord injury. He is past president of the Association of Academic Physiatrists and the American Academy of Physical Medicine and Rehabilitation, and past chairman of the American Board of Physical Medicine and Rehabilitation. He is currently a member of the Advisory Committee for Injury Prevention and Control of the Centers for Disease Control and president of the American Spinal Injury Association.

JOSEPH T. ENGLISH is chairman of psychiatry at St. Vincent's Hospital and Medical Center of New York and professor of psychiatry and associate dean of New York Medical College. Prior to joining St. Vincent's, Dr. English was the first president and chief executive officer of the New York Health and Hospitals Corporation. He has also served as chief psychiatrist of the Peace Corps, director of health programs for the Office of Economic Opportunity in the Executive Office of the President, and administrator of the Health and Mental Health Services Administration of the Department of Health, Education, and Welfare. For the past two years, Dr. English has been chairman of the Professional and Technical Advisory Committee for the Hospital and Accreditation Program of the Joint Commission on Accreditation of Health Care Organizations; since 1975, he has served as chairman of the Mental Health/Substance Abuse Service Committee of the Greater New York Hospital Association. He was also the first Chairman of the Council on Economics of the American Psychiatric Association and now chairs its Task Force on Prospective Payment.

Dr. English is a fellow of the Institute of Medicine, National Academy of Sciences, American Psychiatric Association, American College of Psychiatrists, New York Academy of Medicine, and the American College of Mental Health Administration. A member of the board of directors of the Kennedy Child Study Center and the board of trustees of Sarah Lawrence College, he is also a Visiting Fellow of the Woodrow Wilson National Fellowship Foundation. He is a member of the editorial board of the *Psychiatric Times* and a consultant to the editorial board of the *American Psychiatric Press*, and has authored more than 100 papers and articles on health-related issues.

DOUGLAS A. FENDERSON is a professor in the Department of Family Practice and Community Health and the School of Public Health of the University of Minnesota, as well as director of the Computer Center and associate director for research of the Department of Family Practice and Community Health. As director of continuing medical education for the University of Minnesota School of Public Health, he helped develop a regional network of accredited continuing medical education sites. He has also served as chief of health services manpower, National Center for Health Services Research; director of the Office of Special Programs, Bureau of Health Professions Education; and, more recently, director of the National Institute of Handicapped Research (now the National Institute on Disability and Rehabilitation Research).

MARGARET J. GIANNINI is presently deputy assistant chief medical director for rehabilitation and prosthetics for the Department of Veterans Affairs and director of the Rehabilitation Research and Development Service. In 1979, she was appointed the first director of the National Institute of Handicapped Research; she also founded and directed the Mental Retardation Institute of New York Medical College and established one of the first university-affiliated facilities at New York Medical College.

Nationally, Dr. Giannini is past president of the American Association on Mental Retardation and the American Association of University Affiliated Programs. She has been actively involved as a member of the National Committee of Children with Handicaps of the American Academy of Pediatrics; she created the Prevention Committee of the American Association on Mental Retardation, and was appointed United Nations Interregional Advisor on Mental Retardation and Developmental Disabilities. She has also been named special consultant to the Mental Retardation Construction Unit of the National Institutes of Health, vice president for medicine of the American Association on Mental Retardation, consultant by special invitation to the President's Committee on Mental Retardation on Early Screening for Prevention, a member of the Scientific Advisory Board of the Kennedy Child Study Center, and a member of the Institute of Medicine. She is a diplomate of the American Board of Pediatrics and a fellow of the American Academy of Pediatrics. Dr. Giannini is the recipient of numerous awards for her professional and humanitarian services and achievements, including the Wyeth Medical Achievement Award, the N. Neal Pike Prize Award for Service to the Handicapped, the Isabelle and Leonard H. Goldenson Award for Technology Application to Cerebral Palsy, and the Distinguished Service Award presented by the President's Committee on Employment of the Handicapped.

MITCHELL P. LaPLANTE is assistant research sociologist and director of the Disability Statistics Program at the Institute for Health and Aging, University of California, San Francisco. While a Social Science Research Council fellow, he received his Ph.D. in sociology from Stanford University and received an award from the American Sociological Association for the best dissertation in medical sociology. He has authored several papers and reports concerned with disability. His research interests include conceptual and definitional issues in disability, the demography and epidemiology of disability, and disability policy.

G. DEAN MacEWEN is chairman and director of education in the Department of Pediatric Orthopaedics at the Children's Hospital in New Orleans. He is also professor and chief of the Section of Pediatric Orthopaedic Surgery, Department of Orthopaedic Surgery, at the Louisiana State University Medical Center, also in New Orleans. Dr. MacEwen is a member of the Société Internationale de Chirurgie Orthopédique et de Traumatologie, for which he serves as first vice president of the executive board and U.S. delegate; the American Academy of Orthopaedic Surgeons; and the American Orthopaedic Association, for which he chairs the Foreign Fellowship Committee. He also chairs the Subcommittee in Pediatric Care of the Louisiana chapter of the American Academy of Pediatrics, and serves as an examiner of the American Board of Orthopaedic Surgery. Dr. MacEwen is a member of the Medical Clinical Care Advisory Board of the National Neurofibromatosis Foundation, and acts as Medical Advisor for the Louisiana-Gulfcoast chapter; he also holds membership in the Pediatric Orthopaedic Society and the Scoliosis Research Society. Before he assumed his present positions, he was medical director of the Alfred I. duPont Institute and past president of the American Orthopaedic Association, the Scoliosis Research Society, and the Pediatric Orthopaedic Society.

ELLEN J. MacKENZIE is assistant director of the Health Services Research and Development Center and associate professor in the Department of Health Policy and Management, Johns Hopkins School of Hygiene and Public Health. She also holds joint appointments in biostatistics and in emergency medicine in the School of Medicine. Her research interests include injury severity scaling and the evaluation of emergency medical and rehabilitation services for preventing death and disability associated with traumatic injury. She has authored several publications in these areas, including a recent report to Congress entitled *Cost of Injury in the United States* (with Dorothy P. Rice and Associates). Ongoing studies for which she is a principal investigator include (1) development and application of methods for evaluating the performance of regionalized systems of trauma care; (2) a multi-institutional, collaborative study of the long-term effects and rehabilitation needs of persons who sustain severe lower-extremity fractures; and (3) development of a functional impairment index for traumatic injuries. Dr. MacKenzie is currently a member of the board of directors of the Association of the Advancement of Automotive Medicine and past chair of the Injury Control/Emergency Health Services Special Primary Interest Group of the American Public Health Association. She also acts as an advisor to private and government agencies involved in the delivery and evaluation of rehabilitation services.

GEORGE L. MADDOX, JR., is professor of sociology and of medical sociology (psychiatry) and chairs the University Council on Aging and Human Development at Duke University. He also directs Duke's World Health Organization/Pan American Health Organization Collaborating Research Center on Aging and the university's Long-Term Care Resources Program. Associated with gerontology and geriatrics since 1959, he served as director of the Duke Center for the Study of Aging and Human Development from 1972 to 1982. He was a founding member of the initial National Advisory Council of the National Institute on Aging, has served as president of the Gerontological Society of America, has chaired the Sociology of Aging Section of the American Sociological Association, and has served as vice president of the Southern Sociological Society. From 1985 to 1989 he served as secretary-general and vice president of the International Association of Gerontology. He is a fellow of the American Association for the Advancement of Science. Dr. Maddox has been awarded the Sandoz International Prize for Research in Aging.

DAVID MECHANIC is director of the Institute for Health, Health Care Policy, and Aging Research at Rutgers University, a University Professor, and the René Dubos Professor of Behavioral Sciences. He is a member of the Institute of Medicine and serves on the National Committee on Vital and Health Statistics of the Department of Health and Human Services and the Health Advisory Board of the General Accounting Office. He chairs the National Institute of Mental Health's Advisory Group on Research Resources in Mental Health Services Research and recently served as vice chair of the Institute of Medicine's Committee for Pain, Disability, and Chronic Illness Behavior. Dr. Mechanic is a member of the National Institutes of Health's National Advisory Council on Aging, chair of the council's Program Committee, and chair of the Section on Social, Economic and Political Sciences of the American Association for the Advancement of Science. He is also the author of numerous books and other publications on health policy and health services research.

JOHN L. MELVIN is professor and chairman of the Department of Physical Medicine and Rehabilitation at the Medical College of Wisconsin and medical director of the Curative Rehabilitation Center of Milwaukee. He is president-elect of the Council of Medical Specialty Societies and past president of the American Congress of Rehabilitation Medicine, the American Association of Electromyography and Electrodiagnosis, the National Association of Rehabilitation Facilities, and the Association of Academic Physiatrists. He is a founding member of the American Board of Electrodiagnostic Medicine and chairman of the American Board of Physical Medicine and Rehabilitation. He has lectured and consulted extensively within the United States and internationally. In addition, he has published regularly on subjects related to physical medicine and rehabilitation.

ARTHUR T. MEYERSON is professor of psychiatry and chairman of the Department of Mental Health Sciences at the Hahnemann University School of Medicine in Philadelphia. Formerly vice chairman and clinical director of the Department of Psychiatry at Mt. Sinai School of Medicine in New York City, he has written extensively in the area of psychiatric disability and chairs the National American Psychiatric Association Committee on Psychiatric Rehabilitation as well as the Task Force on Social Security Income/Social Security Disability Insurance. He has served as chairman of the Mental Health Standing Committee of the President's Committee on Employment of the Handicapped and as an advisor to the last four commissioners of the Rehabilitation Services Administration. Currently, he is conducting studies supported by the National Institute of Mental Health in the prevention of deterioration in a population of severely mentally ill and disabled persons.

DOROTHY P. RICE is professor-in-residence in the Department of Social and Behavioral Sciences, School of Nursing, University of California, San Francisco, with joint appointments in the university's Institute for Health and Aging and Institute for Health Policy Studies. From 1977 to 1982 she served as director of the National Center for Health Statistics. Previously she was deputy assistant commissioner for research and statistics of the Social Security Administration. She is a member of the Institute of Medicine and the Committee on National Statistics, a fellow of the American Statistical Association and the American Public Health Association, and a member of the American Economic Association, the Population Association of America, and the Gerontological Society of America. She holds a bachelor's degree in economics from the University of Wisconsin and was awarded an honorary doctorate by the College of Medicine and Dentistry of New Jersey. Her major interests include health statistics, disability, chronic illness, aging, cost of illness studies, and the economics of medical care.

JULIUS B. RICHMOND is John D. MacArthur Professor of Health Policy (Emeritus) at the Division for Health Policy Research and Education at Harvard University. He received his M.D. and M.S. degrees from the University of Illinois at Chicago. At the State University of New York at Syracuse, he chaired the Pediatrics Department and was dean of the Medical School. In 1965 he was called to Washington to direct the Head Start Program and later served as director for health affairs, initiating the Neighborhood Health Centers Program for the Office of Economic Opportunity. In 1971 he was appointed professor of child psychiatry and human development at Harvard Medical School and became director of the Judge Baker Guidance

Center and chief of psychiatry at the Children's Hospital in Boston. From 1977 to 1981 he served as assistant secretary for health, U.S. Department of Health and Human Services, and surgeon general of the U.S. Public Health Service. Under his leadership, the Public Health Service published *Healthy People: The Surgeon General's Report on Health Promotion and Disease Prevention*. Dr. Richmond has received the Martha May Eliot Award of the American Public Health Association, the Ronald McDonald Children's Charities prize, and the Gustav Lienhard Award of the Institute of Medicine, among others.

MAX J. STARKLOFF is the founder and president of Paraquad as well as co-founder and elected president (in 1983, 1984, and 1985) of the National Council of Independent Living. In the past he chaired the Peer Review Panel for the Title VII Independent Living Grant and Independent Living Program applications and served as an advisor to the National Council on the Handicapped. In August 1985 Mr. Starkloff was one of fifteen delegates to the First Annual Japan-USA Conference of Persons with Disabilities held in Tokyo and Osaka, Japan. Currently, he serves as a member of the advisory committee to the Rehabilitation Research and Training Center in the Prevention and Treatment of Secondary Complications in Spinal Cord Injury at Northwestern University's Rehabilitation Institute of Chicago. Mr. Starkloff has received numerous awards in recognition of his work, including the Commissioner's Distinguished Service Award, from the Commissioner of the Rehabilitation Services Administration, a commendation from the National Council on the Handicapped, and an honorary doctorate of humane letters from the University of Missouri-St. Louis.

DEBORAH A. STONE holds the David Pokross Chair in Law and Social Policy at the Heller Graduate School of Brandeis University. She received a Ph.D. in political science from Massachusetts Institute of Technology (MIT) and has held faculty appointments in political science and public policy at Duke University, MIT, and Brandeis University. She has been a Guggenheim Fellow and a Fellow in Liberal Arts at Harvard Law School. Her research interests include health insurance in the United States and Europe, disability policy, and preventive medicine. She is the author of numerous articles as well as three books: *The Limits of Professional Power: National Health Care in the Federal Republic of Germany*; *The Disabled State*; and *Policy Paradox and Political Reason*.

S. LEONARD SYME is professor of epidemiology at the School of Public Health, University of California, Berkeley. He received his Ph.D. in medical sociology from Yale University in 1957. His research has focused on the social, psychological, and cultural factors that increase the risk of such diseases as coronary heart disease, stroke, and cancer among particular population groups (his studies have included Japanese immigrants to the United States, bus drivers in San Francisco, and civil servants in London). He has also been involved in the design and conduct of community projects to prevent these diseases as well as community studies of smoking cessation, early detection for cancer, and programs to help people reduce disease risk factors. His current research interest is the importance of the early years of life to the development and prevention of disease risk. Dr. Syme's recent publications have dealt with the topics of social support, socioeconomic status, and control of destiny.

JOHN E. WARE, JR., is senior scientist at the Institute for the Improvement of Medical Care and Health at the New England Medical Center Hospitals. He is also principal investigator for the Medical Outcomes Study, which assesses variations in physician practice style and outcomes for patients with chronic conditions treated in different systems of care. Formerly senior research psychologist at the RAND Corporation, he was the principal architect of the surveys of health outcomes and patient satisfaction used in RAND's Health Insurance Experiment. Dr. Ware's current research and consulting activities focus on the development and validation of more practical measures of functional status, well-being measures of process and outcomes in health policy evaluation, health care management, clinical research, and medical practice.

Index

Abortion, 333, 334-335, 336, 338
  see also Family planning, Prenatal services
Academic research, 144, 145, 146, 259, 331
Access issues, 10, 27, 68, 94, 280-284, 329
  aged persons, 208, 210
  assistive technologies, 226, 271
  blind, 257
  delivery strategies, 4, 27-28, 196, 210-
    211, 224-225, 272, 282-283
  developmental disability and, 130-131,
    139, 141, 145
  education, children with disabilities, 130-
    131
  historical trends, 54, 56
  medical/preventive services, 15, 24-26,
    27, 31, 101, 139, 141, 252-258, 268
  national agenda, 15, 31, 268
  prenatal care, 25, 280-281
  public facilities, 33, 87, 88, 94, 233, 330
  transportation facilities, 33, 131, 225, 251,
    330
  vocational services, 27-28, 284
  see also Discrimination
Activities of daily living, 1, 42, 44, 45-56,
    77, 121, 312, 317
  aging and, 44-45, 187, 192-193, 194
  causes of limitation, 56-61, 75, 104
  gender factors, 46, 74
  life tables, 61-67, 74
Acute care, 164-168, 176-179, 209
  emergency services, 165, 168, 174-176
  spinal cord injuries, steroids, 33-34, 177
Administration for Developmental
    Disabilities, 141
Adolescents, 26, 154, 191
Advisory committees, 18-19, 268, 271

Advocacy and advocates, 29-30, 132, 225, 243,
    244, 252, 331
Age factors, 49, 54, 55, 58-59, 245-246
  adolescents, 26, 154, 191
  assistive technologies, 192
  caregivers of aged persons, 209
  chronic conditions, general, 191
  cost of care, 71, 72
  within elderly population, 195
  life tables, 61-67, 74
  mental adjustment to disability, 221, 222
  personal assistance services, 192-193
  young adults, 2, 74-75, 153, 154
  see also Adolescents; Children; Young
    adults
Agency for Health Care Policy, 234
Aging and aged persons, 13, 54, 190, 209,
    210
  access issues, 208, 210
  activity limitations, 44-45, 187, 192-194
  attitudes about, 194-196, 198, 211-212
  attitudes of, 206
  chronic diseases, 2, 13, 32-33, 56, 59, 60,
    100-101, 106, 184-213
  cognitive impairments, 194, 210
  cost of care, 67-68, 210
  drugs, 201, 202, 213
  education of elderly, 195
  epidemiology, 12, 44-46, 48, 50-53, 56,
    59, 67-68, 100-101, 186-193, 195, 199-
    200, 208, 261
  evaluation of services, 196, 198, 213
  family caregivers, 209-210, 256
  gender differences, 192, 195
  health promotion for, 185, 189, 199
  injuries, 201, 206

life course perspective, 38-39, 193-195
mental health and illness, 206, 207-208
multidisciplinary approach, 195, 209, 261
preventive measures, 32-33, 185, 189, 195-213
professional education on, 201, 212-213
projections, 56, 193, 209-211
psychological factors, 195, 210
public education, 185, 201, 211-212
quality of life, 189, 190, 196, 198, 199, 208, 209, 210-211, 212
risk factors, 86, 185, 193, 198, 200, 202-205
social factors, 195, 199, 206, 210-211
see also Medicare
AIDS, see Human immunodeficiency virus
Alcohol abuse, 88, 101, 160, 161, 164, 284
driving while intoxicated, 159-161, 330
fetal alcohol syndrome, 11, 114-115, 138
Allied health professionals, 28, 29-30, 231-232, 286, 331
see also Personal assistance services
American Academy of Pediatrics, 25, 145, 280
American Foundation for the Blind, 257
American Medical Association, 312, 313
Americans with Disabilities Act, 14, 33, 88, 91, 182, 267, 271, 329
Assistive technologies, 10, 14, 17, 107, 177, 271
access to, 226, 271
age factors, 192
cost factors, 226-227, 237, 283
definitional issues, 226
developmental disabilities, 131, 132
fall prevention, 226, 227, 228
insurance coverage, 14, 27, 227, 228, 233, 257
secondary conditions, prevention, 215, 224-229, 232-234, 237, 239, 240
transportation, 251
Association for the Care of Children's Health, 129
Attitudes, 87
about aged persons, 194, 195, 196, 198, 211-212
of aged persons, 206
about people with disabilities, 30, 70, 230, 233, 245, 264
self-perceptions, 48, 90, 194, 206, 219-220, 236-237
Automobiles, see Motor vehicles

Beneficiary Rehabilitation Program, 249-250
Blindness, 257
Bipartisan Commission on Comprehensive Health Care, 25, 280
Birth defects, 65, 134-135

gestational, 113, 114-116, 125-126, 138
hereditary, 86, 112, 113, 115, 125, 330
Birth Defects Monitoring Program, 134-135
Birth weight, 26, 130, 263, 281
Black Americans, 46, 64-65, 114
Brain, 136, 153
cerebral palsy, 117
fetal, 89
fetal alcohol syndrome, 11, 114-115, 138
trauma, 12, 116, 151-153, 155, 156-183
Bureau of Maternal and Child Health and Resources Development, 136-137

Canada, 184, 275
Census Bureau, 43, 102, 276, 327
see also Survey of Income and Program Participation
Census Disability Survey, 276
Centers for Disease Control, 16-17, 18, 34, 102, 241, 269-270, 271, 332-333
developmental disabilities, 122, 134-136, 146
Disabilities Prevention Program, 16, 34, 260-261, 269, 338
injury programs, 156, 183, 260-261
study sponsorship, 332-333, 336-338
Central nervous system, see Brain; Spinal cord injuries
Cerebral palsy, 117, 122
Children, 70, 121, 281
American Academy of Pediatrics, 25, 145, 280
assistance requirements, 192
chronic conditions, general, 191, 284
comprehensive services, 26, 129-131
day care, 129-131
developmental disabilities, acquired, 116, 126-127
educational interventions, 129-131
elementary/secondary education, 121-122, 129-131, 211
epidemiology, 48, 50, 54, 116-117
multidisciplinary approaches, 129, 284
insurance, 25, 280
special education, 121-122, 248, 330
state programs, 284
well-child care, 124, 128
see also Adolescents; Birth defects; Birth weight; Developmental disabilities
Chronic diseases, 6, 12-13, 65, 74, 253
adolescents, 191
aging process and elderly, 2, 13, 32-33, 56, 59, 60, 100-101, 106, 184-213
children, 191, 284
epidemiology, 12, 44-46, 48, 50-53, 56, 59, 67-68, 100-101, 186-193, 195, 199-200, 208, 261
multiple, 60, 191-192

prevention measures, persons with, 39, 106, 196-199
protocols, 208, 213
public education, 185, 201, 211-212
quality of life, 189, 190, 196, 198, 199, 208, 209, 210-211, 212
see also Developmental disabilities
Classification, 255, 273-274, 321-327
injuries, 157-158, 159
severity of disability, 179
WHO international system, 5-6, 20-21, 76-78, 97, 158, 273, 319-320, 325, 327
see also Definitional issues; Models
Cognitive impairments, 178-179
aged persons, 194, 210
learning disorders, 117, 330
mental retardation, 112, 114-115, 118, 119, 133
Commission on Chronic Illness, 311-312
Committee on Employment of People with Disabilities, 78
Communication limitations, 118, 119, 121, 178, 179, 223, 226, 229
Community-based programs
access issues, 27
aged persons, 210
databases, 137-138
demonstration projects, 283-284
developmental disabilities, 130, 143
educational programs, 130
federal coordination, 16, 34, 262, 263
injury rehabilitation, 181, 183
independent living centers, 30, 94, 180, 225, 232
local activities and governments, 262, 282, 283
mental health services, 208
private sector cooperation, 263-264
secondary condition prevention, 238
state regulation of, 263
Comprehensive approaches, 4-14, 242-266
age-related disabilities, 199, 211
injuries, 164-183
prenatal and child care, 26, 129-131
research, 22-23
secondary conditions, prevention, 223-233
vocational, 28, 248, 249-251, 263, 284
see also Multidisciplinary approach
Computers and computer science
case management, 212-213, 225
injury surveillance, 157-158
Conceptual issues, *see* Definitional issues; Models
Coordination, *see* Organization and coordination
Cost and cost analysis, 281
affordable care, 14, 25-26, 182, 253, 280-283

age factors, 71, 72
aged persons, care, 67-68, 210
assistive technologies, 226-227, 237, 283
child care, 70, 139
developmental disabilities, 11, 110
disability-related, general, 1, 24, 67-73, 75, 242, 248, 310, 337
gender factors, 68
health care, general, 25-26, 252, 256
historical perspective, 67-73
injury-related, 11, 12, 147, 148-150, 153, 160, 163, 164, 174, 183
insurance, 27
long-term care, 282
medical services, 69-73, 139
prenatal care, 26, 280-281
secondary conditions, 220
transfer payments, 69, 70, 310
vocational rehabilitation, 250
Cost of Injury in the United States, 163, 183

Day care, 129-131
Definitional issues, 76-83, 97, 268, 273-274
assistive technologies, 226
brain injury, 159
disability, 1, 35-37, 78, 81-83, 118, 121-122, 230, 235, 273-274, 309-327
developmental disability, 109, 118
disabling process, 91-92
evaluation, 35
functional limitation, 5, 7, 35-36, 74, 76, 77, 79, 80, 118, 119-121, 312, 313, 314-315, 321, 325
handicap, 6, 77-78, 118, 320, 324, 325
impairment, 7, 35-36, 79, 80, 118, 121, 312, 314, 319-320, 321
international classification system, 5-6, 76-78
pathology, 7, 35-36, 79-80, 313-314, 319
prevention, 35, 36-37, 97
quality of life, 89-90
rehabilitation, 214
risk factors, 37-38, 84-89, 99
secondary condition, 13, 35, 214, 235
social limitations, 6, 42, 74, 77
Demography, 70, 98, 100, 193
educational attainment, 92-94, 195, 222
projections, 56, 193, 209-210
urban/rural, 11, 12, 131, 153, 233
see also Epidemiology; Gender factors; Racial/ethnic factors; Socioeconomic status
Demonstration projects, 262-263, 283-284
preventive, elderly, 199, 211
Dental health, 203, 206
Department of Education, 137, 248, 250, 263
Department of Health and Human Services, *see specific constituent agencies*

Department of Labor, 102
Department of Veterans Affairs, 259-260
Dependence/independence, 4, 33, 90-91,
  107, 249, 265, 266
  advocacy and, 243, 244
  aged persons, 206
  case study, 219-220
  gender differences, 67
  independent living centers, 30, 94, 180,
    225, 232
  institutionalized persons, 47, 206, 210
  see also Activities of daily living;
    Assistive technologies; Functional
    limitations; Mobility limitations
Depression, 33, 40, 205, 206, 215, 219, 221,
  222, 238, 240
Developmental disabilities, 10-11, 109-146
  access issues, 130-131, 139, 141, 145
  acquired, 116, 126-127
  assistive technologies, 131, 132
  CDC, 122, 134-136, 146
  coordination of services, 34, 132-133,
    139, 141, 143, 144-145
  costs of, 11, 110
  definitional issues, 109, 118
  epidemiology, 11, 21, 109-122, 131, 134-
    139
  federal programs, general, 141, 142, 145
  functional limitations, 118, 119-121
  historical perspective, 122-123
  local community activities, 130, 143
  mental retardation, 112, 114-115, 118,
    119, 133
  models, 118-122
  multidisciplinary approach, 129
  poverty and, 141-142, 145
  preventive measures, 11, 34, 118, 122-146
  private sector, 143-144
  professional education on, 132, 146
  research, 138-139
  risk factors, 122, 123, 125-127
  screening, 122-123, 128-129
  secondary conditions, 122, 123
  state government action, 34, 131, 133,
    137-138, 141, 143, 144-145
  toxicology of, 11, 114-115, 124, 131, 134
Developmental Disabilities Act, 109
Diabetes, 196, 197
Disabilities Prevention Program (CDC), 16,
  34, 260-261, 269, 338
Disability conceptualization, 320-327
Disabling process, 91--92
Discrimination, 33, 87, 182, 223, 263-264,
  329
Down syndrome, 115
Drug abuse, 88-89, 164, 207, 284
  see also Alcohol abuse
Drug labeling, 201

Drugs, prescribed, 86
  aged persons, 201, 202, 213
  secondary conditions, 228, 229, 236
  spinal cord injuries, 33-34, 177

Economic factors, see Cost and cost
  analysis; Employment and unemployment; Income maintenance; Productivity, losses; Socioeconomic status
Educational attainment, 92, 93-94, 195, 222
Education and training
  childhood, 121-122, 129-131, 211
  families of people with disabilities, 29-30,
    87
  family planning, 26-27, 128-129, 338
  learning disorders, general, 117, 330
  mental retardation, 112, 114-115, 118,
    119, 133
  of people with disabilities, 117, 177-178,
    213-233, 248, 287
  preventive, 105, 129-131
  special, for children with disabilities, 121-
    122, 248, 330
  see also Professional education; Public
    education; Vocational rehabilitation
Education for All Handicapped Children
  Act, 330
Elderly, see Aging and aged persons;
  Medicare
Emergency medical services, 165, 168, 174-
  176
Employee Retirement and Income Security
  Act, 254
Employment and unemployment, 17, 78, 87,
  94, 102, 251
  brain damage and, 152-153
  discrimination, 33, 87, 182, 223, 263-264,
    329
  insurance provide by employer, 24, 253,
    254
  occupational risk factors, 84, 157, 330
  quality of life and, 33, 172-173
  productivity losses, 68, 69, 148, 163
  spinal cord injuries, 154, 220
  SSDI, 52, 248, 249-252, 257, 310, 313
  vocational services, 27-28, 93-94, 165,
    172, 179-183, 244, 248, 249-251, 263,
    284, 311
  women, 64
  work limitations, 43, 50, 51, 54, 56, 64,
    74, 154, 220, 221-223, 233, 253-254,
    257-258, 316
Environmental factors, 86-88, 224, 233, 237
  preventive measures, 105, 131-132, 233
  public facilities, access, 33, 88, 87, 94,
    233, 330
  secondary conditions, 224, 233, 235, 237
  toxic agents, 98, 131

transportation facilities, access to, 33, 131, 225, 251, 330
urban/rural, 11, 12, 131, 153, 233
weather, 94, 233
see also Assistive technologies; Safety equipment; Social factors
Epidemiology, 1, 4, 32, 34, 41-75, 95-104, 337
children, 48, 50, 54, 116-117
chronic diseases and aging, 12, 44-46, 48, 50-53, 56, 59, 67-68, 100-101, 186-193, 195, 199-200, 208, 261
data sources, 34, 41-45, 97-104, 134-138, 274-276
developmental disabilities, 11, 21, 109-122, 131, 134-139
disability indexes, general, 103-104, 179, 276-277, 315
functional limitations, 21, 40, 42-44, 45, 49-50, 51
injuries, 12, 22, 32, 39, 147-159, 176, 179
life expectancy, 1, 56, 61, 64-65, 67, 184, 185, 208
life tables, 61-67, 74
longitudinal, 22-23, 99, 102, 193-194, 200, 261, 277-279
national program, 15, 20, 21-22, 31, 268, 243, 245-246, 268, 274-277
prevalence data, general, 1, 4, 32, 41, 45-56, 101-102, 309
secondary conditions, 22, 137, 218, 220, 240
see also Risk factors
Ethical issues, 252
Europe, 251-252
Evaluation, 39, 68, 159, 337
advocacy, 331
age-related disease prevention, 196, 198, 213
community-based, 283-284
definitional issues, 35
disability conceptualization, 320-327
government assistance programs, 68, 182
injury prevention, 160
injury rehabilitation, 181, 182-183
national program, 273, 283
preventive measures, general, 247, 278-279, 284
public assistance programs, 68, 102
rehabilitation programs, 245, 279
secondary conditions, prevention, 223, 234-335
Exercise
as primary prevention, 86, 200, 205, 229-230, 248
for people with disabilities, 177-178, 229-230, 235

Fall injuries, 149, 150, 155, 157, 160, 164, 201, 206
assistive/safety devices, 226, 227, 228
Families/informal caregivers, 222, 223, 232, 256, 271
aged people with disabilities, 209-210, 256
developmental disabilities, poverty, 141, 145
education of, 29-30, 287
Family planning, 26-27, 128-129, 281-282, 338
abortion, 333, 334-335, 336, 338
Federal government, 14-31, 248-258
age-related disabilities, 185
developmental disabilities, 141, 142, 145
disability-related expenditures, general, 24
home care programs, 255-256
injury prevention, 260-261
interagency coordination, 19-20, 24, 102, 133, 241, 243, 258-259, 263, 267, 271-274
local coordination by, 16, 34, 262, 263
national objectives, 15, 31, 245-247, 249, 268
rehabilitation research, 259-260
state cooperation with, 16, 34, 131, 133, 141, 145, 248, 250, 261, 262, 311
see also Laws, specific federal; National Disability Prevention Program; *specific departments, agencies, and programs*
Fetal alcohol syndrome, 11, 114-115, 138
Firearms, 150, 154, 157, 330, 338
Follow-up, 179-183, 225
Foreign countries, 65, 76, 184, 251-252, 275, 279, 310
Fragile X syndrome, 112
Framingham Study, 102
Functional electrical stimulation (FES), 177, 179
Functional limitations, 32, 90, 196
defined, 5, 7, 35-36, 74, 76, 77, 79, 80, 118-121, 312, 313, 314-315, 321, 325
developmental disabilities, 118, 119-121
epidemiology, 21, 40, 42-44, 45, 49-51
injury-related, 171-172
spinal cord injuries, drugs, 33-34, 177
see also Activities of daily living

Gender factors, 54, 62-63, 64, 67, 256
activity limitations, 46, 74
aged persons, 192, 195
disability costs, 68
injuries, 12, 153
Genetics, 86, 112, 113, 115, 125, 330
preventive interventions, 123-124, 128-129, 330

screening, 330, 333, 334
Glasgow Coma Scale, 151-152
Government role
    developmental disabilities, 11, 110
    private sector coordination, 17-18, 261-
        264, 270-271, 331
    see also Community-based programs;
        Federal government; Public assistance;
        State governments
Guide to Clinical Preventive Services, 247-
    248

Handicap, 6, 77-78, 118, 320, 324, 325
Head injuries, see Brain
Head Start programs, 129-130, 145, 284
Health Care Financing Administration, 44,
    102, 138, 145, 199, 263
Health care professionals
    allied, 28, 29-30, 231-232, 286, 331
    associations, 25, 145, 280, 312
    attitudes of, 245
    physicians, 27, 29, 222, 231, 232, 245,
        285-286, 331
    see also Personal assistance services;
        Professional education
Health promotion, 38-39, 105, 245-247, 283
    aged persons, 185, 189, 199
    models, 38-39, 227, 283
    secondary conditions and, 215, 224, 227-
        230
Health services delivery, 4, 27-28, 196, 210-
    211, 224-225, 272, 282-283
    secondary conditions, 224-225
Healthy People 2000, 185, 246-247
Hearing, see Communication limitations
Hispanics, 136
Historical perspectives, 2
    access issues, 54, 56
    conceptualization of disability, 311-327
    costs of disability, 67-73
    developmental disabilities, 122-123
    employer-provided insurance, 254
    injuries, 32, 155-156
    prevalence of disabilities, 53-56
Home care, 210, 233, 255-256
    see also Families/informal caregivers;
        Personal assistance services
Homelessness, 207, 262
Housing, 220, 225
Human immunodeficiency virus, 88, 96, 107
    perinatally acquired, 115-116

Impairment
    defined, 7, 35-36, 79, 80, 118, 121, 314,
        319-320, 321
    injury-related, 171-172
    see also Multiple impairments; specific
        impairments

Income maintenance, 310
    Social Security Disability Insurance, 52,
        248, 249-252, 310, 313
    Supplemental Security Income, 52, 141,
        248, 310
Independence, see Dependence/independence
Independent living centers, 30, 94, 180, 225,
    232
Indexes of disabilities, general, 103-104,
    179, 276-277, 315
Informal caregivers, see Families/informal
    caregivers
Injury, 11-12, 147-183
    aged persons, 201, 206
    brain damage, 12, 116, 168-183
    CDC, 156, 183, 260-261
    classification, 157-158, 159
    computer surveillance, 157-158
    coordination of services, 157-158, 164,
        183
    cost of, 11, 12, 147, 148-150, 153, 160,
        163, 164, 174, 183
    education on, 164, 182
    epidemiology, 12, 22, 32, 39, 147-159,
        176, 179
    evaluation of interventions, 159, 160, 181,
        182-183
    firearms, 150, 154, 157, 330, 338
    functional limitations/impairments, 171-
        172
    gender factors, 12, 153
    historical perspectives, 32, 155-156
    local efforts, 181, 183
    medical services, 147, 155, 165, 168, 174-
        176
    mobility limitations, 176-177, 178, 179
    multidisciplinary approach, 182
    prevention, 37-38, 39, 159-164, 183, 201,
        226, 227, 228, 260-261, 330
    productivity losses, 148, 163
    psychological factors, 151, 152, 165, 173,
        179-183
    quality of life, 172-173, 182
    risk factors, 84, 157, 330
    secondary conditions, 164, 168, 174-176
    social factors, 151, 152, 163, 173-174,
        179-183
    traumatic brain injury, see Brain
    urban areas, 12, 153
    young adults, 74-75, 153
    work-related, 84, 157, 330
    see also Brain; Fall injuries; Motor
        vehicles; Spinal cord injuries
Injury Control and Disabilities Prevention
    Programs, 260
Institute of Medicine, 26, 39, 200, 281, 332,
    333, 335
Institutionalized persons, 47, 206, 210

Instrumental activities of daily living, *see* Activities of daily living
Insurance, 17, 24-25, 211, 252-257, 271, 280, 282
    assistive devices, 14, 27, 227, 228, 233, 257
    eligibility criteria, 14, 26-27, 139, 182, 227, 228, 233, 254-257, 280, 313
    employer-provided, 24, 253, 254
    family planning/prenatal services, 25, 26-27, 139, 280
    injuries, rehabilitation, 182
    Medicaid, 24, 248, 255, 257
    Medicare, 24, 44, 199, 209, 229, 255-257
Injury in America, 39, 163, 183
Injury Prevention, 183
Interagency Committee on Disability Research, 258, 259
Interagency Council on Disability Prevention, 19, 272
Interagency Forum on Aging-Related Statistics, 53
International Center for the Disabled, 43, 48, 244, 250
International perspectives, 65, 76, 184, 251-252, 275, 279, 310
    see also World Health Organization
International Classification of Impairments, Disabilities, and Handicaps, 5-6, 20-21, 76-78, 97, 158, 273, 319-320, 325, 327

Laws, specific federal, 242, 243
    Americans with Disabilities Act, 14, 33, 88, 91, 182, 267, 271, 329
    Developmental Disabilities Act, 109
    Education for All Handicapped Children Act, 330
    Employee Retirement and Income Security Act, 254
    Medicare Catastrophic Coverage Act, 256
    Occupational Health and Safety Act, 330
    Rehabilitation Act, 313
    Social Security Act, 249
    Vocational Rehabilitation Act, 311
Lead toxicity, 11, 116-117, 131
Learning disabilities, 117, 330
    mental retardation, 112, 114-115, 118, 119, 133
    special education, 121-122, 248, 330
Legal issues
    discrimination, 33, 87, 182, 223, 263-264, 329
    driving while intoxicated, 161
    injury reporting, mandatory, 159
    see also Laws, specific federal
Life course perspective, 38-39, 193-195, 235
    aged persons, 185

Life expectancy, 1, 56, 61, 64-65, 67, 184, 185, 208
Lifestyle risk factors, 88-89, 228, 248
Life tables, 61-67, 74
Local activities and governments, 262, 282, 283
    see also Community-based programs
Longitudinal studies, 22-23, 99, 102, 275-276, 277-279
    aging and chronic diseases, 193-194, 200, 261
Longitudinal Study of Aging, 44-45, 67
Long-term care, 4, 194, 243, 244, 265, 282, 285
    insurance, 27, 255-257
    national survey, 44, 53, 194, 200, 209
    nursing homes, 46, 149, 206, 210, 219, 256
Louis Harris and Associates, 43
    International Center for the Disabled, 43, 48, 244, 250

Maternal and Child Health Bureau, 129
Maternity Outreach Services, 262-263
Medicaid, 24, 248, 255, 257
Medical services, 4, 14
    access issues, 15, 24-26, 27, 31, 101, 139, 141, 252-258, 268
    acute care, 164-168, 176-179, 209
    costs, 69-73, 139
    emergency services, 165, 168, 174-176
    injury-related, 147, 155, 165, 168, 174-176
    model of disability, traditional, 27, 36-37, 104, 244-245, 339
    secondary conditions, 224-225
    see also Health care professionals
Medicare, 24, 44, 199, 209, 229, 255, 256, 257
Medicare Catastrophic Coverage Act, 256
Mental health and illness, 207, 208
    adjustment to disability, age factors, 206, 207-208, 221, 222
    aged persons, 206, 207-208
    chronic, 5, 40, 207-208
    coordination of services, 263
    depression, 33, 40, 205, 206, 215, 219, 221, 222, 238, 240
    secondary conditions, 5, 33, 216, 219, 221-223
    work limitations, 51, 251-253
    see also Alcohol abuse; Cognitive impairments; Drug abuse; Psychological factors
Mental retardation, 112, 114-115, 118, 119, 133
    special education, 121-122, 248, 330

Metropolitan Atlanta Congenital Defects
Program, 134
Metropolitan Atlanta Developmental
Disabilities Study, 135
Minority groups, 1, 12, 45, 46, 64-65, 114,
136, 153
Mobility limitations, 2, 65
developmental disabilities, 118, 119
injury-related, 176-177, 178, 179
public facilities, 33, 87, 88, 94, 233, 330
transportation facilities, 33, 131, 225, 251,
330
weather-related, 94, 233
young persons, 74-75
see also Paralysis
Models, 97
acute care and rehabilitation, 164-183
demonstration projects, 199, 211, 262-
263, 283-284
developmental disability, 118-122
disability, general, 4, 5-10, 76, 83-108,
193-195, 196, 309-327
health promotion, 38-39, 227, 283
injuries, response, 164-183
medical, traditional, 27, 36-37, 104, 211,
244-245, 339
protocols, 13, 208, 213, 234-241, 259
secondary conditions, 215-223
spinal cord injuries, 154
Motor vehicles, 38-39, 149-150, 153, 157,
161-162
driving while intoxicated, 159-161, 330
safety equipment, 38, 157, 161-163, 339
spinal cord injuries, 11, 154, 155
Multidisciplinary approach, 259, 265, 266,
285, 321
aged persons and aging, 195, 209, 261
child-focused programs, 129, 284
developmental disabilities, 129
injury-related disabilities, 182
secondary conditions, 234
Multiple impairments, 94-95, 121, 218
drugs, multiple, 201
chronic, 60, 191-192
injury-related, 174
risk factors, 234
see also Secondary conditions

Nagi, Saad, 4, 7, 76, 77, 81-82, 83, 95, 309-
327
National Accident Sampling System, 156
National Center for Health Services
Research, 136, 138
National Center for Health Statistics, 102,
135-136, 156-157
National Center for Medical Rehabilitation
Research, 261

National Coalition for the Prevention of
Mental Retardation, 133
National Committee for Injury Prevention
and Control, 160
National Council on Disability, 16, 34, 43,
78, 133, 243, 269, 331
National Council on the Handicapped, see
National Council on Disability
National Crime Survey, 156
National Disability Prevention Program, 4-
31 (passim), 34, 267-287, 332, 337
aged persons, 190-191
agenda, 15, 31, 268
education, 15, 31, 268
epidemiology, 15, 20, 21-22, 31, 268,
243, 245-246, 268, 274-277
evaluation, 273, 283
objectives, 15, 31, 245-247, 249, 268
preventive measures, 4-14, 17, 18, 32-33,
245-247, 267-273, 284
research, 15, 31, 268, 272, 277
National Electronic Injury Surveillance
System, 156
National Handicapped Sports and Recreation
Association, 229-230
National Health and Nutrition Examination
Surveys, 136
National Health Interview Survey, 42-43, 44,
45-48, 50-51, 53, 60, 61, 64, 66, 73,
74, 75, 95, 102, 276
aging and chronic diseases, 186, 189, 191-
192
developmental disabilities, 118, 135
injuries, 156-158
secondary conditions, 218
Supplement on Aging, 44-45, 60, 67, 192
National Hospital Discharge Survey, 156-
158
National Institute of Child Health and
Human Development, 261
National Institute on Aging, 102, 261
National Institute on Disability and
Rehabilitation Research, 78, 102, 137,
146, 166, 241, 258-259
National Institute of Mental Health, 263
National Institutes of Health, 136, 146, 259
National Long-Term Care Survey, 44, 53,
194, 200, 209
National Maternal and Infant Health Survey,
136
National Medical Care Expenditures Survey,
136
National Medical Care Utilization and
Expenditure Survey (1980), 110, 135-
136
National Research Council, 39, 103, 220
National Spinal Cord Injury Data Base, 155
Native Americans, 114

New Jersey, 262-263
Nursing homes, 46, 149, 206, 210, 219, 256
Nutrition, 86, 136, 138, 200, 201, 204, 229, 235, 248

Occupational Health and Safety Act, 330
Occupational disabilities
  risk factors, 84, 157, 330
  work limitations, 43, 50, 51, 54, 56, 64, 74, 154, 220, 221-223, 233, 253-254, 257-258, 316
Office of Disease Prevention and Health Promotion, 133
Office of Human Development Services, 145
Organization and coordination, 14-19, 31, 258-266, 267-273
  acute care, 165
  advisory committees, 18-19, 268, 271
  aging and chronic disease, 195, 208-211
  developmental disabilities, 34, 132-133, 139, 141, 143, 144-145
  injury-related disabilities, 157-158, 164, 183
  interagency, 19-20, 102, 133, 241, 243, 258-259, 263, 267, 268, 271-274
  local, 282
  local-federal, 16, 34, 262, 263
  national agenda, 15, 31, 268
  private sector, 17-18, 261-264, 270-271, 331
  research, 19, 22-23, 277
  secondary conditions, 224-225, 241
  state-federal, 16, 34, 131, 133, 141, 145, 248, 250, 261, 262, 311
  see also Comprehensive approaches; Multidisciplinary approach

Paralysis, 2, 95, 154, 176-177
  paraplegia/quadraplegia, 35, 154, 155, 177, 215, 219-220
Pathology, 7, 35-36, 79-80, 234, 313-314, 319
Personal assistance services, 271
  age factors, 192-193
  attendants, education, 29-30, 232, 287
  federal insurance for, 254-255
  see also Assistive technologies; Families/ informal caregivers
Physicians, 222
  access to, 27
  education, 29, 231, 232, 285-286, 331
Peer influence, 132, 173, 225
Political factors, 163, 328
  advocacy and advocates, 29-30, 132, 225, 243, 244, 252, 331
  see also Public opinion
Poverty, 1, 24-25, 47, 48, 92, 253, 280
  developmental disabilities, 141-142, 145

Head Start programs, 129-130, 145, 284
homelessness, 207, 262
Medicaid, 24, 248, 255, 257
prenatal care, 26, 262-263, 281-282
  see also Public assistance
Pregnancy termination, *see* Abortion; Family planning; Prenatal services
Prenatal services, 26-27, 37, 101, 124, 128-129, 281-282, 333, 337-338
  abortion, 333, 334-335, 336, 338
  access to, 25, 280-281
  comprehensive, 26, 262-263
  cost factors, 26, 280-281
  drug abuse, 88-89
  family planning, 26-27, 128-129, 281-282, 338
  fetal alcohol syndrome, 11, 114-115, 138
  insurance coverage, 25, 26-27, 139, 280
  poor women, 26, 262-263, 281-282
  state program, 262-263
Preventing Low Birthweight, 26, 281
Preventive measures, 1, 40, 104-108, 242-266, 330-331, 337
  access to, 24-26, 139, 141, 252-258, 268
  age-related chronic disabilities, 32-33, 185, 189, 195-213
  chronic disabilities, persons with, 39, 106, 196-199
  comprehensive, 4-14
  definitional issues, 35, 36-37, 97
  developmental disabilities, 11, 34, 118, 122-146
  educational, 129-131, 286-287
  environmental factors, 105, 131-132, 233
  evaluation, general, 247, 278-279, 284
  genetic, general, 123-124, 128-129, 330
  injury, 37-38, 39, 159-164, 183, 226, 227, 228, 260-261, 330
  insurance coverage, 25, 26-27, 139, 211, 227, 228, 233
  life course perspective, 38-39, 193-195
  model of, 102-103, 104-108
  national, 4-14, 17, 18, 32-33, 245-247, 267-273, 284
  private sector, 40
  research, 24, 278-279
  secondary conditions, 3, 7, 14, 27, 164, 214, 215, 223-241
  social factors, 4, 23-24, 237-238
  standards, 103
  see also Health promotion; Prenatal services; Risk factors; Safety equipment; Screening; Well-child care
Private sector, 331
  advocacy, 29-30, 132, 225, 243, 244, 252, 331
  developmental disabilities, 143-144
  employment programs, 251

government coordination of, 17-18, 261-
264, 270-271, 331
insurance, 14, 17, 24-25, 26-27, 139, 182,
211, 227, 228, 233, 253, 252-257, 271,
280, 282
local cooperation, 263-264
preventive measures, 40
Productivity, losses, 68, 69, 148, 163
Professional associations, 25, 145, 280, 312
Professional education, 28-29, 31, 146, 264-
265, 268, 284-286
on aged persons, 201, 212-213
developmental disabilities, 132, 146
national agenda, 15, 31, 268
researchers, 279, 331
secondary conditions, 231, 232, 239-240
see also Vocational rehabilitation
Projections, aging population, 56, 193, 209-
211
Prosthetics, see Assistive technologies
Protocols, 13, 208, 213, 234-241, 259
Psychological factors, 23-24, 92-93, 94, 98-
99, 278
aged persons, 195, 210
injuries, 151, 152, 165, 173, 179-183
rehabilitation, related to, 206, 207-208,
221, 222, 236-237
see also Mental health and illness
Public assistance, 248, 253, 282
developmental disabilities, 141
eligibility criteria, 56, 249-250, 256, 257,
263, 313
evaluation, 68, 182
housing, 220, 225
Medicaid, 24, 248, 255, 257
Medicare, 24, 44, 199, 209, 229, 255,
256, 257
people with mental disabilities, 208
Social Security Disability Insurance, 52,
248, 249-252, 310, 313
Supplemental Security Income, 52, 141,
248, 310
see also Medicaid; Medicare
Public education, 15, 17, 28, 31, 230, 264,
268, 283, 286-287
aging process, 185, 211-212
chronic diseases and aging, 185, 201, 211-
212
family planning, 26-27, 128-129, 281-282
injury-related disabilities, 164, 182
national agenda, 15, 31, 268
secondary conditions, 224, 230-233
Public facilities, access to, 33, 87, 88, 94,
233, 330
transportation, 33, 131, 225, 233, 330
Public Health Service, 245-246
Public opinion, 4, 94
about aging, 194, 195, 196, 198, 211-212

about people with disabilities, 30, 70, 230,
233, 264

Quality of life, 1, 2-3, 4, 8, 20, 32, 34, 74,
105, 245, 265-266
aging and chronic diseases, 189, 190, 196,
198, 199, 208, 209, 210-211, 212
central nervous system injury, 172-173,
182
disability model, factor in, 85, 89-91
employment and, 33, 172-173
handicap, defined, 78
secondary condition prevention, 235
standard of living, 84, 90
WHO, 89-90
see also Activities of daily living;
Dependence/independence

Racial/ethnic factors, 1, 12, 45, 46, 64-65,
114, 136, 153
blacks, 46, 64-65, 114
Hispanics, 136
Native Americans, 114
Regulations
alcohol and drug abuse, 161, 164
environmental toxins, 131
labeling, 201
see also Standards
Rehabilitation, 3, 107, 214
concept of, 311
evaluation of, 245, 279
geriatric, 194-195
independent living centers, 30, 94, 180,
225, 232
injuries, systems approach, 164-183
models, 164-183
professional education on, 231
psychological factors, 206, 207-208, 221,
222, 236-237
research, 24, 258-260, 278-279
secondary conditions, prevention, 214,
215, 236-237
Social Security Disability Insurance, 52,
248, 249-252, 310, 313
vocational, 27-28, 165, 179-183, 244, 248,
249-251, 263, 284, 311
Rehabilitation Act, 313
Rehabilitation Services Administration, 263
Research, 22-24, 75, 100, 268, 277-279
aging and disease, 189, 193-194, 208
brain, 136
coordination, 19, 22-23, 277
developmental disabilities, 138-139
injuries, 163, 164, 176, 179
national program, 15, 31, 268, 272, 277
preventive measures, 24, 278-279
rehabilitation, 24, 258-260, 279
risk factors, 4, 33, 86, 98-99, 164, 277-278

secondary conditions, 234, 240-241
social factors, 278
socioeconomic status, 23-24, 278
training for, 279, 331
university-based, 144, 145, 146, 259, 331
see also Demonstration projects;
Epidemiology; Evaluation
Retirement History Survey, 102
Risk factors, 4, 8, 12-13, 20, 80, 84-89, 91-
92, 94, 96, 101, 228, 248
aged persons, 86, 185, 193, 198, 200,
202-205
assistive technologies and, 226
brain injury, 153
definitions, 37-38, 84-89, 99
developmental disabilities, 122, 123, 125-
127
epidemiological research, general, 4, 22,
33, 98-99
injuries, 163, 164, 165
insurance classifications, 255
multiple impairments, 234
occupational, 84, 157, 330
research, 4, 33, 86, 98-99, 164, 277-278
secondary conditions, general, 214, 215,
226, 234, 235
sexual activities, 88, 96, 107, 248
see also Screening; *specific factors*
Robert Wood Johnson Foundation, 263
Rural areas, 131

Safety equipment, 163-164, 330
fall injuries, prevention, 226, 227, 228
motor vehicles, 38, 157, 161-163, 339
Schizophrenia, 207
Screening, 106, 107, 247-248, 257
developmental disabilities, general, 122-
123, 128-129
employer-provided insurance, 254
federal support, 145
genetic, 330, 333, 334
Secondary conditions, 13-14, 94-95, 214-241
assistive technologies and, 215, 224, 225-
229, 232, 233, 234, 237, 239, 240
CDC, 241
coordination of services, 224-225, 241
cost, 220
defined, 13, 35, 214, 235
depression, 33, 40, 205, 206, 215, 219,
221, 222, 238, 240
developmental disabilities and, 122, 123
drug treatment, 228, 229, 236
environmental factors, 224, 233, 235, 237
epidemiology, 22, 137, 218, 220, 240
evaluation of interventions, 223, 234-335
health promotion interventions, 215, 224,
227-230
injury-related, 164, 168, 174-176

learning disabilities, 330
local intervention, 238
medical interventions, general, 224-225
mental/emotional, general, 5, 33, 216,
219, 221-223
multidisciplinary approach, 234
prevention, 3, 7, 27, 33, 34, 107, 164,
207, 223-241
professional education on, 231, 232, 239-
240
protocols, 13, 234-241
public education, 224, 230-233
rehabilitation and, 214, 215, 236-237
research, 234, 240-241
risk factors, 214, 215, 226, 234, 235
social factors, 223, 235, 237-238
Sensory limitations, 118, 119, 121, 178, 179,
203, 216, 228
Sex differences, *see* Gender factors
Sexual activity
family planning, 26-27, 128-129, 281-282
of people with disabilities, 222
as risk factor, 88, 96, 107, 248
Smoking, 88, 101, 200, 205, 248
Social factors, 75, 86-87, 98-99
aged persons, 195, 199, 206, 210-211
disability definitional issues, 6, 42, 74,
77, 315-317, 320, 321, 324, 325
injuries, 151, 152, 163, 173-174, 179-183
international comparisons, 252
limitations, defined, 6, 42, 74, 77
peer influence, 132, 173, 225
preventive interventions, 4, 23-24, 237-
238
research, 278
and secondary conditions, 223, 235, 237-
238
support networks, 4, 99, 132, 206, 223,
224-225, 237-238
see also Demography; Public opinion
Social Security Act, 249
Social Security Administration, 102, 138,
249
Social Security Disability Insurance, 52,
248, 249-252, 257, 310, 313
Socioeconomic status, 47, 101
brain injury epidemiology, 153
in disabling process, 23-24, 84, 92, 93, 94
prenatal care, 281-282
research on, 23-24, 278
see also Poverty
Speech, *see* Communication limitations
Special education, 121-122, 248, 330
Spinal cord injuries, 12, 150-151, 153-183,
215
adolescents and young adults, 154
employment issues, 154, 220
motor vehicles, 11, 154, 155

paraplegia/quadraplegia, 35, 154, 155, 177, 215, 219-220
protocols, 236, 259
steroids, 33-34, 177
Sports and athletics, 154, 229-230
Standards
accreditation, professional education, 231
chronic disease, protocols, 208, 213
disability indexes, general, 103-104, 179, 276-277, 315
disability measures, 20-21, 179, 273-274
insurance eligibility, 14, 26-27, 139, 182, 227, 228, 233, 254-257, 280, 313
national objectives, 15, 31, 245-247, 260, 268
prevention criteria, general, 103
public assistance, eligibility, 56, 249-250, 256, 257, 263, 313
secondary conditions, protocols, 13, 234-241
spinal cord injuries, protocols, 236, 259
see also Classification; Definitional issues; Quality of life
Standards of living, 84, 90
State governments, 262
aged persons, data, 190
blind, services, 257
child-focused programs, 284
databases, 137-138, 190-191
developmental disabilities, 34, 131, 133, 137-138, 141, 143, 144-145
federal cooperation with, 16, 34, 131, 133, 141, 145, 248, 250, 261, 262, 311
home care programs, 255-256
injuries, mandatory reporting, 159
local activities, regulation, 263
prenatal care, 262-263
rehabilitation programs, 311
vocational rehabilitation, 248, 250
Statistical programs and activities, see Cost and cost analysis; Epidemiology
Steroids, 33-34, 177
Substance abuse, see Drug abuse
Supplemental Security Income, 52, 141, 248, 310
Supplement on Aging (NHIS), 44-45, 60, 67, 192
Surgeon General, 184-185, 333
Surveillance, see Epidemiology
Survey of Income and Program Participation, 43-44, 49-53, 74, 75, 102, 253

Survey of Occupational Injuries and Illnesses, 156

Technical assistance, 34
Technology, see Assistive technologies; Safety equipment
Therapy, see Rehabilitation
Toward Independence, 243, 260
Toxicity
environmental, general, 98, 131
developmental disabilities, 11, 114-115, 124, 131, 134
lead, 11, 116-117, 131
Training, see Education and training
Transfer payments, 69, 70, 310
Transportation facilities
access to, 33, 131, 225, 233, 330
assistive devices, 251
Traumatic Brain Injury, 180
Traumatic brain injury, see Brain; Injury
Traumatic injury, see Injury

Uniform Hospital Discharge Set, 157
University programs, 144-146, 259, 331
Urban areas, 233
brain injuries, 12, 153
lead poisoning, 11
Utilization of services, 27, 68

Veterans, 52, 259-260, 310
Vocational rehabilitation, 27-28, 93-94, 165, 172, 179-183, 244, 248, 249-251, 263, 284, 311
Vocational Rehabilitation Act, 311

Weather, 94, 233
Well-child care, 124, 128
Women, 64, 256
see also Gender factors; Prenatal services
Work issues, see Employment and unemployment
World Health Organization, 4, 7, 76, 83
ICIDH classification system, 5-6, 20-21, 76-78, 97, 273, 319-320, 325, 327
quality of life, 89-90
World Institute on Disability, 256

Young adults, 2
injuries, 74-75, 153
spinal cord injuries, 154
see also Adolescents